Change Through Time in Psychoanalysis

I0888239

Change Through Time in Psychoanalysis presents a new stage of the work done through the IPA Committee on Clinical Observation between 2014 and 2020—the advances in our method, the Three Level Model (3-LM), and our clinical thinking.

In this new volume, ideas on observational research, clinical narratives based on 3-LM group discussions, and adaptations of the model for training candidates show more experience, more depth, more answers, and, of course, new questions. Contributors from three regions of the IPA have written extended case studies of 10 psychoanalyses, rich in verbatim session material, focusing on the main dimensions of the patient's psychic functioning, specific changes in the analytic process, and related interventional strategies.

The reader will find, in the method and in the clinical narratives, new and clarifying points of view in the observation of transformations in patients in psychoanalysis and of the analysts' techniques, useful both in professional development and in teaching candidates.

Margaret Ann Fitzpatrick Hanly, PhD, is a training and supervising analyst of the Canadian Institute of Psychoanalysis, Chair of the IPA Committee on Clinical Observation, past Director of the Toronto Institute of Psychoanalysis, and a member of the Executive Editorial Board of the *Psychoanalytic Quarterly*.

Marina Altmann de Litvan, PhD, is a Child and Adolescent Psychoanalyst (IPA) and a training and supervising analyst of the Uruguayan Psychoanalytical Association. She is Chair of the Clinical Research Subcommittee and former Chair of the Clinical Research Subcommittee of the IPA (2010–2017).

Ricardo Bernardi, MD, PhD, is an Honorary Member of the Uruguayan Psychoanalytical Association, Emeritus Professor of the School of Medicine, full member of the National Academy of Medicine of Uruguay, and Vice-Chair of the IPA Research Committee.

Psychoanalytic Ideas and Applications Series

IPA Publications Committee

Gabriela Legorreta (Montreal), Chair and Series Editor; Dominique Scarfone (Montreal); Catalina Bronstein (London); Larry Brown (Boston); Michele Ain (Montevideo); Carlos Moguillanski (Buenos Aires); Udo Hock (Berlin); Christine Kirchhoff (Berlin), Gennaro Saragnano (Rome) Consultant; Rhoda Bawdekar (London), Ex-officio as IPA Publishing Manager; Paul Crake (London), Ex-officio as IPA Executive Director

Recent titles in the Series include:

Psychoanalytic Studies on Dysphoria
The False Accord in the Divine Symphony
Marion M. Oliner

Contemporary Perspectives on the Freudian Death Drive
In Theory, Clinical Practice and Culture
Edited by Victor Blüml, Liana Giorgi and Daru Huppert

Permanent Disquiet
Psychoanalysis and the Transitional Subject
Michel de M'Uzan

Psychoanalytic Work with Families and Couples
Clinical Perspectives on Suffering
Susana Kuras Mauer, Sara Moscona, and Silvia Resnizky

Narcissistic Fantasies in Film and Fiction
Masters of the Universe
Ilany Kogan

Psychoanalytic Reflections on Writing, Cinema and the Arts
Facing Beauty and Loss
Paola Golinelli

"This book is a relevant contribution to clinical, technical, and theoretical psychoanalysis. The Three-Level Model was already introduced in the first volume of the Committee on Clinical Observation, and this volume shows how the group has continued to deepen their work with this method in a quite remarkable way. While the aim is still to observe psychic change by studying clinical materials in groups, this time an important achievement has been made through the application of the model to different fields, such as child analysis, and clinical cases presented by candidates. The latter contribute significantly towards fostering Psychoanalytic Education. The authors deal with sensitive and difficult subjects such as the notions of impasse, common ground or pluralism, among others, without eluding controversy, thus promoting a sincere dialogue between different theoretical approaches. The book is a must-read for all those truly interested in contemporary psychoanalysis."

Virginia Ungar, MD, IPA President

"The authors have woven clinical thinking together with rich verbatim material and systematically documented how psychoanalysts can illustrate how change takes places in psychoanalysis. Their methods are original, rigorous, and creative. The book is inspirational in that the methodology is uniquely suited to illustrate how psychoanalysts and analysands work together and the subtle, and not so subtle, changes that occur over time through their interactions. The material can be studied by many groups of clinicians allowing for replication of ratings, which permits an establishment of reliability. Clinicians will recognize vivid accounts of how patients grow and change over time. Both clinicians and researchers will be impressed by the development of a method that retains the complexity of clinical work. The book provides psychoanalysts with a way to teach present and future psychoanalysts how to practice in, and study, our field."

Judith L. Kantrowitz, PhD, training and supervising analyst, Boston Psychoanalytic Society and Institute; author of *The Role of the Patient-Analyst March in the Process and Outcome of Psychoanalysis*

"*Change Through Time in Psychoanalysis*, by a high-powered international team of respected psychoanalytic clinicians, researchers, and epistemologists, is a major contribution to the current endeavour to develop new methods for studying psychoanalytic processes, bringing together psychoanalysts working from different theoretical models. They are the first in this new field to look at what kinds of changes actually take place in psychoanalysis and how these come about, using an original and clinically meaningful combination of careful in-depth psychoanalytic exploration of detailed cases, together with more systematic forms of assessment. Their work on metaphors as anchor points for evaluating change is one particularly interesting example of how this kind of research remains rooted in, and contributes to, psychoanalytic thinking. I congratulate these excellent colleagues whose book is important reading for all of us who feel responsible for evaluating and validating what we really do and how and why patients can benefit from psychoanalysis."

Bernard Reith, President of the Swiss Psychoanalytical Society, past Chair of the EPF Working Party on Initiating Psychoanalysis, Co-Chair for Europe of the IPA Working Parties Committee

Change Through Time in Psychoanalysis

Transformations and Interventions, The Three Level Model

Edited by
Margaret Ann Fitzpatrick Hanly,
Marina Altmann de Litvan, and
Ricardo Bernardi

Routledge
Taylor & Francis Group
LONDON AND NEW YORK

First published 2021
by Routledge
2 Park Square, Milton Park, Abingdon, Oxon OX14 4RN

and by Routledge
52 Vanderbilt Avenue, New York, NY 10017

Routledge is an imprint of the Taylor & Francis Group, an informa business

© 2021 selection and editorial matter, Margaret Ann Fitzpatrick Hanly, Marina Altmann de Litvan, and Ricardo Bernardi; individual chapters, the contributors

The right of Margaret Ann Fitzpatrick Hanly, Marina Altmann de Litvan, and Ricardo Bernardi to be identified as the authors of the editorial material, and of the authors for their individual chapters, has been asserted in accordance with sections 77 and 78 of the Copyright, Designs and Patents Act 1988.

All rights reserved. No part of this book may be reprinted or reproduced or utilised in any form or by any electronic, mechanical, or other means, now known or hereafter invented, including photocopying and recording, or in any information storage or retrieval system, without permission in writing from the publishers.

Trademark notice: Product or corporate names may be trademarks or registered trademarks, and are used only for identification and explanation without intent to infringe.

British Library Cataloguing-in-Publication Data
A catalogue record for this book is available from the British Library

Library of Congress Cataloging-in-Publication Data
Names: Hanly, Margaret Ann Fitzpatrick, 1948– editor. | Altmann de Litvan, Marina, editor. | Bernardi, Ricardo, editor.
Title: Change through time in psychoanalysis : transformations and interventions, the three level model / Margaret Ann Fitzpatrick-Hanly, Marina Altmann de Litvan, Ricardo Bernardi.
Description: Milton Park, Abingdon, Oxon ; New York : Routledge, 2021. | Includes bibliographical references and index. |
Identifiers: LCCN 2020042195 (print) | LCCN 2020042196 (ebook) | ISBN 9780367560911 (paperback) | ISBN 9780367560904 (hardback) | ISBN 9781003096382 (ebook)
Subjects: LCSH: Psychoanalysis—Case studies.
Classification: LCC BF173 .C438 2021 (print) | LCC BF173 (ebook) | DDC 150.19/5—dc23
LC record available at https://lccn.loc.gov/2020042195
LC ebook record available at https://lccn.loc.gov/2020042196

ISBN: 978-0-367-56090-4 (hbk)
ISBN: 978-0-367-56091-1 (pbk)
ISBN: 978-1-003-09638-2 (ebk)

Typeset in Palatino
by Apex CoVantage, LLC

Contents

Contributors

Marina Altmann de Litvan, PhD. Psychoanalyst, full member and training analyst of the Uruguayan Psychoanalytic Association. Chair Clinical Research Subcommittee of the IPA. Former Chair, IPA Clinical Observation Committee (2010–2017). Consultant 2017–present). APU Education Committee (2010–2013). Co-Chair of the Education-Research Subcommittee (2007–2009). Research fellow, University College London, Third Annual Training Programme (1997). Visiting professor, University College London, IPA Research Training Programme (2005, 2006, 2016). Sigourney Award (2017). Raquel Andreucci Gomes Psychologist by PUC / SP. Psychoanalyst IPA, Associate Member of the Psychoanalysis Brazilian Society of São Paulo (SBPSP). Graduated in Child Psychoanalysis from SEDES SAPIENTIAE Institute; and from the Rorschach Society of São Paulo – Aníbal da Silveira. Participant in Clinic 0 to 3 – Initial parent/baby interventions at the Psychoanalytic Service Center of SBPSP. Participant in the SBPSP Autism Study Group.

Raquel Andreucci Gomes, Psychologist by PUC / SP. Psychoanalyst, IPA. Associate Member of the Psychoanalysis' Brazilian Society of São Paulo (SBPSP). Graduated in Child Psychoanalysis from SEDES SAPIENTIAE Institute.

Ricardo Bernardi, PhD. MD. Psychiatrist at Facultad de Medicina, Universidad de la República, UdelaR, Uruguay. Psychoanalyst for the Uruguayan Psychoanalytic Association. Past Chief in Medical Psychology at the Medicine School (UdelaR). FEPAL (1992), 2° award from the National Academy of Medicine (1997). Mary S. Sigourney Award. Regional Editor for Latin America of the *International Journal of Psychoanalysis* (2008–2011). Vice Chair IPA Research Board (2009–present). Member of the IPA Clinical Observation Committee (2009–2017). Official IPA Consultant (2017–present).

Beatriz de León de Bernardi. Full member and training analyst, Uruguayan Psychoanalytic Association (APU). Past President of the APU. Regional Editor for Latin America for the *International Journal of*

Psychoanalysis. Past representative, Latin America IPA Board. Member of the IPA Education Committee. Published papers and books on patient–analyst interaction and the analyst's contribution to the analytic process, the concept of countertransference in Latin America (IJP, 2000).

Nancy Delpréstito. Uruguayan Psychoanalytical Association (APU). Associated member (APU). Training analyst and supervisor of Psychoanalytical Psychotherapy – Psychiatric Clinic, Hospital de Clínicas (2007–2015). Faculty, University Institute of Psychoanalysis of the Asociación Psicoanalítica del Uruguay (2013–present). Member of the Latin American group of Clinical Observation Groups (2011–present).

Carolyn S. Ellman, PhD. Adjunct Clinical Professor and supervisor, NYU Postdoctoral Program in Psychotherapy and Psychoanalysis. Training and supervising analyst and faculty, Institute of Psychoanalytic Training and Research. Training and supervising analyst, Contemporary Freudian Society. Member of the IPA and CIPS. Senior Editor of *The Modern Freudians: Contemporary Psychoanalytic Technique* (2000) and *Omnipotent Fantasies and the Vulnerable Self* (1997).

Mayela Falvy, PhD. Clinical psychologist, Pontificia Universidad Católica del Perú (PUCP). Psychoanalyst Didact of the Peruvian Society of Psychoanalysis (SPP). Private practitioner. IPA member. FEPAL member. Board member of the Institute of Psychoanalytic Psychotherapy Inter-Cambio. Moderator, Clinical Observation and Transformation Committee, the Three Level Model, Lima, Peru.

Margaret Ann Fitzpatrick Hanly, PhD. Training and supervising psychoanalyst for the Canadian Institute of Psychoanalysis. Chair of the IPA Committee on Clinical Observation. Past President of the Canadian Psychoanalytic Society. Past Director of the Toronto Institute of Psychoanalysis. Chair of the IPA Committee on Clinical Observation (2017–present). Executive Editorial Board, *The Psychoanalytic Quarterly*, editorial boards of the *International Journal of Psychoanalysis* and *Canadian Journal of Psychoanalysis*.

Liliana Fudin de Winograd, Lic. Training and supervising psychoanalyst at the Argentine Psychoanalytic Society. Founding member and past President of the Argentine Psychoanalytic Society (SAP). Past Director of the Institute of Psychoanalysis de Argentine Psychoanalytic Society. Ex-Professor of Mental Health, Facultad de Medicina, Universidad de Buenos Aires.

Natalia Goungian. Psychoanalyst at the Uruguayan Psychoanalytical Association (APU). Associated member of the APU. Child and adult psychoanalyst (2020). Graduated from the University of Psychology of the UDELAR Montevideo, Uruguay.

Siri Erika Gullestad, PhD. Training and supervising analyst of the IPA. Professor Emeritus of Clinical Psychology, Department of Psychology, University of Oslo, Norway. Past Chief of the Clinic for Dynamic Psychotherapy. Past President of the Norwegian Psychoanalytic Society. Past Head of the Department of Psychology. Author of many books and articles within the psychoanalytic field. Member of the IPA Clinical Observation Committee (2012–present).

Charles Hanly, PhD. Training and supervising analyst of the IPA. Toronto Institute of Psychoanalysis. Professor Emeritus (philosophy) at the University of Toronto. Author of four books and many theoretical and applied papers and chapters in journals and books. Served two terms as President of the International Psychoanalytical Association.

Mette Hvalstad. Child and adolescent psychiatrist. Chief Physician, psychoanalyst, snf board member at the Norwegian Association of Psychoanalysis. Practices in Oslo and Inland Hospital.

Juan Pablo Jiménez, MD, PhD. Psychoanalyst at the Santiago Psychoanalytic Association (APSAN). Professor for Psychiatry, University of Chile. Director, Millennium Institute for Research in Depression and Personality, Santiago, Chile.

Bernadette Kovach, PhD. Board-Certified Fellow in Child, Adolescent & Adult Psychoanalysis by the American Board of Psychoanalysis. In private practice in Farmington Hills Michigan. Faculty of the Michigan Psychoanalytic Institute. Chair of the Child and Adolescent Psychoanalysis Program. Co-Chair of the Candidate Progression Committee. Member of the Curriculum Committee and Educational Committee. Clinical supervisor for Authority Health, University of Detroit Mercy, University of Michigan, and Wayne State University.

Marianne Leuzinger-Bohleber, Prof. Dr. Phil. Past Director of the Sigmund-Freud-Institut in Frankfurt am Main, Germany. Professor Emeritus of psychoanalysis at the University of Kassel. Training analyst, German Psychoanalytical Association. Member of the IPA and the Swiss Psychoanalytical Society. Chair of the IPA Research Subcommittee on Conceptual Research (2001–2009). Vice Chair of the Research Board of the IPA (2010–present). Research fields: clinical and extra-clinical research in psychoanalysis, psychoanalytical developmental research, prevention studies, interdisciplinary dialogue between psychoanalysis and literature, educational sciences, and neurosciences. Member of and Consultant at the IPA Clinical Observation Committee (2009–present).

Luisa Pérez Suquilvide, MD. Psychiatrist and psychoanalyst. Co-Chair of the Teaching Faculty of the University Institute of Psychoanalysis of the Uruguayan Psychoanalytical Association. Member of the Clinical Observation Committee of the IPA. Practices in Montevideo, Uruguay.

Pilar Raffo de Lavalle, Adult, Adolescent, and Child Psychoanalyst in private practice. Member, the Lima Psychotherapy Center. Master's degree in Gender, Sexuality and Public Policy from the Mayor National University of San Maroos, Peru. Psychotherapist and supervisor in the Psychosocial Care Center in Lima, treating clients affected by political and social violence.

Griselda Revella, PhD. Psychoanalyst, Uruguayan Psychoanalytical Association (APU). Associated member (APU). Member of clinical research group in child psychoanalysis (APU, 2013–present). Co-coordinator of APU Child Department (2007–2008). Member of the Child Department of APU (2002–2014). Supervisor at the Individual Psychoanalytical Psychotherapy – Psychiatric Clinic, Hospital de Clínicas (2007–2016). Faculty at the Asociación de Psicoterapeutas del Uruguay (AUDEPP-IUPA). Faculty at the University Institute of Psychoanalysis of the Asociación Psicoanalítica del Uruguay.

Andrea Rodríguez Quiroga de Pereira, PhD Psychology, Buenos Aires Psychoanalytic Association, Adult and Child analyst. Member of the IPA Research Committee. Professor of Research Methodology at the Universidad del Salvador (USAL). Professor of Psychotherapies at the Pontificia Universidad Católica Argentina (UCA). Research Fellow of the University College of London (IPA, 2001). Co-coordinator and Substitute Chair of the (FEPAL) Research Committee (2013–2015). Research in psychodynamic psychotherapy, specifically single cases, and training and ethical practice in adult and child psychotherapy.

Bruno Salesio, MD. Full member of the Pelotas Psychoanalytic Society and of the Brazilian Psychoanalytic Society of Rio de Janeiro. Training and supervising analyst in the Pelotas Institute of Psychoanalysis. Member of the IPA Clinical Observation Committee. Reviewer for the *International Journal of Psychoanalysis* and the *Brazilian Psychoanalytic Review of Psychoanalysis*. Published several papers on psychoanalysis in Portuguese, Spanish, and English.

Patricia Singer, Lic. Member of the Uruguayan Psychoanalytical Association. Treasurer of the e-journal *Psychoanalysis Today* (2017–present), Member of the Uruguayan Exchange Center of the Psychoanalytical Association. Member of the Theory and Clinic Psychoanalytical Group, APU.

Beth Steinberg, PhD. Training and supervising analyst, faculty, Chair of the Psychoanalytic Psychotherapy Education division, Co-Chair for psychoanalytic training outreach, and the Curriculum Chair for the Psychoanalytic Psychotherapy training program at the San Francisco Center for Psychoanalysis. Practices in San Francisco.

Robert White, MD. Western New England Institute for Psychoanalysis. Member of the IPA Clinical Observation Committee. Director of Western New England Studies in Psychoanalytic Psychotherapy. Assistant Clinical Professor of Psychiatry at Yale University. Published papers and book chapters on Bion and intersubjectivity.

Introduction

Margaret Ann Fitzpatrick Hanly,
Marina Altmann de Litvan, and
Ricardo Bernardi

It is with great excitement that we present here a new stage of the work done through the IPA Clinical Observation Committee between 2014 and 2020—the advances in our method and thinking. In the first publication of this committee, edited by Marina Altmann de Litvan, *Time for Change: Tracking Transformations in Psychoanalysis—The Three-Level Model* (2014), the authors described the development of the Three-Level Model, and its questions: To what extent has the patient clinically improved (or worsened) during analysis? What are the main dimensions of psychic functioning in which the changes have, or have not, occurred? What hypotheses can best explain the changes observed, such as changes in the use of the analyst and the analyst's interpretations, and changes in the patient's capacity for symbolization? What problems observable in the verbatim sessions were not addressed? What alternative hypotheses, referring to a patient's problematic functioning, appearing repeatedly in the session material, could account for the absence of change?

Contributors to this book propose that the attitude adopted in making more systematic clinical observations guided by the questions of the 3-LM can complement the analytic attitude of free-floating attention or "goallessness." Moreover, the voice of the analyst when reading the sessions, as well as the way participants/analysts return to resonant moments in the analysis as they become immersed in the language of the patient and the analyst, brings the analytic unconscious into the work of the groups. In order to understand the challenge of psychoanalysis in bringing about "profound personality change" (Wallerstein, 1965), moderators of groups (the writers of these chapters) have focused on analytic listening, together with better-defined concepts for formulating the presenting pathology. Moderators attend to the shifts in the functioning of the patient and of the analytic couple, and they study the therapeutic action facilitated by the interventions.

Over the past several years of work (see Altmann, Fitzpatrick Hanly, & Leuzinger-Bohleber, 2012), the committee has made gains in understanding the analyst's implicit and explicit theories and in valuing the combinations of analytic techniques used in different psychoanalytic cultures (Canestri, 2006; Tuckett et al., 2008). "To facilitate transformations in our patients through the therapeutic process leading to changes in their inner worlds is a goal shared by all psychoanalysts" (Altmann de Litvan, 2014).

> The task is not to unify the psychoanalytic theory or validate clinical observations. It is to explore how to gain a better knowledge of individual patients to facilitate beneficial functional changes in them. The term used to denote the activities of these IPA workgroups is "enquiry," a term that includes the developing knowledge and understanding that any adequate analyst gains in the course of analytic work with patients, which the analyst uses to make therapeutically mutative interpretations, and which will form the foundations of a more unified evolving psychoanalytic theory.
>
> (Hanly, 2011, p. 2)

We reported that "more than 1,000 analysts have already participated in groups working with this model in many cities in different regions: Buenos Aires, Mendoza, São Paulo, Pelotas, Campo Grande, Lima, Montevideo, New York, San Francisco, Toronto, Frankfurt, Tel Aviv, and Prague" (Altmann de Litvan, 2014, p. xxviii). Now we can report on the participation of over 1800 psychoanalysts from these cities in which 3-LM groups have met again, as well as in Boston, Detroit, Chicago, Austin, Los Angeles, Lima, Rio, Lisbon, Oslo, Madrid, London, and Vienna in recent years.

In this new volume our approaches and clinical narratives show more experience, more depth, more answers, and, of course, new questions. Experience has confirmed that when a small group of psychoanalysts share a "clinical text" (with numbered lines facilitating a shared reading), they observe the analytic couple together, developing a deeper understanding of the presenting problems and suffering of the patient, consolidating the "anchor points" (or landmarks) from which change can be observed later in the clinical narrative (Fitzpatrick Hanly, 2014). This immersion in a shared text, with the voice and the presence of the analyst, creates a space in which to articulate different theoretical approaches in a manner that feels safe and provides an opportunity for open discussion of technique such that members of the group can better understand what may have seemed like a "foreign" concept. The second level of the model aims to identify the main dimensions of change and is based on the concepts that define psychic functions, which are used by contemporary psychodynamic diagnostic systems: the *Operationalized Psychodynamic Diagnosis* (*OPD-2*) (OPD Task Force, 2008), the *Psychodynamic Diagnostic Manual* (PDM-2 Task Force, 2015), and the Level of Personality Functioning Scale (American Psychiatric Association, 2013). In the third level discussion, the foci of the analyst's interventions are reviewed. Hypotheses on the analyst's theory of therapeutic action, as reflected in the analyst's interventions, are discussed by the participants. The 3-LM group reviews the interventions that fit with, or could account for, the transformations or absence of transformations in the patient and the process. This exploration of session material is a bottom-up inferential process, since it starts from the clinical data and ordinary language and advances towards more abstract alternative theoretical hypotheses.

While the "second look" is a term applied to the analyst's recognizing and thinking about a period of impasse in an analysis, "the moments in which one abandons one's attitude of 'suspended attention' and proceeds to the 'second look,' questioning oneself as to what is happening in the analytic situation" (Baranger, Baranger, & Mom, 1983), the combined processes of the Three-Level Model constitute a "third look" at the analytic process. The "third look" of the 3-LM clinical thinking extends the questioning attitude and engages the group process to read the session material and to consider the evidence of change, with the multiple theories and approaches of participants, and the long-term temporal dimension, taking a double perspective: progressive and *après-coup* or *a posteriori*.

In writing the chapters for this new book, contributors have engaged in a second 3-LM "expert" group process in which committee members, moderators, and consultants look at the first 3-LM report and re-examine selected aspects of the case material to answer specific questions on change and mechanisms of change. This volume presents new accounts of psychoanalyses, focusing on specific dimensions of the patient's psychic functioning, specific changes in the analytic process, and specific interventional strategies. It is our hope that the reader will find these clinical narratives, rich in verbatim, new and clarifying points of view in the observation of transformations in the patients and of the analysts' technique, useful both in professional development and in teaching candidates.

Our journey with the 3-LM has clarified obstacles too, and challenges to the method, some of which have shed new light on issues that we see as having value for psychoanalysts.

> Today it is not simple to determine to what degree . . . different theoretical approaches are coincidental, contradictory, or complementary, or if they are incommensurable because they refer to different aspects of clinical facts. . . . The central question is no longer a prescriptive

> one—how an analysis has to be—but rather a factual one: what effect does analysis produce in the analyst's real practice?
>
> (Bernardi, 2014, pp. 4–5)

We continue to ask: What is the nature and reliability of our clinical research? The preface to *Time for Change* stated, "[Q]uestioning of the objectivity of clinical observation . . . has had a long history beginning with the problems . . . raised by Freud" (Hanly, 2014). Our experience with the 3-LM over 10 years brings tentative findings:

> When clinical discussions follow an inferential process that starts with the clinical material and progresses toward theoretical hypotheses, "windows" open where it is possible to develop a fecund communication. The first of these windows . . . relies on the internal resonance generated by certain fragments of the material, which triggers a process of associations in the entire group. This process enriches participants' understanding of the material. A second field where communication may be productive is that of the conceptualization of basic clinical phenomena tied to the patient's transformations.
>
> (Bernardi, 2016, pp. 4–5)

A third window is created by examining what the analyst's interventions address in the patient's mind, and difficulties (the foci of interventions) and changes in those interventions over time, linked with ideas on how they facilitated changes in the patient (or did not). Also, in the third-level deliberations, a fruitful communication takes place when participants discover their consensus on the implicit theories and operational models of the presenter, despite their theoretical differences (Bernardi, 2016). However, the analyst's intention in making an interpretation may be different from the effect it has on the patient, and third-level discussions aim to explore actual mechanisms of change (see Chapter 15). The evolution of the model is grounded in the challenging goal to use session material to observe "links between the analyst's interpretations (and the theories implied in them), and the change (and no change) in the patient, in order to create hypotheses on therapeutic action in the analysis backed by clinical data" (Fitzpatrick Hanly, 2019, p. 1033).

> New Initiatives offer psychoanalysts needed continuing opportunities for professional development to improve the quality of clinical work and theorizing. The development of methodologies to improve and test clinical observation and theory building will provide psychoanalysis with the capability for evidence-based clinical practice, that

will enhance its ability to compete with other therapies and possibly restore something of its earlier place in the health sciences.

(Hanly, 2011, p. 4)

Organization of the book

Part I: Clinical thinking in psychoanalysis

Chapter 1, "A common ground in clinical discussion groups," focuses on "intersubjective resonance and implicit operational theories." The chapter proposes that clinical discussion groups based on the Three-Level Model for Observing Patient Transformations (3-LM) enable us to reflect on the clinical common ground shared by psychoanalysts who have different theoretical frameworks (Ungar, 2014; Bernardi, 2017). The very existence of this common ground is controversial; however, in their controversy Wallerstein (2005) and Green (2005) proposed an observational procedure that might clarify this matter. This procedure bears great similarity to the one used by clinical discussion groups that apply the 3-LM.

Chapter 2 presents a detailed illustration of how reflecting on the patient's presenting problems in the language and enactments of the first sessions allows the analyst to see how these crucial problems unfold, shift, and change over time. The patient, a young professional woman, moved from a dangerous polyamorous lifestyle to a married life with a baby. In her internal life, she had identified with her depressed mother, with split-off memories of early trauma and repressed conflicts over dependency and over Oedipal and sibling rivalries. Ms C's metaphors for her painful female bodily experiences, with affective states from which she was dissociated, were addressed by the analyst, often in the transference, and led to improvements observed in her psychic functioning. Chapter 3, "Bodily metaphors as anchor points in facilitating change," illuminates how the bodily metaphors in Ms C's associations vividly portray the traumatic and depressive experiences as well as unconscious conflicts as they enter the early sessions. Images referring to central aspects of the patient's subjectivity appear as key metaphors that embody corporal representations and emotions, and, in the course of the analysis, the shift in the metaphors shows transformations in the intrapsychic experience and patterns of relationship in the analytical process.

Part II: Change in metaphors and dreams

Chapter 4, "Changes and no changes in the representation of self and others through images and metaphors," describes how a patient with panic attacks experiences herself through metaphors and images in her dreams, which are extremely disturbed by negative emotions, particularly fear, as she struggles to stabilize her self-representation. The discussion by Ricardo Bernardi explores the strengths and limitations of the clinical evidence in the material, giving an illustration of his thinking about a tentative framework to assess the weight of the evidence in a clinical narrative. Chapter 5, "Changes in dreams in the psychoanalysis of traumatized, chronically depressed patients in the frame of the LAC depression study applying the 3-LM," brings to life the evolution of a patient, beautifully observed through the changes in his dreams over the years. A detailed discussion appreciates the changes in associations and the dreams in this analytic process and shows how they reveal the patient's painful conflicts and survivor guilt, implied in the role the patient's brother has in his internal world and in his dreams.

Part III: Foci of the analyst's interventions, mechanisms of change

Two chapters take up central questions concerning how we can observe the analyst's interventions as they facilitate specific processes of change. Chapter 6, "'I don't want to be like my mother': Exploring changes in identity using the analyst as model," illustrates how a 24-year-old daughter of immigrants uses her analyst as a new object and as a model, facilitating changes in unconscious identity-defining internal objects. The function of the analyst as model adds to the concept of the internalization of the analytic function. Chapter 7, "Sequence of changes and interventions in the analysis of a violent patient," describes in detail a sequence of remarkable changes in the analysis of a very difficult violent patient. When John started treatment, he was addicted to alcohol, marijuana, and cocaine; he physically assaulted and humiliated his companions. He was responsible for organizing physical punishments for anyone who dared to damage the family business. His father didn't accept him as a legitimate son, and he was repeatedly exposed as a child to the sexual life of his parents. The analyst worked on these severe difficulties in the transference interpretations to allow him to feel legitimate as a person, as a son, and as a brother. John responded positively, stopped using drugs, approached his father and half-brothers (by whom he was eventually recognized), had children, and improved his sex life with his wife. Bernardi's discussion shows that the clinical material allows the reader to track the sequence of changes in the way John understands and integrates his problems and traumatic experiences.

Part IV: Impasse

Part IV underlines the importance of examining why there is so little change in some analyses. In Chapter 8, "Three hypotheses on impasse in the case of Janine," each of three authors develops a hypothesis in assessing the factors at work in a partial impasse in an analysis: (1) object relations approach to impasse; (2) a plea for affirmation in the treatment; (3) understanding the patient's anal narcissism in the impasse. Chapters 8 and 9 explore a crucial matter in our model's capacity to observe and understand both change and no change in long-term psychoanalyses. The clinical material presented in 3-LM groups may reveal chronic enactments and partial impasse. These tend to appear more often when the basic psychopathology is more primitive, organized at borderline or psychotic levels, or when the degree of the deficit in certain mental capacities seems to have led to a pressure for enactment, and to imply a lack of capacity for differentiation and representation, and the primary anxiety of fragmentation (Killingmo, 1989). In this type of process, the analyst may not have recognized his or her participation in an enactment so that it becomes difficult to see how either party could pull out of the interaction. In some psychoanalyses studied by the 3-LM, the analyst's self-exploration of counter-transference reveries (Baranger, Baranger, & Mom, 1983), a second look when outside the sessions (De Bernardi, 2000), or consultation with a third party has helped to work through an impasse. Chapter 9, "Change and impasse in a systematic case study: Foci of the analyst's interpretations," asks what difficulties are, and are not, addressed in the analysis. The patient was a struggling creative writer who came to analysis suffering from bouts of suicidal depression and severe obsessional symptoms. His life improved, he was able to use his talent as a writer in a different field, and he showed some positive changes. The paper tracks absence of change in important dimensions of his internal dynamics that remained unchanged, and presents details from the verbatim (taped and transcribed) sessions, about the way an impasse developed in the analytic process. The discussion compares the observations in two 3-LM reports with the findings from systematic clinical research, and shows remarkable correspondences between the systematic research and the observational clinical research in assessing his difficulties at the beginning of the analysis, and in describing what changed and what did not, what was addressed in the patient's material, and what was not addressed.

Part V: New uses of the 3-LM in the transmission of psychoanalysis and in professional development

This section addresses our work on the core mandate within the IPA community: professional development and candidate education. The authors of Chapter 10, "The 3-LM's contribution to developments in analytical treatment," describe creative adaptations of the 3-LM format for use in IPA Institute training programs. The authors initiated new seminars in their institutes, using 3-LM questions to help candidates make clear formulations backed by rich clinical data, in composing their clinical reports and clinical papers for graduation. Chapter 11, "A dialogue between 3-LM presenters and moderators," brings to life the voices of our presenters, to whom we owe a great debt. They tell us about their experiences in preparing session material and presenting to 3-LM groups. They tell us about insights they took from the experience back to their clinical work, adding to their thinking in ongoing analyses. Committee members and moderators have interspersed brief commentaries, giving context to the insights of presenters, together elucidating many details in our methods, and the thinking underlying them.

Part VI: Clinical observation groups and the psychoanalyses of children

This section of the book presents the clinical observation of children using the 3-LM by the members of the IPA Clinical Observation Committee. The 3-LM methods were adapted to study the analysis of children by Altmann de Litvan, Miller, and Bernardi, presented in our first book, *Time for Change: Tracking Transformations in Psychoanalysis—The Three-Level Model* (2014). In this second book, we thought it would be of interest to present two clinical narratives with analytic material on child patients, which provide and reflect on the evidence of transformations the children underwent through their analytic processes. The first clinical narrative presents a detailed presentation and discussion of the analysis of a 5-year-old girl, at the three levels. The second clinical narrative is about the case of a 5-year-old boy who lost his mother at a very young age; here the group focused on observing what the young patient could teach us about his early mourning. Do children go through the mourning process? If so, what are its distinctive features?

Part VII: Improving clinical evidence

Chapter 14, "Assessing strengths and limitations of clinical evidence in a psychoanalytic clinical material," proposes a tentative framework to assess the weight of evidence in a clinical narrative. The chapter argues that clinical papers need to ground their hypotheses on change in psychoanalysis in clinical observation and should include a "Discussion" section that explains the strengths, limitations, biases, and omissions in the clinical data to ensure the traceability and conceptual reproducibility of their conclusions.

Finally, this new book reflects the many fruitful dialogues among committee members and consultants from the three regions of the IPA on these crucial topics in psychoanalysis. We do not hold to the idea that anything goes, but try to discover which concepts and theories are most coherent, and which have most explanatory power, for a particular psychoanalytic process. We have had to learn to reflect on the differences in our theories and cultures, to take the time to understand our differences as we explore detailed clinical materials together.

Part VIII: Three-Level Model

In Chapter 15, "Guidelines for organizing 3-LM groups," the authors present the current thinking behind each step of the Three-Level Model for Observing Patient Transformations, articulating the rationale for this method of clinical observation, and the aims for the group discussion at each of the three levels. The Guidelines describe in detail how to prepare the clinical material for a 3-LM group (for adult and child psychoanalyses), and describe the roles and procedures of the presenter, the moderator, the group, and the reporter.

References

Altmann, M., Fitzpatrick Hanly, M.A., & Leuzinger-Bohleber, M. (2012). Project Committee on Clinical Observation Panels. *International Journal of Psychoanalysis, 93*(3), 748–750.

Altmann de Litvan, M. (Ed.). (2014). *Time for change: Tracking transformations in psychoanalysis—The Three-Level Model*. London: Karnac.

American Psychiatric Association (2013). Level of Personality Functioning Scale.

Baranger, M., Baranger, W., & Mom, J. (1983). Process and non-process in analytic work. *International Journal of Psychoanalysis, 64*, 1–15.

Bernardi, R. (2014). The Three-Level Model (3-LM) for observing patient transformations. In M. Altmann (Ed.), *Time for change: Tracking transformations in psychoanalysis—The Three-Level Model* (pp. 3–34). London: Karnac.

Bernardi, R. (2016). La formulación clínica del caso: su valor para la práctica clínica [The clinical formulation of the case: Its value for clinical practice]. In *La formulación psicodinámica de caso. Su valor para la práctica clínica* [*The psychodynamic formulation of the case: Its value for clinical practice*] (pp. 25–44). Montevideo: Grupo Magro Editores, Universidad Católica del Uruguay.

Bernardi, R. (2017). A common ground in clinical discussion groups: Intersubjective resonance and implicit operational theories. *International Journal of Psychoanalysis, 98*(5), 1291–1309.

Canestri, J. (2006). Implicit understanding of clinical material beyond theory. In J. Canestri (Ed.), *Psychoanalysis: From practice to theory* (pp. 13–28). Chichester: John Wiley & Sons.

De Bernardi, B. D. (2000). The countertransference. *International Journal of Psychoanalysis, 81*(2), 331–351.

Fitzpatrick Hanly, M. A. (2014). A traumatized patient in analysis: Observing patients' transformations. In M. Altmann (Ed.), *Time for change: Tracking transformations in psychoanalysis—The Three-Level Model* (pp. 187–208). London: Karnac.

Fitzpatrick Hanly, M. A. (2019). Panel on "Transformations in female bodily experiences and bodily metaphors." *International Journal of Psychoanalysis, 100*(5), 1031–1033.

Green, A. (2005). The illusion of common ground and mythical pluralism. *International Journal of Psychoanalysis, 86*, 627–632.
Hanly, C. (2011). Memo to IPA Board. Unpublished.
Hanly, C. (2014). Preface. In M. Altmann de Litvan (Ed.), *Time for change: Tracking transformations in psychoanalysis—The Three-Level Model* (pp. ix–xxiv). London: Karnac.
Killingmo, B. (1989). Conflict and deficit: Implications for technique. *International Journal of Psychoanalysis, 70*, 65–79.
OPD Task Force (2008). *Operationalized Psychodynamic Diagnosis (OPD-2)*.
PDM-2 Task Force (2015). *Psychodynamic diagnostic manual*. New York: Guilford Press.
Reith, B., Lagerlöf, S., Penelope, C., Møller, M., & Skale, E. (Eds). (2012). *Initiating psychoanalysis: Perspectives*. Abingdon: Routledge.
Tuckett, D., Basile, R., Birksted-Breen, D., Böhm, T., Denis, P., Ferro, A., Hinz, H., Jemstedt, A., Mariotti, P., & Schubert, J. (2008). *Psychoanalysis comparable and incomparable: The evolution of a method to describe and compare psychoanalytic approaches*. Abingdon: Routledge.
Ungar, V. (2014). Tracking patient transformations: The function of observation in psychoanalysis. In M. Altmann (Ed.), *Time for change: Tracking transformations in psychoanalysis: The Three-Level Model* (pp. 97–121). London: Karnac.
Wallerstein, R. S. (1965). The goals of psychoanalysis: A survey of analytic viewpoints. *Journal of the American Psychoanalytic Association, 13*, 748–770.
Wallerstein, R. S. (2005). Dialogue or illusion? How do we go from here? Response to André Green. *International Journal of Psychoanalysis, 86*, 633–638.

Part I

Clinical thinking in psychoanalysis

Chapter 1

A common ground in clinical discussion groups

Intersubjective resonance and implicit operational theories[1]

Ricardo Bernardi

Introduction

In this chapter I discuss the nature of the dialogue among analysts who employ different theoretical frameworks. I focus on the conditions that facilitate fruitful exchanges. The fact that this dialogue can actually take place is relevant to elucidating the epistemological status of our discipline and to laying the foundations for the development of true scientific controversies. Such controversies generate more favourable conditions for the progress of clinical practice and psychoanalytic education and research.

The features and effects of pluralism continue to interest our discipline. First, the word *pluralism* denotes a fact: there is a plurality of theoretical and technical ideas in psychoanalysis. Second, it suggests the existence of a collective agreement that enables the coexistence of these diverse ideas within the same institutional framework. This was, for instance, the result of the well-known controversies between Freud and Klein (King & Steiner, 1991), which took place in the British Society between 1941 and 1945. These controversies ended with a "gentlemen's agreement" that made it possible for different schools of thought to coincide in one society.

Yet the idea of pluralism involves a more ambitious aspiration, namely the existence of a space for sharing ideas and experiences among the various schools. The aim is not just to achieve consensus but, more essentially, to develop an interaction that will favour the growth of the discipline. Such interaction includes both agreement and the clarification and explanation of dissent. Nonetheless, the conditions that render this exchange fruitful are rarely found. The Freud-Klein controversies did not lead to the development of such a space. Neither did pluralism help meet this goal in the Río de la Plata (Bernardi, 2001). Widlöcher (2008) has wondered, with good reason, if psychoanalysts know how to debate. Without debate, pluralism may easily cease to be a shared argumentative field where alternative hypotheses can compete and interact and become a "plurality of orthodoxies" (A. Cooper, 2008), resulting in the fragmentation of the field.

A common ground is needed for an enriching interaction to occur. In the philosophy of language, the expression *common ground* or *grounding* refers to the "mutual knowledge, mutual beliefs, and mutual assumptions that are essential for communication between two people" (Clark & Brennan, 1991, p. 127). Communication includes productive agreements and disagreements and brings into play not only content-related issues but also questions tied to the exchange itself. In this chapter I pay particular attention to communication that brings to light a clinical common ground and ways in which this common ground may favour a fertile pluralism.

First, I examine the nature of the difficulties posed by theoretical and clinical communication in psychoanalysis. Wallerstein and Green engaged in a key debate on the existence of a clinical common ground in 2005. Both concluded that an exercise or procedure should be developed to determine whether or not this common ground exists. My analysis is based on the experience of IPA clinical discussion groups that applied the Three-Level Model for Observing Patient Transformations (3-LM). Second, starting from these group experiences, I look at the features of the clinical common ground in each of the three levels making up the model: phenomenological observation, clinical conceptualization, and theoretical explanation. Finally, I present conclusions about the relevance of the clinical common ground for psychoanalytic training and scientific dialogue among analysts.

Pluralism: Theoretical integration or incommensurability?

Is it difficult to achieve a conceptual integration of conflicting theoretical approaches? The same word can denote different things, depending on the theoretical framework, and each school may designate the same phenomenon, or aspects of it, with a different name. For this reason, a "top-down" conceptual integration, which starts from universally accepted metapsychological premises or assumptions, is not feasible; axiomatic postulates or assumptions vary. Theoretical diversity, moreover, results in diverse ways of perceiving clinical phenomena. Consequently, it is hard to determine to what extent the various theories speak of the same phenomena and/or conceptualize them in a compatible or commensurable way.

When I started teaching at my institute, I attempted to compare Freud's interpretation of the Wolfman's major dream (Freud, 1918) with the reinterpretation of this dream by authors such as Melanie Klein (1932/1964) and Jacques Lacan (1966), discussed by Serge Leclaire (1958). I was powerfully struck by the fact that, while the three approaches considered the dream in similar ways and used similar theoretical terms, the clinical facts they identified as relevant and their metapsychological postulates were clearly different. We should hence ask ourselves if there is a space of shared meaning among these approaches or if, following Kuhn (1962) and Feyerabend (1962), they have adopted incommensurable perspectives. Or, to put it more simply, do different analysts see the same wolves (Bernardi, 1989)?

Freud chose the sexual content of the dream; Klein based her interpretations on the aggressive oral aspects (the wolf's open mouth); and Lacan and Leclaire focused on the formal determinants (V, W, M. . .), that is, the signifiers. As a result, the aspects deemed relevant are not the same. The three approaches use similar words—*unconscious, Oedipus, transference*, and so on. Yet the semantic and pragmatic contexts differ. The Lacanian concept of Oedipus must be understood in connection with notions such as the real, the imaginary, and the symbolic. This is not the case with Freud. At the same time, the Kleinian view of the Oedipus complex is part of a network that includes concepts such as positions, early anxieties, unconscious phantasy, and part-objects.

When we base our observation on certain theoretical premises, we choose phenomena that agree with our premises. It is, therefore, very difficult, if not impossible, to achieve conceptual integration on this basis. The attempt by the IPA Project Committee on Conceptual Integration (Bohleber et al., 2013; Bohleber et al., 2015) shows how hard this task becomes when it involves basic concepts such as enactment and unconscious phantasy. Integration is questionable because it is not practically possible to include all the relevant versions of these notions used by different psychoanalytic cultures or to offer a conceptual definition that encompasses them all.

Neither is it feasible to offer clinical examples that are universally accepted. When we start from conflicting theoretical premises, it is hard to find common clinical models. Different theories describe different phenomena. For example, Kohut describes self-objects; Klein, part-objects; and Lacan, *objet (petit) a*. Rather than unobserved or neglected, the phenomena that are left out are unobservable from certain theoretical frameworks. This situation forces us to wonder if we are in the presence of what Hacking (1999) calls "interactive kinds" or "classes," where concepts intended to describe reality actually modify it.

Summing up, the situation we find is similar to what philosophers have called *semantic holism*. This approach claims that a certain part of a language can be understood only in terms of its relationship with this language as a whole. Consequently, a gap is opened between psychoanalytic theories that resembles the deep, gestaltic change in people's world view described by Kuhn as a paradigm shift, which generates a relation of incommensurability between theories (Kuhn, 1962). Quine's (1960) holism suggests the inability to prove a specific hypothesis when it is considered in isolation from the rest of the theory. This hypothesis is part of a network of assumptions and auxiliary hypotheses that are being simultaneously tested.

From this perspective, rather than aspiring to speak the same language, psychoanalysts, like many other scientists, must learn to be polyglots. We will thus be able to communicate with colleagues who use a different theoretical language and allow them to speak the language of their favoured theory. The scenario actually becomes more complex if we consider dialects, that is, different versions or interpretations of the same author—a common occurrence within a region or among the followers of this author. Such intra-theoretical differences give rise to debates that are no less passionate or uncompromising than inter-theoretical dissension. For this reason, while areas of intersection or convergence have been found between theories (Kernberg, 1993; G. Gabbard, 1995; Filho, 2003), it does not seem possible to assert that a common language has been achieved.

In general, training in pluralistic institutions responds to the polyglot model. Analysts are taught to use a variety of theoretical languages, and the accent is placed on using them in a way that is consistent with the metapsychological postulates of each. Nevertheless, this should be just the first step. Psychoanalytic training should place a similar emphasis on transmitting ways of creating a fruitful dialogue among theories and of checking them against each other or developing alternative hypotheses that may be compared when tackling clinical problems. Without this second step, we reinforce semantic holism, and each analyst ends up speaking his or her own language and expecting it to encompass the totality of psychoanalysis.

In my opinion, the logical and semantic barriers that stand between theories are not insurmountable. These barriers develop when the clinical material is examined on the basis of theoretical principles that are viewed as the only admissible ones. "Top-down" deductive reasoning prevails, and phenomena that do not fit into the theoretical framework are excluded. As a result, certain metapsychological agreements must be attained for clinical-level agreements to develop. In actuality, however, attaining such agreements is not a necessary or legitimate requirement, nor does it reflect the spontaneous reasoning that unfolds in clinical practice. Furthermore, the detailed study of some current psychoanalytic controversies suggests that rather than as the effect of a real situation of incommensurability, the barriers thus generated may be viewed as defensive strategies to prevent the clinical material from challenging metapsychological premises (Bernardi, 2002).

The clinical common ground

The key question is whether communication can rely on a clinical common ground that is shared by analysts with differing theoretical perspectives.

If so, this clinical common ground should serve as a starting point for a "bottom-up" inference process that would make it possible to progress upward from shared clinical experiences toward theoretical explanations of a higher level of abstraction.

The presence or absence of a clinical common ground was the focus of a well-known controversy between Wallerstein (2005) and Green (2005). Reaffirming earlier statements (Wallerstein, 1988, 1990), Wallerstein claimed that, despite their varying theoretical and technical positions, analysts share a common ground at the clinical level. Green strongly questioned this claim. From a perspective close to semantic holism, he argued that theoretical and clinical concepts were inseparable and challenged the analytic community to show the presence of this mythical common ground in scientific papers, congresses, or psychoanalytic debates.

Interestingly, Green suggests an empirical procedure that might be useful to identify a kinship among theories. He states that such kinship should be demonstrated through a long-enough series of discussion sessions among analysts with different theoretical and technical approaches. "Now, to my knowledge, this exercise has never been attempted," adds Green (2005, pp. 628–629). Wallerstein agrees with this procedure and considers it an example of empirical research. He also indicates the potential existence of "differences in our conception of the necessary steps in the process of this demonstration (or determination)" (Wallerstein, 2005, p. 637), but does not elaborate on this point. Nonetheless, I believe it is critical to identify these steps so as to show where and under what conditions the common ground may be revealed.

We may view the procedure or exercise proposed by Green as an extremely useful and interesting observational study or natural experiment concerning the nature and scope of the clinical common ground. The standard situation would involve communication failures among analysts with different affiliations, which tend to occur, following Green, in scientific exchanges or controversies involving metapsychological differences. Such controversies show, as Green claims, that "most of the time psychoanalysts speak only one language in psychoanalysis, their own" (Green, 2005, p. 631).

The above-mentioned "experiment" suggests, instead, exploring a different path that may provide a basis for communication that will prevent failure. To this end, we must search for the common ground in the immediate effect of the material on analysts' minds, regardless of the way they will interpret it later, and then identify points of contact, step by step, in the inference process that goes from this first impression to descriptive concepts to theoretical descriptions. A "bottom-up" process of this sort starts at the experiential level, granting this level a consistency of its own, despite the potential influence of analysts' previous theories and experiences.

The Three-Level Model for Observing Patient Transformations as a tool to explore the common ground

There is a growing interest in regions of the IPA in conducting group discussions of clinical material with an array of methodologies. The Working Party on Comparative Clinical Methods (Tuckett, 2006; Tuckett et al., 2008) focuses on the study of analysts' "explanatory model" of working. Other groups emphasize different aspects of psychoanalytic work, such as the way we listen (Faimberg, 1996), the specificity of psychoanalysis, or other topics of similar clinical relevance. These groups show that analysts with different theoretical and clinical traditions can discuss clinical material together.

I will refer specifically to the Three-Level Model for Observing Patient Transformations (3-LM) (Altmann de Litvan, 2014; Bernardi, 2014a, 2014b) because the ascending inference process discussed earlier plays a key role in this model, and we can, therefore, inquire into the clinical ground that supports theoretical interpretations. In 2011, I submitted the 3-LM to the IPA Clinical Observation Committee for its implementation with clinical discussion groups. The model constitutes a heuristic guide or tool to observe patients' changes and transformations through three successive levels of analysis. As Green and Wallerstein requested, these groups are made up of analysts with different theoretical frameworks who discuss a large quantity of clinical material selected by the analyst. The material belongs to different periods in a considerably long analysis. Discussions usually take 10 to 12 hours—three or four for each level. Close to 1,000 analysts from various regions have participated in these groups to date (2016).

The first level of observation is phenomenological. Group participants are invited to listen to the material with the "third analytic ear" (Reik, 1968) and to share what resonates with them. They are asked to defer the formulation of interpretations and, instead, to discuss those aspects of the material that, in their view, stand out in relation to patient transformations. Transformations comprise changes in patients' lives and in analysis, more particularly, in the ways in which patients "use" both the analyst (in Winnicott's sense) and their own mental and bodily resources. At the same time, group members are asked to point out which fragments had the greatest impact on them regarding the suggestion of unconscious meanings, even if they cannot yet clearly identify these meanings. They are requested to pay attention to those metaphors or images that most resonate with them. These fragments become *anchor points* from which subsequent changes can be traced, and lead to new associations in other participants. The shared resonance, in turn, opens new paths of inquiry for the group.

At this point I would like to go back to the Wolfman. I would like to imagine how this first level of analysis would have unfolded with the Wolfman's material if we had had a literal transcription of the analysis. Obviously, we do not have it. Nevertheless, while it is not fully equivalent, we can conduct the exercise by adding to the original account of Freud's case history what the Wolfman himself wrote in his memoir and what his next analyst, Ruth Mack Brunswick, has related (Gardiner, 1971). Doubtless, Freud did not underestimate the resonance of the material or the need to render it carefully in the patient's words.

Freud writes,

> I was struck by the fact that from time to time he [the Wolf Man] turned his face towards me, looked at me in a very friendly way as though to propitiate me, and then turned his look away from me to the clock. . . . A long time afterwards the patient . . . recalled that [in a tale] the youngest of the seven little goats hid himself in the case of the grandfather's clock while his six brothers were eaten up by the wolf. So what he had meant was: "Be kind to me! Must I be frightened of you? Are you going to eat me up? Shall I hide myself from you in the clock-case like the youngest little goat?"
>
> (Freud, 1918, p. 40)

When Freud says "I was struck," he is talking about his internal resonance. Let us imagine now what would happen if we asked ourselves what other fragments resonate with us when we hear these words. I would like to talk about my own associations. In his memoirs, the Wolfman, Sergei Pankejeff, recalls a photograph of a wolf standing straight with its mouth open in a book that had scared him. He says that when he was 4 years old, his sister announced that she would show him an image of a pretty girl. Instead, she showed him the photograph of a wolf, which terrorized him, and he reacted with a temper tantrum. Yet he adds an interesting comment: he believes that the actual cause of this reaction was not so much his fear of the wolf as his disappointment and anger because his sister had teased him.

We do not know to what extent this anecdote constitutes a screen memory. In any case, in my listening I would focus on the resonance of emotions such as anger and humiliation, which are not dominant affects in Freud's narration of the case. Such emotions lead me to remember the patient's paranoid episode when, years after ending his first analysis, he sought Ruth Mack Brunswick's help upon Freud's advice. Sergei felt that the treatment provided by a doctor (whom Ruth Mack Brunswick, in this new analysis, linked to Freud) had damaged his nose, and that he wanted to kill that doctor.

This type of suspended attention aimed at the entire material does not seek to obtain direct support for a particular theory or interpretation. Obviously, there is no observation free of theory. When discussing "the use of the analyst" or "the patient's transformations," participants tend to evoke the ideas of authors such as Winnicott or Bion. Nonetheless, in the first level, the focus is not on these ideas. Rather, the latter are used only to point in the direction in which observations should be made. The discussion is intended to remain in a nebulous pre-interpretive level that resorts to group members' conceptual frameworks to make it easier for certain traces of the material to stand out on their own merit. For instance, patients' emotions such as rage or humiliation appear in new signifying contexts that are different from those of the above-mentioned interpretations (based on sexuality, oral aggression, and so on). Rather than certainty, this open form of listening aspires to offer greater complexity and new questions in order to reach a deeper understanding of the material.

Looking at the groups' work, we can see the usefulness of this broadened approach, which involves the interlinking of manifold perspectives. In this way, unilateral or rushed interpretations are avoided, and the complexity of the interconnections that are present in the material comes to light. When the material resonates with participants, "lines of force" can be drawn in it and "theory-phantasies" can be evoked (Nieto et al., 1985), thus opening the path for the emergence of new meanings.

The language used by the group plays a key role. For reflection to unfold, the discussion must be held in a spontaneous language, free from technical jargon. Participants should allow themselves to achieve a state of daydreaming or "transformation in dreaming" of their listening. Many contemporary authors highlight this issue, among them, Antonino Ferro (2009). At the same time, participants are asked to add a "second look" (Baranger, Baranger, & Mom, 1983) to this flow of spontaneous associations. This look critically examines what may be happening between patient and analyst at this time and what may happen concurrently in the discussion group. In this way, participants are alert not only to the effect of the material on them but also to what happened in the session and what is happening in the group. They should seek to open manifold perspectives or vertices from where to examine the material. They are always invited to point out which specific parts of the material support their observations or occurrences so as to compare them with the observations and occurrences of the other participants. (At the beginning of the discussion session every participant receives a copy of the material with line numbers.)

Let us look at the other levels of analysis of the 3-LM. In the second level, the discussion aims to identify the major dimensions of change. Concepts used must be objectifiable, on the basis of operationalized categories or dimensions. This procedure involves a change in perspective and, therefore, a complementary, binocular look at clinical phenomena.

The questions that guide group discussions are inspired by the dimensions provided by current psychoanalytic diagnostic systems such as the *Psychodynamic Diagnostic Manual*, the Level of Personality Functioning Scale (LPFS) of the *DSM-5*, Section III, and, particularly, the *Operationalized Psychodynamic Diagnosis* (*OPD-2*) (OPD Task Force, 2008). These systems, especially *OPD-2*, offer dimensions such as "Experience of Illness, Relational Patterns, Conflicts and Defenses, Structural Functions" (identity and self and other perception, affect regulation, symbolization, and bonding). These dimensions require that first-level clinical intuitions be supplemented with a research attitude that is highly alert to validity, reliability, and bias prevention.

The third level of the 3-LM invites participants to compare the analyst's implicit or explicit hypotheses with other potential theoretical hypotheses and to discuss possible interpretive strategies and examine the extent to which these hypotheses are consistent with the clinical material. In this way, each of the three levels allows us to explore the clinical common ground from a different angle.

Level 1: Shared resonance

I would like to illustrate the shared resonance phenomenon occurring in the first level with a case that was simultaneously discussed by four groups of analysts with different theoretical frameworks.

Roy started a psychoanalytic psychotherapy two years ago. He sought help because he was suffering from depression and was beset by ideas of death. Repeated failures and significant losses in different areas of his life prompted him to stop embarking on new projects. His life was progressively deteriorating. The group discussed the material during several hours and compared members' conclusions at the end of the day. It is worth pointing out that participants' overall clinical judgments concur to a great extent. The group largely agreed that in these two years Roy had improved in important areas of his life. He was progressively able to make better use of the analyst and of his own resources to achieve some changes. These changes, however, were incipient and precarious.

Determining the level of agreement is important because it provides a basis to establish consensus among experts. Many 3-LM groups have recently started to answer questionnaires before and after discussions, and research funded by the IPA's Research Committee is being conducted to identify the degree of consensus among assessments of change (Garbarino, personal communication). Besides agreement on certain clinical intuitions or judgments, another process tends to confirm the existence of a common ground and is particularly significant from a psychoanalytic standpoint. I am referring to the shared resonance mentioned above: a certain fragment or image that resonates with one participant triggers in other participants associations with other parts of the material that, in turn, reverberate in such a way that enrich the understanding of the first fragment.

Let us turn now to the clinical material.

P: *It's as if after [my mother's death] I'd been a robot, something like that.*
A: *Robots don't have a mother, or a father, or feelings. They don't have a life or a death.*

The discussion of this image of a robot led some participants to recall metaphors from other sessions:

P: *My car's clutch broke. You can only shift gears if you do it at the right moment. Braking is the problem. . . .*
A: *[Repeating] You can only shift gears if you do it at the right moment. . . .*
R: *People and cars are so similar!*
A: *And the risk is hitting the gas and trying to change everything at once, and then not being able to brake.*

These metaphors, whereby Roy offers a mechanical representation of himself, drove participants to evoke other fragments of the material that might be connected to them. Their evocation, in turn, suggested unexplored dimensions of the underlying phenomena. For example, at a certain point the analyst presenting the case remembered a dream the patient had had. In this dream Roy found out that his car had been stolen and could not find it. The dream gave the group new clues about the patient's difficulties in taking ownership of his own life.

While group members listen from the perspective of their own theories, resonance is not primarily declarative. What they share, rather, is the effect of unconscious communication on analytic listening, hence the evocative power of metaphors or language tropes. These images retain some ambiguity or indetermination that enables participants to examine the unconscious material in a better way than do abstract theoretical terms. *Robot* or *car* expresses aspects of Roy's experiences that facilitate the exploration of his relationship with himself (mind and body) and with others. They thus provide a richer basis for second-level conceptualizations and theoretical hypotheses, which are discussed in the third level. Freud claims that the analyst "must turn his own unconscious like a receptive organ towards the transmitting unconscious of the patient. He must adjust himself to the patient as a telephone receiver is adjusted to the transmitting microphone" (Freud, 1912, pp. 115–116).

In the first level of the 3-LM, participants also let resonate in them the ways in which other group members listen to the material and the expressions of these various modes of listening. These expressions transcend verbal language to include tone of voice and bodily gestures. Mutual resonance, however, does not mean identical resonance. In physics, resonance happens when a vibrating system leads another system to oscillate with greater amplitude within a certain frequency. In this sense, discussion groups act as a resonator. They favour a multiplying effect while acknowledging that each participant reacts according to his or her personal equation. For this reason, participants' theories and experiences do not necessarily act as an obstacle. Instead, they may be enriching, especially when a dialectic spiral is triggered that makes group members see the material from a new perspective in each step.

Just as in an analysis the new associations provoked by an interpretation are more important than patients' explicit agreement with it, so are chain resonances generated in participants highly valuable for discussion groups. Shared resonance phenomena are not essentially different from counter-transference reactions, even if they occur in different contexts. Gabbard (1995) has pointed out that understanding and using counter-transference in clinical practice constitutes an emerging path toward the creation of a common ground among analysts.

The reliance of psychoanalysis on an emotional, embodied, and situational form of knowledge that is, therefore, subjective has long been its epistemological Achilles heel. Paradoxically, however, this weakness is also its strength. Psychoanalysts are privileged to have this mode of deep emotional intersubjective understanding at our disposal. Empathy is our best tool to scan others' emotions. A similar resonance may thus be observed in therapists with very diverse theoretical training or technical criteria. The role psychoanalysis assigns to unconscious emotional phenomena in communication would not surprise an ethologist, nor a neuroscientist like Damasio. As Frans De Waal (2013) notes, empathic understanding is an evolutionary acquisition that has allowed our species and neighbouring species to survive. Psychoanalysis uses and furthers this potential, which is highly developed in humans.

We may conclude that in this first level of discussion the clinical common ground is manifested, above all, in the mutual resonance produced in different group participants by certain fragments of the clinical material. Such resonance expands the network of associations and enriches the understanding of the material.

Level 2: From empathetic resonance to the conceptualization of diagnostic dimensions

New challenges arise when we shift from intuitive and metaphoric observations in the first level, to conceptualizing the dimensions of therapeutic change in the second. Participants have to identify these dimensions and determine the significance of the change. To do so, they must reach a basic agreement on the relevant psychodynamic factors that are at the heart of the patient's psychopathology and on how much they have changed.

Let us return to the robot metaphor. The groups agreed that this image reflected one consequence of the patient's paralyzed or frozen mourning processes. Moreover, they also concurred that it could be inferred that certain structural functions had been affected, among them, the sense of self, the sense of agency, affect regulation, the processing of bodily emotions and experiences, and internal and external object relations. Do these agreements point to the existence of a common ground at this level as well? Yes and no.

The answer may be affirmative because the discussion shows an appreciable consensus on certain dimensions that describe patient change. Furthermore, consensus would increase if we used operationalized categories and previous training, as suggested in the *OPD-2*. Still, it is hard to make progress on this topic as a result of the appearance of divergences that may be categorized in two groups. For many analysts, operationalization is both acceptable and desirable. It involves the ability to find an agreed-upon definition of the dimensions of psychic change that we observe in analysis and serves as the basis for the formulation of more consistent theoretical concepts that are better anchored in clinical experience.

Other colleagues, by contrast, radically disagree with this path, as they consider that it makes us lose sight of the truly psychoanalytic essence of these concepts. Operationalization leads to taking into account what the *OPD-2* graphically calls the "smallest common multiple" among theoretical concepts belonging in different theories (OPD Task Force, 2008, p. 14). Many analysts think that, although these dimensions may have some validity, they fail to capture what is really significant from a psychoanalytic point of view.

Consequently, as we move from the first to the second level, the agreement becomes partial or problematic when defining the observed phenomena. For instance, Roy's "robot" experience does not hamper communication in the first level. In the second level, by contrast, while some participants agreed that an essential aspect of this experience could be defined as a loss of the "sense of agency," others believed that it was better expressed as failures in the "subjective position of the subject." We thus encounter once again the problem of semantic holism I described earlier. This problem is not necessarily linked to a specific term but to the fact that resorting to this expression entails making use of the entire set of terms of the theoretical language from which it derives.

The most radical stances, which reject any form of diagnostic conceptualization for impeding our psychoanalytic understanding of patients' uniqueness (e.g., Hoffman, 2009), evince the reappearance of the dichotomy that forces psychoanalysis to opt between the scientific and hermeneutic traditions. From my perspective, this is a false dilemma; given human complexity, psychoanalysis needs the contribution of both hermeneutics and natural science to answer the questions arising from its practice. Our discipline is not in limbo between science and hermeneutics. Rather, it seeks answers that may require either relying on its own clinical method, or resorting to scientific tradition in some cases, and to hermeneutic tradition in others (Bernardi, 2015).

Metaphors, like all creations of the arts and humanities, enrich our understanding of human experience. In the same way, to answer other questions, such as those about validity, reliability, and bias, or about causal relations, we must have recourse to scientific methodologies, more particularly, to statistics and neurosciences. The critical question is not whether one method is better than the other, but which is the most suitable to answer a certain type of question. Usually, we need to combine different perspectives. Like sailing and the social sciences, psychoanalysis benefits from the triangulation of its knowledge by comparing methods and perspectives. Moreover, it is interested in the consilience of its ideas and the contributions of other disciplines.

In sum, at the level of the description and conceptualization of clinical phenomena, our experience with the 3-LM shows that it is possible to reach an agreement among analysts with different theoretical affiliations. Still, there is no unanimity on the scope of this agreement and its relevance for psychoanalysis. The answer to these questions depends to a great extent on the value assigned to the search for consilience of psychoanalytic knowledge and the knowledge derived from other methods and sources.

The common ground at the level of theoretical explanations

We would expect the greatest differences among analysts with diverse theoretical frameworks to appear at the third level, when explanations for patient changes are discussed. Surprisingly, however, that is not the case. Discussions show frequent agreement among analysts with varied theoretical backgrounds on the most convincing hypotheses that explain the presence or absence of change in patients. Such agreement is possible due to the nature of the questions and of the answers offered by the group. Discussion in the third level is not aimed at answering general, abstract questions linked to psychoanalytic theory but at solving specific clinical problems identified in the previous levels. For instance, in the case of Roy, the questions focused on changes happening in mourning processes—in traumatic situations that might have affected the patient's evolution, his structural vulnerabilities, and so on.

Answers to such questions do not rely on specific metapsychological principles but, more directly, on participants' implicit personal theories.

Implicit or private theories (Sandler, 1983; Canestri, 2006, 2012) are conscious-preconscious theories developing in the interface between public or official theories and analysts' personal experience. They lie at the core of the conceptual, referential, and operational framework (Pichon-Rivière, 1998) that guides every analyst's work. The metapsychological premises that we actually use in our practice are dramatic, situational, and dialectic and seek to reflect the link between patient and analyst (Bleger, 1969; Bernardi & de León Bernardi, 2012). For this reason, while they are necessarily related to the general metapsychological systems upon which analysts rely, they express, above all, analysts' personal way of working, in keeping with their own personal and professional development.

We are not clones who apply theory in similar ways. We receive manifold influences, which we shape according to our experience. These implicit theories can incorporate the material's internal resonance and formulate it in an operational way in relation to our work with patients. They hence bring into play the analyst as an actual person and thus, paradoxically, strengthen the common ground. It is at the level of personal models where communication among analysts becomes more fluid and more dialectically fruitful, even if their theoretical frameworks differ.

The thorough discussion that develops in the first and second levels reveals the complexity of each clinical case, thus discouraging the use of theoretical clichés. Group members usually point out the incomplete or partial nature of the suggested theoretical explanations. At the same time, since the theoretical hypotheses discussed are personal mini-models, they need not be meticulously linked to the general theories from which they stem. These hypotheses often feed on elements from different theoretical traditions that are used flexibly. At the end of one discussion group, one participant stated that it was the first time that he could not clearly identify the theoretical background of the other group members after many hours of conversation.

This reaction is common in discussion groups, because what participants' interventions show is not so much the theory that inspires them but the ways in which they use this theory in practice. While, ultimately, they complement each other, clinical situation thinking and formal discourse differ. According to Zimmer (2014), the former seeks to respond to demands posed in the session by "multiple phenomena occurring simultaneously and to make an intervention in the moment which is useful in any number of ways." Contrariwise, as we can appreciate when reading a paper, writing about clinical theory responds "to the demands of formal intellectual discourse selecting out a single phenomenon and, often, considering that phenomenon through the lens of a single theoretical perspective and describing it with that perspective's particular vocabulary" (Zimmer, 2014, n.p.).

I would add that the difference between the two tends to blur when authors pose questions about or explore similarities among several approaches to a specific clinical situation (S. H. Cooper, 2015). Similarities will appear that may be more easily perceived in a "bottom-up" clinical reasoning than in an analysis that pays attention to authors' theoretical background. Deductive processes play a useful role at the clinical level when, on the basis of general theoretical principles, they suggest hypotheses or metaphors that enhance our understanding of the clinical material. Critically comparing diverse theoretical perspectives helps perceive nuances and different approaches that sharpen our clinical understanding. Nonetheless, if certain theoretical principles become absolute and exclusive and do not admit comparisons or challenges, they lose their usefulness and may hamper our understanding of the material. Clinical discourse may thus become apodictic or rhetorical-persuasive (as defined by argumentation theory) instead of critical and inquiring.

The complexity of clinical situations requires a different type of inference. When we face these situations, which can be understood from different perspectives or vertices, analysts look for the formulation that will best grant consistency and meaning to the multiplicity of elements before us. This inference leap toward the hypothesis that offers the best explanation resembles the abduction process described by C. S. Peirce. "Best explanation" is not the explanation that is most in accordance with a certain theoretical approach. It is the one that has the greatest clinical richness and heuristic capacity, generates a productive consensus, and is clinically useful.

Abductive reasoning is similar in many ways to eliminative inductivism, advanced by Edelson (1988). Following this approach involves progressively dismissing the least-grounded hypotheses and retaining the most convincing ones. Internal resonance guides in this path, and triangulation strengthens the conclusions reached. Triangulation shows convergence with information that stems from diverse theoretical perspectives and research methodologies.

Despite the ideal promoted by logical empiricism, clinical observations cannot be linked to metapsychological principles through a rigorous system of deductions and inductions. There are too many leaps in the inferential clinical process. At the epistemological level, there is an under-determination of theory by evidence that is not exclusive to psychoanalysis but can be easily noticed in our discipline. We have already mentioned holistic under-determination, which makes it difficult to verify a certain hypothesis separately from the rest of the theory. In addition, contrastive under-determination (Stanford, 2013) is common in psychoanalysis, because clinical material usually admits several interpretations that are sometimes complementary but, at other times, represent mutually exclusive hypotheses. As we have seen, the same clinical situation may be understood in different ways, depending on the perspective adopted. Moreover, new and better hypotheses may emerge that will prove the current ones inadequate (transient under-determination).

Under-determination makes it very hard to determine the overall superiority of a psychoanalytic theory over others or test particular statements that derive from this theory's general principles. Yet it is important to point out that it does not mean total indetermination or radical relativism. On the contrary, it forces us to examine very carefully the reasons that drive us to favour certain hypotheses over others (Laudan, 1990).

I referred earlier to the abductive processes, or reasoning based on eliminative inductivism, that guide clinical thinking. Clinical research can also be supplemented with qualitative or quantitative research procedures. I have already mentioned the study of the reliability of clinical judgments. We can progress through this path in search of consensus among experts on crucial issues for our discipline. Yet we can also take other paths. Participants in discussion groups found it useful to compare conclusions reached with the 3-LM in the initial phase of an analysis with conclusions drawn a few years later with the addition of new material (Hernández Romillo, 2014). In this way, we can further the study of the predictive validity of observations made with this model.

Identifying which opinions are confirmed and which are not as the analysis evolves has great educational value, as I can attest by my own experience. We can also design procedures to study concurrent validity by comparing the conclusions reached by the discussion group through an evaluation scale or instrument that is applied to the material discussed. This has been done in some groups, which compared their opinions with the Levels of Personality Functioning Scale (*DSM-5*, Section III) mentioned above (Altmann, personal communication).

In short, at the level of theoretical explanation, a clinical common ground may be achieved, thanks to a shared space where participants can examine and compare different explanatory hypotheses in relation to a clinical material. The aim is to determine to what extent these hypotheses are consistent with the material and their potential contribution to patient transformation.

Conclusions

As Green claims, it is very hard to prove the existence of a common ground at the level of verbal interpretations formulated according to different metapsychological premises. Nevertheless, we can find a common ground at the level of the inferential processes brought to play by analysts in their actual psychoanalytic practice in their effort to understand the material. Finding a common ground becomes possible when group discussion progresses from the bottom up, that is, from immediate experience to higher levels of theoretical abstraction. In this way, participants may shed light on the shared knowledge, beliefs, and assumptions making up a common ground that facilitates fruitful communication. These conclusions arise from numerous experiences with the 3-LM with the participation of analysts from various regions and psychoanalytic cultures. Clinical observation groups that use other methodologies may reveal other aspects of this issue.

Green's question in his debate with Wallerstein aimed to inquire into "the kinship between two different theories" (Green, 2005, p. 628). The conclusions of our exercise or "natural experiment" show an essential kinship among analysts' clinical thought processes rather than among theories as such. We are dealing, therefore, with in vivo theories as they exist and operate in analysts' mind and practice.

When clinical discussions follow an inferential process that starts with the clinical material and progresses toward theoretical hypotheses, windows open where it is possible to identify a fecund communication. The first of these windows, as shown above, relies on the internal resonance generated by certain fragments of the material, which trigger associations in the entire group. This process enriches participants' understanding of the material. A second field where communication may be productive is that of the conceptualization of basic clinical phenomena tied to the patient's transformations. Yet in this case the scope of agreement is limited by the epistemological and methodological controversies I discussed earlier. Finally, at the level of interpretive hypotheses, we have seen that communication becomes particularly fertile when, rather than focusing on metapsychological formulations, the discussion centres on participants' implicit theories. These theories are of personal and operational and address specific clinical problems identified in the previous discussion levels.

Through these windows, we can identify some components of the clinical common ground that are extraordinarily valuable for scientific exchange and psychoanalytic education. Furthermore, they will render pluralism into a space for productive exchange. Additionally, the focus of the 3-LM on transformations during analysis highlights the significance attached in our discipline to benefiting our patients. A clinical common ground makes it easier to reach clinical consensus among experts on the outcomes of psychoanalysis and on the best paths to achieve them. In this way, clinical data supplement information gathered by systematic empirical research.

A basic issue in pluralistic institutions is promoting the sharing of ideas and experiences at levels where such a sharing is truly effective. The 3-LM shows that this is the case with unconscious communication, as is reflected in intersubjective resonance and in the dialectic exchange that emerges when analysts' personal operational models are brought into play. It is hence useful for scientific and training activities to include group discussion sessions where analysts can expound on the reasons that led them to consider that certain hypotheses are the most convincing. Learning based on the study of clinical problems should be encouraged.

Scientific communication in psychoanalysis improves when it starts from specific clinical situations and brings into play the internal resonance of the material as well as analysts' personal operational frameworks. In this context, overarching metapsychological systems should be taken into consideration as a source for these frameworks rather than as incontrovertible great narratives. Clinical discussion groups, such as the one studied here, offer an effective path to promote both personal and institutional growth by making it easier for analysts to find their own voice (Gabbard & Ogden, 2009).

Lastly, the fact that discussion groups also reveal unanswered questions or clinical discrepancies that have not been solved should not be viewed as a drawback. Contrariwise, it helps develop analysts' "negative capability," that is, their ability to tolerate ignorance, uncertainty, and doubt (Bion, 1970). This ability is also an essential component of the clinical common ground in our pluralistic age.

Note

1 Published as A. Bernardi (2017), A common ground in clinical discussion groups: Intersubjective resonance and implicit operational theories, *International Journal of Psychoanalysis, 98*(5), 1291–1309. An earlier version of this paper (Bernardi, 2016) was published as "Investigación conceptual en psicoanálisis: ¿Tenemos conceptos universales o términos multívocos? [Conceptual research in psychoanalysis: Do we have universal concepts or multivocal terms?]." *Revista de Psicoanálisis de la Asociación Psicoanalítica Argentina, 73*(2–3), 168–178.

References

Altmann de Litvan, M. (Ed.). (2014). *Time for change: Tracking transformations in psychoanalysis—The Three-Level Model.* London: Karnac.

Baranger, M., Baranger, W., & Mom, J. M. (1983). Process and non-process in analytic work. *International Journal of Psychoanalysis, 64,* 1–15.

Bernardi, R. (1989). The role of paradigmatic determinants in psychoanalytic understanding. *International Journal of Psychoanalysis, 70 (Pt 2),* 341–357.

Bernardi, R. (2001). The need for true controversies in psychoanalysis: The debates on Melanie Klein and Jacques Lacan in the Rio de la Plata. *International Journal of Psychoanalysis, 83,* 851–873.

Bernardi, R. (2002). La necesidad de controversias en Psicoanálisis. Los debates sobre M. Klein y J. Lacan en el Río de la Plata. In *Psicoanálisis. Focos y aperturas* (pp. 44–73). Montevideo: Psicolibros.

Bernardi, R. (2014a). The assessment of changes: Diagnostic aspects. In M. Altmann de Litvan (Ed.), *Time for change: Tracking transformations in psychoanalysis—The Three-Level Model* (pp. 263–278). London: Karnac.

Bernardi, R. (2014b). The Three-Level Model (3-LM) for observing patient transformations. In M. Altmann de Litvan (Ed.), *Time for change: Tracking transformations in psychoanalysis—The Three-Level Model* (pp. 3–34). London: Karnac.

Bernardi, R. (2015). What kind of discipline is psychoanalysis? *International Journal of Psychoanalysis, 96*, 731–754.

Bernardi, R. (2016). Investigación conceptual en psicoanálisis: ¿Tenemos conceptos universales o términos multívocos? [Conceptual research in psychoanalysis: Do we have universal concepts or multivocal terms?]. *Revista de Psicoanálisis, 73*, 165–178.

Bernardi, R., & de León de Bernardi, B. (2012). The concepts of Vínculo and dialectical spiral: A bridge between intra- and intersubjectivity. *Psychoanalytic Quarterly, 81*, 531–564.

Bion, W. R. (1970). *Attention and interpretation*. London: Tavistock.

Bleger, J. (1969). Teoría y práctica en psicoanálisis. La praxis psicoanalítica [Theory and practice in psychoanalysis: Psychoanalytic practice]. *Revista Uruguaya de Psicoanálisis, 11*, 287–303.

Bohleber, W., Fonagy, P., Jiménez, J. P., Scarfone, D., Varvin, S., & Zysman, S. F. P. (2013). Towards a better use of psychoanalytic concepts: A model illustrated using the concept of enactment. *International Journal of Psychanalysis, 94*, 501–530.

Bohleber, W., Jiménez, J. P., Scarfone, D., Varvin, S., & Zysman, S. (2015). Unconscious phantasy and its conceptualizations: An attempt at conceptual integration. *International Journal of Psychoanalysis, 96*, 705–730.

Canestri, J. (Ed.). (2006). *Psychoanalysis: From practice to theory*. London: John Wiley & Sons.

Canestri, J. (Ed.). (2012). *Putting theory to work: How are theories actually used in practice?* London: Karnac.

Clark, H. H., & Brennan, S. E. (1991). Grounding in communication. In L. B. Resnick, J. M. Levine, & S. D. Teasley (Eds), *Perspectives on socially shared cognition* (pp. 127–149). Washington, D.C.: American Psychological Association.

Cooper, A. M. (2008). American psychoanalysis today: A plurality of orthodoxies. *Journal of the American Academy of Psychoanalysis and Dynamic Psychiatry, 36*, 235–253.

Cooper, S. H. (2015). Clinical theory at the border(s): Emerging and unintended crossings in the development of clinical theory. *International Journal of Psychoanalysis, 96*, 273–292.

De Waal, F. (2013). *The bonobo and the atheist: In search of humanism among the primates*. New York and London: W. W. Norton & Company.

Edelson, M. (1988). *Psychoanalysis: A theory in crisis*. Chicago: The University of Chicago Press.

Faimberg, H. (1996). Listening to listening. *International Journal of Psychoanalysis, 77*, 667–677.

Ferro, A. (2009). Transformations in dreaming and characters in the psychoanalytic field. *International Journal of Psychoanalysis, 90*, 209–230.

Feyerabend, P. (1962). Explanation, reduction and empiricism. In *Scientific explanation, space, and time* (Vol. 3, pp. 28–97). Minneapolis: University of Minnesota Press.

Filho, P. D. (2003). Recent theoretical convergences in psychoanalysis and their epistemological importance. *International Journal of Psychoanalysis, 84*, 1189–1202.

Freud, S. (1912). Recommendations to physicians practicing psycho-analysis. *S.E. 12* (pp. 109–120) [Consejos al médico sobre el tratamiento psicoanalítico. *Obras completas: Tomo 12* (pp. 107–119). Buenos Aires: Amorrortu].

Freud, S. (1918). From the history of an infantile neurosis. *S.E. 17* (pp. 1–124).

Gabbard, G.O. (1995). Countertransference: The emerging common ground. *International Journal of Psychoanalysis, 76*, 475–485.

Gabbard, G. O., & Ogden, T. H. (2009). On becoming a psychoanalyst. *International Journal of Psychoanalysis, 90*, 311–327.

Gardiner, M. M. (Ed.). (1971). *The Wolf-Man by the Wolf-Man*. New York: Basic Books.

Green, A. (2005). The illusion of common ground and mythical pluralism. *International Journal of Psychoanalysis, 86*, 627–632.

Hacking, I. (1999). *The social construction of what?* Cambridge, MA: Harvard University Press.

Hernández Romillo, S. (2014). Leticia: The emergence of questions about herself. In M. Altmann de Litvan (Ed.), *Time for change: Tracking transformations in psychoanalysis—The Three-Level Model* (pp. 35–50). London: Karnac.

Hoffman, I. Z. (2009). Doublethinking our way to "scientific legitimacy": The desiccation of human experience. *Journal of the American Psychoanalytic Association, 57*, 1043–1069.

Kernberg, O. F. (1993). Convergences and divergences in contemporary psychoanalytic technique. *International Journal of Psychoanalysis, 74*, 659–673.

King, P., & Steiner, R. (Eds). (1991). *The Freud-Klein controversies 1941–1945* (Vol. 11). London and New York: Tavistock-Routledge.

Klein, M. (1932). *The psycho-analysis of children*. London: Hogarth [*El psicoanálisis de niños*. Buenos Aires: Hormé, 1964].

Kuhn, T. S. (1962). *The structure of scientific revolutions*. Chicago: The University of Chicago Press.

Lacan, J. (1966). *Écrits: A selection* (Trans. Alan Sheridan). New York: Norton, 1977 [*Écrits*. Paris: Seuil].

Laudan, L. (1990). Demystifying underdetermination. In C. Wade Savage (Ed.), *Scientific theories*. Minnesota Studies in the Philosophy of Science (Vol. 14, pp. 267–297). Minneapolis: University of Minnesota Press.

Leclaire, S. (1958). A propos de l'épisode psychotique que présenta "l'homme aux loups" [Concerning the psychotic episode presented by "the Wolfman"]. *Psychanalyse, 4*, 108–135.

Nieto, M., Bernardi, R., Altmann, M., Bouza, G., Cárdenas, M., & de León, B. (1985). Investigando la experiencia analítica: una propuesta [Inquiring into the analytic experience: A proposal]. *Revista Uruguaya de Psicoanálisis, 83*, 117–135.

OPD Task Force (Ed.). (2008). *Operationalized Psychodynamic Diagnosis (OPD-2): Manual of diagnosis and treatment planning*. Cambridge, MA: Hogrefe & Huber Publishers.

Pichon-Rivière, E. (1998). *El proceso grupal. Del psicoanálisis a la psicología social* [The group process: From psychoanalysis to social psychology]. Buenos Aires: Nueva Visión.

Quine, W. (1960). *Word and object*. Cambridge, MA: The MIT Press.

Reik, T. (1968). Theodor Reik speaks of his psychoanalytic technique. *American Imago, 25*, 16–20.

Sandler, J. (1983). Reflections on some relations between psychoanalytic concepts and psychoanalytic practice. *International Journal of Psychoanalysis, 64*, 35–45.

Stanford, K. (2013). Underdetermination of scientific theory. In *The Stanford Encyclopedia of Philosophy*. http://plato.stanford.edu/archives/win2013/entries/scientific-underdetermination/.

Tuckett, D. (2006). The search to define and describe how psychoanalysts work: Preliminary report on the project of the EPF Working Party on Comparative Clinical Methods. In *Psychoanalysis: From practice to theory* (pp. 167–200). West Sussex: Wiley.

Tuckett, D., Basile, R., Birksted-Breen, D., Böhm, T., Denis, P., Ferro, A., Hinz, H., Jemstedt, A., Mariotti, P., & Schubert, J. (2008). *Psychoanalysis comparable and incomparable: The evolution of a method to describe and compare psychoanalytic approaches*. Abingdon and New York: Routledge.

Wallerstein, R. S. (1988). One psychoanalysis or many? *International Journal of Psychoanalysis, 69*, 5–21.

Wallerstein, R. S. (1990). Psychoanalysis: The common ground. *International Journal of Psychoanalysis, 71*, 3–20.

Wallerstein, R. S. (2005). Dialogue or illusion? How do we go from here? Response to André Green. *International Journal of Psychoanalysis, 86*, 633–638.

Widlöcher, D. (2008). *Les psychanalystes savent-ils débattre?* Paris: Odile-Jacob.

Zimmer, R. (2014). Discussion of Cooper, S. H. (2015). Clinical theory at the border(s): Emerging and unintended crossings in the development of clinical theory. *International Journal of Psychoanalysis, 96*, 273–292.

Chapter 2

Underlying clinical thinking on change and therapeutic action

Marina Altmann de Litvan,
Margaret Ann Fitzpatrick Hanly,
and Robert White

Introduction

This chapter will show the relationship between psychoanalytic research and clinical work, using the Three-Level Model (3-LM) through an example of the case of a patient showing transformations in her life as well as in her inner world. These observations are the result of the discussion of the same clinical material in 12-hour sessions by 40 analysts in three different clinical observation groups held in San Francisco and in Boston in 2015, using reports from these groups (two of us, Altmann and Hanly, served as moderators or reporters for the groups).

We will start with the more general results along the course of the analysis, following with some vignettes from the verbatim clinical material from the analysis, in order to get access to how this analyst helped in the transformation of this particular patient. Although different psychoanalytic cultures use the 3-LM in different ways, we found that main ideas about the clinical material in the first phenomenological level show remarkable convergences. As Bernardi (2014, p. 9) points out, "The experiences undergone with the 3-LM show a high degree of group consensus in the estimation of the changes in the patient, especially at the first and second levels."

The chapter contains the following sections:

1 The global change of the patient, according to reports based on group discussions and a questionnaire filled out by each participant.
2 A discussion of "anchor points," scenes, or images that had a deep impact on the group and are used to compare the initial moments with subsequent moments in the treatment. These anchor points are referred to in tracking changes in the patient during the analysis, and they emerge in the discussion of Level 1.
3 Two specific dimensions in Level 2 concerning the observation of change or absence of change using specific vignettes from the analysis.

The dimensions selected are relational patterns (outside the analysis and with the analyst) and structural aspects of mental functioning.

4 The foci of the analyst's interventions and explicit and implicit theories of the analyst about therapeutic action are discussed in Level 3.

5 Conclusions regarding the clinical material observed and the group discussion.

Clinical material

The patient has been in psychoanalytic treatment for eight years. She started treatment once a week, then twice a week in the second year, and finally four times a week and on the couch in the third year. She came to therapy because she felt "incapable of handling" her life and "vulnerable." The analyst presented six sessions: the first twice-a-week session one year after starting treatment, two sessions after two years, one session after four years, and two sessions after seven years. The patient, Ms C, is a middle-aged, single woman, half-Asian, half-Jewish, trained as a social worker. She is attractive but often appears to dress in a sexually provocative style and, in the analyst's mind, seems "like a child trying to look like an adult." She provokes in the analyst a wide range of feelings, "from very protective to disgusted." She describes herself as having a polyamorous lifestyle, reporting very risky behaviours involving sex and drugs. She reports that, during the first years of her life, her mother was depressed and both parents were distant. The family moved from Europe to the United States when she was 7 years old and then moved within the country shortly thereafter. Her mother was hospitalized several times when Ms C was 10 as a result of medical problems, possibly following a hysterectomy. Some family members on her mother's side (not close) were possibly killed in the Holocaust. Her father and his extended family are from Asia; some still live there.

Level 1: Global change in the patient

Group members were asked to fill out questionnaires about assessment of global change before the group discussions, reflecting on their individual reactions to the patient materials, and after the group discussions, reflecting on the influence of the group. Prior to the group discussions, most group members (8 of 11) found important global changes in the patient, moderate changes (7 of 11) in the patient's use of the analyst and his or her interpretations, and important changes (7 of 11) in the patient's use of her own mental and bodily resources in the analysis. In the reports written after the group discussions, groups often tended to focus on different aspects of the complicated dynamic picture. In this patient, some groups emphasized external changes, other groups internal changes, and still others observed it from different transferential positions of patient and analyst.

One report emphasized external change but saw more work to be done on internal change: "Dramatic changes in external life, from dangerous sexualized behavior to marriage and motherhood: missing a mother, finding a mother (analyst), becoming a mother." However, the group asked what the indicators of changes in the internal functioning, the dynamics, and defences were: "The patient is able to acknowledge her need for the analyst and is beginning to fight with/differentiate from her analyst rather than comply or flee."

Another report emphasized similar changes in the internal dynamics and in the relationship with the analyst:

> Transformational hours reflect a significantly greater capacity to depend upon the analyst and make use of the analyst's facilitation so as to be able to think, link, and understand rather than act out. . . . Good progress was noted, given this is the mid-phase of analysis—but the hope would be for deeper and more substantial internalization in the future of this treatment.

A third report also emphasized internal changes:

> The group observed changes in the patient's capacity to love, to be cared for, and in her psychosexuality (infantile-libidinal). Ms C entered analytic treatment talking of her polyamorous and risky sexual behaviors with men, women, and couples. After several years in analysis, she was married and had a baby, taking a year off work to be with the baby. In addition, changes were observed in the relationships with her mother and father, with more capacity to observe what her parents were actually like. . . . Ms C felt and showed "disconnectedness" in early sessions; while she can speak about her worries about "dissociation" in later sessions.

Anchor points to track changes in the patient

Naked lunch

After the material is read aloud by the analyst, the group starts a free discussion about the changes or transformations they can observe in the materials (Level 1: Phenomenological Description of Transformations). The group listens to the unconscious voice of the patient: "Resonance of the material among participants adds a new dimension to the clinical process, which could be named 'observation of observations'" (Bernardi, 2014,

p. 11). This resonance allows the group to track "lines of force" and evoke "theoretical fantasies" about the material (Nieto et al., 1985). It is important, in a clinical observation group, when the resonance of the material for each participant triggers a series of exchanges from diverse theoretical perspectives, shedding new light on the analytic process (Bernardi, 2014, p. 10). When they listen to the clinical material, the mental state of the participants in the group is a state of floating attention. Nevertheless, the clinical observations must be connected back to the evidence in the clinical material (Bernardi, 2014, p. 8). The group is asked to identify two or more "anchor points," images, metaphors, or affect states that appear to capture a key dynamic conflict in the opening hours. The group then looks for evidence of these anchor points in the later hours, comparing before and after for transformations.

An example of an anchor point in the clinical material might be helpful here. The group came back many times to one of Ms C's descriptions (hour 1, 2009) of a lunch with a current boyfriend (M) after a romantic night: "Intimate lovemaking and nice walk . . . things were positive, serene." Then she told him that she was thinking of having a second "naked lunch" with an older colleague and friend. She had no idea why her boyfriend got angry. She said she'd had a "hysterical reaction to M yelling" at her, "just feeling overwhelmed"; "I panicked." It was clear that she provoked anger without realizing what she was doing. The analyst intervened, showing how she made her boyfriend angry. The patient insisted that "the nudity wasn't sexual. He's married, he's much older—why is this such a huge problem?" M replied, "I don't believe you. Did you want to sleep with him?"

P: *He went on and on. Things get calm, and then he comes over and it's the same old thing. He understands that he's overly possessive. I have this fear of another man looking at my body. When I start crying, he comforts me but then gets angry again. The only way to get him to not be angry is to go to this extreme. I kept going back to: how do I feel this way when this morning was like bliss?*

A: *It is interesting that you said that to him, because I think you know that having had lunch naked with someone would upset him.*

P: *I get this feeling of being dishonest, like if there's an interaction with a man. . . . I do think I was wondering if it was okay. It wasn't feeling uncomfortably intimate, but I think we both felt really opened up and intimate. . . . This is maybe a strategy I use at times without being thoughtful about it.*

A: *Aware of it.*

P: *Yes, aware of it. . . . Yes, this feels helpful to think about it that way. I mean I guess what it brought up for me . . . I was thinking more . . . I was trying to look at what was going on with . . . having easy connections, not sexual, but he was a radical type social worker and Burning Man, and the idea of getting so intimate does seem odd to me now—also makes me think about what kind of things I was doing at that time.*

A: *I also feel aware that you have said a few times that you want to talk about what's going to happen with us and both times you wanted to do that, you came in a crisis. . . .*

P: *I'm feeling able to admit that it feels scary to do that.*

The analyst also noted that this session took place when the patient was making the transition to twice a week, but it was unclear if the analyst made this connection to the patient.

What meaning did the group find in this anchor point, the naked lunch? Was there a voyeuristic pleasure? A need for another man to look at her naked body? A need for self-assurance? Was she genuinely confused by her boyfriend's reaction and/or unconsciously trying to provoke him? She became quite anxious when he reacted with anger. She was emotionally quite fragile, with rapidly shifting states:

P: *When things feel on a good path, and then something happens, and then some feeling like too happy or too opened-up, and then something goes wrong, and I feel overwhelmed by it . . . the more I put into something, the more risk and pain is involved.*

The analyst reflected, "One minute it's bliss, and the next minute everything is falling apart." The patient also observed that she was "not totally knowing the boundaries with myself." The analyst also noted, "It seemed that she had no boundaries." The group identified fragile self-esteem with rapid shifts in affect and poor ego boundaries. Only after the analyst's intervention could she think about what she did and reflect on ideas of honesty and dishonesty. This was surprising, because the patient was a social worker and appeared to operate at a higher developmental level. For her, intimacy was the presence of two naked bodies; it was not psychic or emotional intimacy. The group thought this indicated dissociated aspects of the patient, linked with the body. When the analyst said, "Aware of it," one member of the group thought of a "mirroring" intervention, reflecting the affect of the patient. The naked lunch allowed her to connect "easily," and she denied the sexual side of nudity: "having easy connections, not sexual." She defended herself by dissociation, disavowal, and acting out.

Six years later (hour 6, 2015), the analyst reported that she saw her on Tuesday, the second session of the week. The patient had called after the previous session, feeling very disturbed by it, so the analyst called her back and left a message.

P: *Now I'm feeling overwhelmed again—like where to start, what's really going on. Just talking about all the sex stuff and not having sex is really bringing a lot up. It's really disturbing some control, something deep, fundamental to how I've operated . . . I don't exactly know what, but the idea of picking up the phone after calling you. . . . I was in a different state . . ., there was this huge feeling of resistance.*

A: *. . . I understand that you didn't necessarily want to talk to me, but you wanted to hear back from me.*

P: *I guess I did imagine you'd call and leave a message—wouldn't a part of me prefer to talk to you?*

A: *I just think having a brief phone conversation is different than hearing back from me. Maybe that's pressure . . . for more contact than you could handle, and this feeling somehow you should be able to handle more contact. Kind of like sex.*

P: *Wanting more contact. . . .*

A: *In here. It's interesting. Maybe the fact is that when you're feeling like you were feeling yesterday morning—cut off, lost, raw, wanting—you'd take almost anything. Like if someone came along and wanted to have sex with you, maybe you would. . . . Because you wouldn't really know, and you'd be so desperate for something, but what you would really want is to be back here with me feeling safe and protected.*

P: *. . . [She says she started to feel more just now, like yesterday—a feeling in her left arm—a "deep" feeling]. To me it feels like something really deep and painful is being touched—it seems like the feeling when I start to cry—like a stinging, sharp. . . . This emotional pain . . . I did have it just now. . . . Then when you said the part about sex, I got a little sidetracked. I think you were feeling raw and vulnerable and lost. . . . I think that's what brought the feelings back.*

She associated this with her 17th birthday, when she lost her virginity with her boyfriend: "You know I deliberately, on my 17th birthday, lost my virginity—with my boyfriend. But the feeling was, I don't really know . . . what sex is for . . . and I don't really know what celebrating my birthday is about."

In hour 5, 2015:

P: *Before that I had a flash of something sexual with you, still in the white tank top. It's right here and I'm pulling you towards me—our mouths. It also felt scary, and unsafe—but I did feel like I was feeling a little arousal and then that flash.*

A: *Maybe what we're seeing is you start to have a feeling in your body, maybe a yearning, a feeling of loss, anger, like when you felt like the clock was turned towards someone else and you imagined me with someone else, and then this fantasy happens, a sexual fantasy, or a sexualized fantasy, that kind of obliterates that, your feelings, that is. [She cries.]*

Level I: Conclusions about change and no change in these vignettes

The patient responded more fully to the analyst in finding her feelings, "using her mind and body" in the analysis when the analyst reminded her that "she wouldn't really know" what she felt, and asked her to see what feeling came, and asked her to stay with her feelings.

Anchor point 2: Hide-and-seek

Three groups underlined a second anchor point they called playing hide-and-seek, connecting it to the "use of the analyst," as noted in the intense counter-transference experiences of the analyst in the early sessions before and after breaks. The analyst felt that she had "to tolerate that all thinking and feeling were collapsing" and that Ms C was experiencing the analyst "as trying to control and hurt her."

In the first period of analysis the analyst comments:

> *Ms C schedules her own vacation without any reference to me. During these times, things would collapse, and Ms C would resort to action and boundaryless sexual goings-on there. . . . It was very difficult to connect these things with the breaks in our meetings or to understand anything about what was going on. Part of my counter-transference at these times was that something dangerous and aggressive was happening and that she felt that she was not being protected. But these feelings would become inaccessible, and I would have to tolerate all my thinking and feeling collapsing while she dissociated.*

In the second year of analysis (hour 3, 2010), when the analysis began at four times a week, Ms C brought memories and a metaphor about hiding and being afraid to be found, from the time after the family moved to the United States from another continent.

P: *Two thoughts about coming in today or in general on Wednesdays—one feeling is like having nowhere to hide, and the other one was it feels really vulnerable, and I guess it feels right now like it's revealing something about me, not sure if it's to you—maybe just to myself—that . . . sort of like I can't be trusted with hiding spaces. . . . Right now, it feels like there is this feeling. . . . I'm remembering this thing when I was 6. We moved to the United States—July 6—summer—a townhouse in San Jose. I don't remember what happened, but I was supposed to say "I am sorry" to my mom and I wouldn't say I was sorry, and so I ran away. I went to cross the street—there were these carports across from each other. I was hiding in some bushes, and it felt scary. It felt scary, like I felt scared she wouldn't find me and that she would.*

That all felt scary. . . . I don't know how that ended. I think she was calling my name. I'm pretty sure she didn't find me. I have some image I came in and got in trouble and maybe I did say sorry, I don't know. . . .

A: *In these images it seems like there is a very ominous or scary feeling about being found—there isn't any sense of relief or something good coming out of it or being taken care of. Just very exposed in a scary way.*

[The analyst returns to the scene that the patient brings and shows her emotions of fear and being scared, but also points out the "relief" of being found, a relief that was not experienced by the patient with her mother. This intervention helps to modulate the experiencing of separation and affect regulation.]

P: *I have no idea what the subject matter was when I was 6 [long silence, the analyst asks what's going on]. I was thinking a little bit about the incident, then thinking about playing hide-and-seek—the image I have of hiding somewhere—it feels totally scary. If someone finds you, it's going to be scary. If someone finds you, they're scared—it just seems clear to me now—I never thought it was fun to play hide-and-seek—hiding alone somewhere and the moment someone finds you, it just seems really scary, it just seems not fun to me.*

Five years later (hour 5, 2015) we found a new meaning of hiding:

P: *Yeah. It's sort of reminding me of what I was saying yesterday about self-satisfaction, being in the back of the car and being in my own world—in that transition, it doesn't feel like you're hiding. Maybe it's that clear reality that you have your own whole reality, like being in the back of the car. There are all these things that'll never be shared. It's private. Not a secret.*

At the beginning of the analysis, the patient reacted to loss and rejection by physical withdrawal, running away, without awareness of her fears or her wish to be found and comforted; she would just collapse, as seen both in the transference during "breaks" or in her description of interactions with her mother. In a dissociated state, she regressed to a paranoid fear of being attacked and controlled. The analyst, too, got pulled into the confusional state and felt paralyzed; neither was able to discuss the interaction or put it into words. By year two, she could start to put into words her fears of humiliation, but she was not aware of wanting to be found, nor could she experience any relief or security in the finding. It was only when the analyst bought up wanting to be found that she could label her feelings "hide-and-seek." By the fifth year, she could appreciate a concept of privacy and a self-identity that is not shared unless you want to. For this anchor point, we see a clear transformation, the ability to name and identify discrete emotions, the ability to describe frightening experiences rather than physically withdraw, and the beginning of identifying needs and wishes, wanting to be found and held. She no longer needed the defence of projection and paranoia.

Level 2: Dimensions of change

Level 2 aims to identify the most important dimensions of transformations in specific dimensions of psychic functioning. This level requires a more focused listening from group participants; it is a secondary process. All group members found changes from the initial moment of the analysis to later moments in every dimension, going from severe limitations of functioning to moderate disturbances, with some limitations on functioning. The dimensions identified as having undergone more changes were "relational patterns with the analyst" and "perception of others, empathy."

Relational patterns[1]

From the anchor points the group selected, we will re-observe the different relationship patterns. We will see how events with significant others were described by the patient in the past and in recent experience, and observe the patient's present interaction with the analyst, including transference and counter-transference.

Relational patterns outside the analysis

Ms C started treatment in a polyamorous lifestyle, with sex and drugs, and dressed in a sexualized and provocative style. She was aggressive and inhibited, she acted out, and she demonstrated very risky behaviours, which she could not regulate.

Six years later (hour 5, 2015), she brought up polymorphous perverse phantasies:

P: *Yeah, when I'm reading—by myself—it's a very familiar feeling of reading—this would be common in any book—when the character is yearning. In this vampire book that I'm reading, the guy is yearning for blood, but it seems sexual.*

A: *Is he yearning for blood or a person? Is he yearning for a person?*

P: *[Talks about the man yearning for a beautiful woman]. It feels very familiar to feel that way while reading—the words are giving me a sense of this person's physical experience—a focus on and warmth in the genital region and a pressure that wants to be relieved, and, if you press it against something, it will be more intense and then be relieved—longing and yearning where the pressure is greater—more arousal—finding something to press up against—I think the arousal comes to the groin area. He could suck her neck, but he'd be pressing up against her. The satisfaction would not be from getting the blood in his mouth. But I was thinking earlier how much safer that is—being by myself reading, feeling these things—than actually doing something sexual.*

At first overwhelmed by "reactions," the patient developed more subjectivity in her phantasies.

Six years later, as a mother, Ms C had developed a good physical and mental contact with the baby, although she said, "I didn't have a very physical relationship with my parents." The patient observed her mother's difficulties in experiencing a relaxed physical contact, when holding her baby. "She was so awkward." She wondered if her mother would be a safe caretaker for her baby: "My mom would be overwhelmed, frantic, and what that would mean about her taking care of him [the baby] in the future." She said, "Now I'm feeling overwhelmed again. Like where to start, what's really going on . . ., just talking about the sex stuff and not having sex is bringing a lot up."

At the beginning of the analysis, Ms C searched for contact with an object, via action and dissociation, as we saw in the scene of the naked lunch. Sex was a way to feel alive, and seduction was a way to control the object. Objects were just bodies to press against and to facilitate discharge of pressure. She could not even imagine oral pleasures in her object or herself. It was only safe to be walled off, solitary, protected, without involvement. These different types of interaction showed the difficulty she had in achieving emotional intimacy with others. Ms C moved from the "Burning Man," the "naked lunch," with a polymorphous and promiscuous acting out, to marriage. A question arose in the group about what kind of object her husband was for her. Did she love her husband? Had he become a more differentiated object for her? The analyst answered that Ms C and her husband dated for two years before getting married. The analyst thought Ms C loved him. They met in an exercise activity, "walking on ropes." Transformation in relational patterns outside the analysis remained uncertain; it was not clear yet what kind of object her husband was to her and what kind of intimacy she could tolerate or enjoy.

Relational patterns with the analyst

At the beginning of the analytic process Ms C seemed to have no recognition of the other, then (November 2010, four sessions a week) she began showing a need for the analyst: "I'd like to hear from you now." She could use the interpretations about the analytic couple: "I definitely looked at the weekend as [self-]sabotage. . . . I felt abandoned by A [her friend]." The analyst interpreted:

A: *I think about you at this party Saturday, or when your cousin touched you, or when you left here Friday, feeling abandoned by me—like out there on your own, and feeling how can this happen and no one's looking out for you.*

P: *I did feel on Friday—we did talk about me going to my cousin's close to the end. I did feel like it was like, "OK . . . good luck." I feel like so much happened yesterday. . . . That statement felt like when I was 6 or 7, if I tell my mom, it's gonna be really unpleasant. I don't want to feel bullied, etc. Or do something just because it'll be easier for him or me. So, I felt really angry about that . . . and then I had a "date" with a guy for an hour—the guy who's half-Asian and half-Jewish, and dinner with H [ex-boyfriend] to talk about work things.*

A: *It sounds like you feel unprotected by and angry at them and me also, and then you turn to men.*

The focus of the analyst's interpretation referred to separation anxieties and her feelings of abandonment (past and present). In her relationship with the mother, abandonment and separation contained unpleasant and rejection feelings, as we saw in the metaphors of "hide-and-seek."

At five years of analysis (December 2014), we can observe the emergence of a different person, with a wider range of affects and remembering, wanting more contact, planning for the future:

P: *Yesterday feeling like I can't believe you're leaving for all this time when I'm so pregnant and so much is going on. . . . I do feel angry about that. I can feel it in my jaw. It's because you're not going to be here that I'm in this state—this really efficient "getting things done, everything kind of working out and convenient" state, that's your doing—like the summer. Whatever excitement on Christmas morning I don't get to come in the next day and tell you. [She talks about the relationships between M and her and D and her]. I feel sad, in all that—family, love, connection, I don't get to have that with you—I don't have the support to feel all the different sides—and I have fear about my dad—and just what it's going to be like to have M more involved . . . [silence]. I am having some feelings about. . . . With my paycheque.*

Ms C noticed more about her relationship with her mother, and that she felt safer and more in contact with the analyst:

P: *I feel very not thought of—like the opposite of feeling tracked. I don't have any clue if she understands or knows where I'm at, and I can't track her either. Yeah, it feels like the opposite of the feeling of when I call you and you call me back. That feels safe. Like I know that you know. I am imagined [sic] you would listen to it soon and that you would know where I was at.*

As with her outside relationships, in the beginning of the analysis, she could acknowledge the loss of the analyst over the weekend, but she was quickly forgotten and replaced by sexual interest in a replacement. The analyst was treated as a thing, reflected in the counter-transference. By the fifth year, she was aware of the continuous presence of the analyst inside her, listening to her, allowing her to "survive." In the closeness there were different proximities that were bearable. Intimacy was constructed through the closeness or touching of bodies, and through different mental spaces that were generated. It was not clear how much she could mentalize the analyst as a separate person with her own concerns and personality differing from hers.

Structural aspects of mental functioning

In the 3-LM, questions on structural functions "aim at exploring further what is described as vulnerabilities, fragilities, deficits, or developmental arrests of the patient. Four dimensions are taken into account, following the OPD-2 criteria" (Bernardi, 2014, pp. 14–15).

The first dimension, "self-perception, sense of identity, and integrity of the self," "refers to the patient's capacity to perceive what occurs in his own mind and to build, based on that, an integrated and differentiated sense of his personal identity and of his capacity to project towards the future" (Bernardi, 2014, p. 15).

The group asked, how capable is the patient of adequately perceiving her own internal states and those of others? And how has that changed? During the first year of treatment Ms C had a very poor grasp of the mental state of her boyfriend, as we observed in the scene of the naked lunch. She had no idea what she was doing. She did not think in the sessions about what her mother's illness had been that caused the hospitalizations, or why her mother had become depressed. When she brought her mother into the session, her thoughts are superficial. The questions "Why did my mother get sick?" or "Why did my mother get depressed?" were never raised. At the beginning of the treatment, when she missed a session, she did not care; time was not so important: "I do not see the future." Ms C was a successful social worker (identified with her successful businessman father), but she showed signs of a strong identification with her depressive mother from when she was a little child. The patient had no "space" for compassion towards or understanding of her mother. First the patient was rather non-verbal: she acted; then, through the course of the analysis, she verbalized more and was able to associate present with past; then, she started giving a place to the past. In the scenes of the naked lunch we see Ms C's difficulty in understanding the thoughts and feelings of others, and how she was challenged by alternative perspectives and became confused about the impact of her actions on others.

In the most recent sessions, she took care of her baby, having decided not to work for the first year, giving "agency and direction to her life"; now she cared about time and the future; she started working on a retirement plan. She also cared about the mother she could become. In this way she was considering the future and time. When she was pregnant, she worried about how delivery would go, and whether she or the baby would die. Being pregnant brought phantasies of a dead mother, and she was defending against them. In the last sessions, she realized that she could become numb (afraid of not feeling things properly), which was different from being dead or completely dissociated. "I am scared not to feel the fear, layers of non-contact."

From being "chill," she became able to depend on someone: a transition from a pathological dependence to an idealizing transference in which she could form a quite profound bond with her analyst. She was tied to the analysis with idealization and dependence. Her core conflictual relationship seemed to be with the "dead mother" (in Green's sense, 1996) (but more needed to emerge in relation to the father). If she depended on this dead mother, she imagined she would die. Therefore, she needed to be self-sufficient—using mechanisms of control and omnipotence. The family reported that she was more able to show conflicts and be naughty before the brother was born, when she was 3 years old, after which she "became happy." She needed her mother, but she could not supply reassurance or meet her needs.

Later, Ms C made important progress in her ability to consider, and have interest in considering others' experiences, although at times it was not easy. In working this through, Ms C theorizesd about others' perspectives, but mostly as they related to possible effects on her. She had been confronting the reality that her analyst had her own world and the implications of that for excluding Ms C. There were references to her sister-in-law and husband, trying to figure out their intentions toward her. At the same time, she showed some empathy and insight toward her mother when the mother was taking care of Ms C's baby, who became fussy. Certainly, there had been progress in empathy, but she was still fairly self-referential in her thinking, understandably, as she grappled with learning more fully her own and others' minds and behaviours (Bender et al., 2011).

The second dimension, "affective regulation," refers to the capacity to regulate impulses, mood affects, and self-esteem, as well as establishing an adequate emotional balance between the needs of oneself and of others. In the beginning hours, she was emotionally quite fragile, with sometimes rapidly shifting states:

P: *When things feel on a good path and then something happens, and then, some feeling like too happy or too opened up, and then, something goes wrong, and I feel overwhelmed by it . . . . The more I put into something, the more risk and pain is involved.*

The analyst reflected, "One minute it's bliss and the next minute everything is falling apart." The patient also observed that she was "not totally knowing the boundaries with myself." The analyst also noted that "it seemed that she had no boundaries." Ms C talked about struggling with feelings of abandonment that came up around a phone message exchange with the analyst. While having a more evolved sense of herself as a separate person, Ms C appeared to be significantly attuned to others to regulate her sense of self and emotional well-being.

We see evidence in the later sessions that Ms C had begun to experience her separateness, but this was frightening because it occurred to her that her analyst had her "own world" that did not include Ms C at times.

The third dimension, "internal and external communication and the capacity for symbolization," is crucial for the psychoanalytic process, because these functions enable the psychic and interpersonal processing of lived experiences and their integration, contributing in this way to mental growth and the elaboration of the psychoanalytic work. At the start of the analysis, Ms C had a poor grasp of the internal world of the other. Later in the analysis, she could get into the internal world of herself and the other, and symbolization (less denial of anxiety and more inner dialogue) appeared.

The fourth and last of the structural functions considered is "the capacity to have deep bonds with internal and external objects," which implies the ability to initiate, preserve, and end relationships, to tolerate separations, and to acknowledge the place of a third. The group observed that the bonds with internal objects were fragile at the beginning of the treatment. Ms C treated others as if they were extensions of herself. Later, she saw the analyst as another, as abandoning her, or trying to set the agenda. The group questioned what would happen with the eventual loss of the analyst.

Regarding her bond with others and intimacy, we observed that at the first year of treatment, Ms C's polyamorous and risky sexual behaviour with many partners represented desperate attempts to connect, while at the same time an acting out, which defended her against knowing about her thoughts and feelings. She tried to cultivate detachment from the analyst to protect herself and was terrified of closeness, dependency, and losing control. Ms C's attempts to connect while failing to cultivate enduring close relationships and her need to ferociously pursue connections and then push people away allowed little genuine mutuality in her relations: "We had this really nice vacation and lovely night with M, close and connected—then he got at me at lunch, and then the contrast was too much."

Intimacy is constructed through the closeness or touching of bodies, and through different mental spaces that are generated. The temperature of the affects in a relationship (cold, mild, warm, or hot) determines the way in which people get along together. This patient described a broad spectrum of scary experiences with difficulties in the modulation of the affects and a loss of impulse control. She had difficulty when she felt "boundaryless": she lost her sense of self and needed someone outside her to help bolster her self-esteem. "I had a chain reaction of bad interactions yesterday . . ., hysterical reactions to M yelling at me, and my clients calling me racist."

People got angry at her, but she did not realize when she had been provocative. When she brought up the naked lunch and the possibility of having another naked lunch, her boyfriend became violent; later she broke up with him. Suddenly something happened and the relationship was broken.

Later, Ms C was clearly motivated to pursue committed relationships, was long past her phase of prodigious sexual acting out, married, and had a baby. In a more recent session, she seemed to be working hard to sort out the nature of closeness. She reflected that except for her baby, "I haven't had any safe physical relationship that wasn't sexual." She talked about a vampire from her book, wondering about the nature of yearning for connection, exploring if it was possible to feel close to someone without being sexually involved. She had a fantasy of doing something sexual with her analyst. She also described her experience of not being thought of or understood by her sister-in-law, her husband, or her mother. She did, however, have some appreciation of being understood and appreciated by her analyst. While there was progress in her work toward understanding and developing fulfilling and reciprocal relationships and in her relationship with her analyst, the clinical material we have suggests that Ms C had not yet fully achieved a higher level (Bender et al., 2011).

Hypotheses of the group

Members of the group observed important changes in the patient and in the analytic process, but noted areas of work still to be done; she was not yet "cured"; "there were problems to be resolved" with her identification with her mother's depression, the meaning of her becoming "happy" when her brother was born, the intergenerational transmission of trauma (Holocaust: several relatives died in concentration camps). Participants thought that the patient identified herself with a depressed mother ("the dead mother"; Green, 1996). She was fighting this depressive mother inside herself, in acting out, and staying "chill," showing no compassion for her mother. However, she was able to develop maternal capacities with her baby (dream). She was able to observe that her mother's behaviour was flat. But she still could not think much about who her mother was. Her perception of herself had developed considerably. She had better reality testing.

Part 2: 3-LM Level 3—Foci of the analyst's interventions and hypotheses about therapeutic action

The background of this case is severe childhood trauma. The analyst reports,

> In her early childhood, Ms C's mother was likely depressed. During these early years, she was not able to respond to Ms C's emotional needs, but rather Ms C precociously began to attune to and look after her emotionally. Her mother described Ms C as unhappy and oppositional until her brother was born when she was 3, when she became "happy." It appears that she started defensively looking at boys in a sexualized way at a very early age. For example, Ms C experienced acute separation anxiety from her mother when she began preschool, and there are many family stories about her having a "boyfriend" at preschool. She also recalls frequently being dropped off for the weekend at her step-grandmother's house and feeling abandoned by her mother even though she loved her grandmother. Ms C recalls being touched inappropriately by her cousin and trying to tell her mother, who seemed herself to be embarrassed by the information and did nothing to help. When Ms C was about 10, her mother began a multiyear medical treatment with multiple hospitalizations for reasons that were never clear. She now imagines it had something to do with her mother's reproductive organs—perhaps a hysterectomy and subsequent complications. In high school, Ms C felt ugly and started using her body to try to get attention and love. She also describes frequently being left alone for weekends by her parents, without anyone checking in on her and without any particular rules. During these times she would have huge parties that involved drinking, drugs, and sex. There seem to have been many situations during high school and beyond that Ms C eventually understood as rape or at least as situations to which she did not consent. Ms C had several unstable relationships in adulthood, most of them with very narcissistic men who wanted to possess and control her, but some of them with people whom she used and then rejected. In the early part of the treatment she had a relationship with a clearly very disturbed man who eventually became violent with her.

This trauma was re-experienced in the first four hours (2009–2010). The patient was very anxious, prone to putting fears into action, mostly seeking out risky erotic encounters with men and using drugs. It seemed that she had no boundaries; she was always scanning, looking, trying to "connect" with people, and having little sense of her interior life or theirs.

As long as she felt "desired," she felt very "on top" rather than vulnerable, scared, and in need of other people. Ms C quickly became a "good" patient, picking up on what she was supposed to talk about, in keeping with her tendency to mould herself to others.

In working with Level 3, we refer back to change observed in Level 1 and ask how change occurred in the defences of projection and paranoia. There was a consistency in the way the analyst worked with the patient in these early hours. Especially in the first two hours, she was helping the patient sort out what was hers from what was not hers. She was identifying feeling states and naming them. She was helping the patient with time sequences. Typical is the "naked lunch" episode in the first hour, where the patient was split between her idealized experience of being with her boyfriend, described as "serene," "settled," "sweet," "beautiful," "perfect," and the jealous rage in her boyfriend when she disclosed a desire to have a naked lunch with an older colleague. The patient was clueless that she precipitated the attack or was provocative in any way. Here is a typical interchange:

A: *It feels like it's coming out of nowhere—like one minute it's bliss and the next minute everything is falling apart—but maybe there's more to understand [referring to the man's jealousy].*

P: *This feeling I can't be happy for too long, but I don't really believe that. I don't know. . . .*

A: *It is interesting that you said that to him, because I think you know that this would upset him and having had lunch naked with someone would upset him.*

P: *[She says she felt upset that she hadn't been more sensitive to how sensitive he is]. It didn't feel that way at the time. I had just gotten an email from him [the lawyer]—I didn't have the sense it had this hotness to it. I don't understand why he has to get so angry.*

The patient and analyst could agree on a pattern of idealized bliss and then catastrophe, but the patient disavowed any personal intent or involvement; it was felt as an outside force. But then there was this exchange:

A: *I'm not focused on how you should be towards him but more whether there is anything to understand about what goes on with you.*

P: *[She remembers something she and I have talked about, how she'll start talking about someone else when things feel intimate.] In some way like maybe. . . . It wasn't feeling uncomfortably intimate, but I think we both felt really opened up and intimate. . . . This is maybe a strategy I use at times without being thoughtful about it.*

A: *Aware of it.*

P: *Yes, aware of it. . . . Yes, this feels helpful to think about it that way.*

The patient had a flash of awareness ("This might be a strategy") after the analyst referred to understanding "what goes on with you." The patient imagined an implied criticism "without being thoughtful about it," but the analyst shifted focus to suggest that Ms C acted without being "aware of it" (provoking jealousy). This helped Ms C recognize (in a more neutral way) that she (unconsciously) "denied the perception" of her acts of provocation. The patient stayed with this non-judgmental recognition: "[Without being] aware of it . . . this feels helpful."

The analyst then referred to the analytic frame (change to two sessions a week), to the transference ("us"), and to the disturbing situation ("crisis"):

A: *You have said a few times that you want to talk about what's going to happen with us [adding the second session], and, both times you wanted to do that you came, in a crisis.*

The analyst was now working in transference by suggesting that the patient's coming "in a crisis" was unconsciously motivated, to avoid talking about "what's going to happen with us." The analyst pointed out a pattern, which she found in the here-and-now, but, in these early hours, the patient did not respond to the transference interpretation.

However, the patient did begin twice-weekly analytic therapy and then three times a week, and, on November 9, 2010, 20 months after the "naked lunch" session, she began at four times a week. In the first Wednesday session (after starting the increased frequency), the patient referred to a childhood trauma. She told the analyst about a family party when an older male cousin, who was at the party, touched her hair in an intimate way. The presenting problem of Ms C's disavowal continued to evolve.

P: *My adult cousin came in and fixed my hair. I had the scarf on, and he got my hair out from under, etc. It felt pretty noticeable. . . . Intimate . . . and familiar. . . . He used to take care of me when I was a kid. I don't know if I felt upset by it. . . . I guess I would've preferred if he hadn't. [She cries]. It makes me more sure, but I still have feelings of doubt that's what happened.*

Ms C described a "doubt," "knowing and not knowing" that the sexual abuse by this older cousin had "happened" in childhood, even while telling the analyst that this "older cousin" touched her in an "intimate" way, without asking, on the weekend.

A: *Maybe you wanted to know that I'm not going to lose track of you and all your feelings as you go on; that this won't be lost, that I'll hold onto it.*

P: *[Crying] Sometimes I feel like if I talk about different things, somehow you think I've forgotten about . . . all the different things. Like I'll be talking about something, and you'll ask me how I feel about coming in tomorrow, and I wonder do you think I've forgotten or I'm not remembering the different things, and the sense that just because I'm not talking about it now, it's not that I'm not thinking about it. I mean sometimes I don't remember. . . . It just felt helpful to hear you say that. . . . I don't know, now I'm feeling a little uncomfortable. . . . I think I'm anticipating how I feel apprehensive telling you about Saturday.*

In this complex association, the patient feared that the analyst doubted Ms C's capacity to "remember" (trying to deny dissociation, the state of mind in which she did not know the abuse happened), then Ms C could admit "Sometimes I don't remember" and was relieved that the analyst knew this scary thing about her mind. One of the scary things about Saturday was that she came in and out of contact with perceptions of danger.

A: *I think about you at this party Saturday, or when your cousin touched you, or when you left here Friday, feeling abandoned by me—like out there on your own, and feeling how can this happen and no one's looking out for you.*

P: *I did feel on Friday—we did talk about me going to my cousin's close to the end. I did feel like it was like, "OK . . . good luck."*

Ms C felt the analyst was sending her away into danger without caring (with a sarcastic "good luck"). At the end of the session, the analyst interpreted the patient's anger at not being protected (by friends, family, and analyst), which led her to turn to men: "It sounds like you feel unprotected by and angry at them [the friend and parents] and me also, and then you turn to men" (end of session).

The focus of the analyst's interpretation was to interpret a sequence of affects and impulses, which implied an intrapsychic dynamic: a mix of compensation, self-harm, and revenge. When the patient felt unprotected by and angry at caretakers, she got into situations where she both attempted to have a "connection," and gratifying attention, but, at the same time, repeated the abuse by picking men who would hurt her, putting her at risk and making the analyst very anxious. The analyst began to help Ms C to recognize and own unconscious affects and impulses, which underlay her unconscious enactments of dangerous situations. The analyst was also working to help Ms C realize that she used crises to avoid talking about "us" meeting twice a week, a closer connection Ms C wanted and feared.

At Level 3, we note that the analyst did not make interpretations about unconscious fantasy scenarios repressed in early childhood, but consistently noted Ms C's lack of safety, sometimes putting it in the here-and-now transference relationship and interpreting her defence in acting out. The patient did not take up the transference directly but used the transference to feel contained and held.

In these early hours in the first year, we can infer from the foci of interventions that the analyst facilitated insight while furthering safety in the therapeutic relationship. Interpretations, which generate insight in the patient, were directed toward clarification of and sorting out basic psychic activities, naming and differentiating affects, observations of self and other, of what is outside and what is inside. On the relationship side, we can infer a kind of containment of anxiety, taking it in, detoxifying, and interpreting. The analyst thereby provided a basic security and steadiness that the patient lacked; the basic analytic task was to detoxify the projected anxieties. By the second year, we start to see interpretation of disavowal, dissociation, and projected fears.

The analyst began to use transference in a more sophisticated fashion by interpreting the wish and fear for more contact with the analyst, which began to give more insight into paranoia and disavowed affects.

Let us turn to an hour eight years after the start of the analysis, first looking at the hour itself.

The hour started off:

A: *[I gave her the bill and she gave me the cheque. This was also a week before I was going away for a week.]*

P: *I slept horribly again. I went to bed, then I woke up—then I felt like there was an earthquake. I was sure my bed was vibrating. I sat up. What do I do now? I was a little panicked, that heartbeat feeling—but feeling doubt too. I even stood up out of the bed. . . . And I did feel like not being able to fall asleep had to do with our break coming up. . . . I had this feeling of stability when I thought of the break. . . . I was trying to hold onto that feeling.*

A: *When were you trying to hold onto it?*

P: *I feel like I am trying to get back to that feeling. No—I want to get to it and explain it and have that feeling be the feeling, I want it to be it. There is probably other feelings [laughs].*

A: *Bummer, I know. Do you know what they are?*

Here we were on familiar ground. The patient had a paranoid fantasy, felt in her body, and started to feel panic anxiety. In the first sessions of the analysis, Ms C was "overwhelmed," totally "panicked," "hysterical" at having angered her boyfriend by making him jealous about the naked lunch; now she was "a little panicked, that heartbeat feeling," but "feeling doubt too about whether the earthquake was real." Yet there were now differences, she could now link her anxiety to the break with the analyst; she could begin to name feeling states and she no longer needed to repeat in action her fears. The analyst made several clarifying remarks, but we can infer that she could just wait.

P: *The feeling I had was anticipating not feeling abandoned by you when you were gone. It was a different feeling of feeling solid, or trusting the whole feeling of taking you for granted that we talked about, and then there was all this anxiety about that . . . and now it seems like the whole sense of that seems shaky, like the bed. Like scared. Like, oh, I can't rely on that feeling—it wouldn't be smart, or safe—I can't trust, I can't rely on you.*

Without the analyst intervening, the patient spontaneously showed her awareness of split transference fantasies, her struggle to keep the analyst as a soothing internal object, and her fears of depending on the analyst. Then, a further revelation:

P: *When I was awake, I was thinking about you [after the earthquake]. I wonder what time she goes to bed? I don't imagine you go to bed at 9:00. I have an image of people who go to bed at 9. I wonder, what time do they eat dinner? How much time do you see your kids and how annoyed do you get if you spend a lot of time with them? [She's quiet].*

The patient showed a curiosity about the analyst, indicating she could now see the analyst as a separate person, with her own concerns and motivations. After several more clarifying questions, the analyst made a long transference interpretation:

A: *Maybe in the middle of the night there was initially some sense of feeling alone and then thinking of me and not knowing what I am doing or where I am, and then maybe that was connected with knowing I am going to be away and . . . some sense of separation and incompleteness. Some area where we are not overlapping. Then that's hard to fathom and that's scary and vulnerable and, then, it becomes more about completing that or doing something to not have that feeling.*

Now we see the analyst gather up several of the patient's points, separation fears, awareness of differentiation, and defensive push to action, all placed in the transference. The patient responded with the insight that she had needed to sexualize her fears, then was aware of new feeling states:

P: *I guess I felt a surge of anger . . . or sadness about you going away, I guess.*
A: *Yeah, what did you feel?*
P: *A flash of oh I could just cry. It was very fleeting. I guess feeling tenderly towards myself for having a hard time having feelings.*

And the patient ended the hour with:

P: *This feeling of absence. We won't be together.*

Moving to an hour in the following week, Ms C came in with a sore throat and runny nose. She shared more paranoid fantasies with the analyst:

P: *This feeling, like being sick, of these invisible, maybe. . . . Like there could be fungus, or something. Thinking about people that are. . . . The feeling of being weak and vulnerable like I'm not going to survive evolution.*

We see a continuation of paranoid states, but she now had the capacity to link her fears to being weak and vulnerable. The change in Ms C's psychic capacities can be observed in the depth and richness of her stories told to the analyst about the paranoid fantasies. The focus of the analyst's interventions remained on the affective states. At this stage, the patient was struggling to talk more openly with her husband (about having sex and his teenage daughter) to be both a mother and sexual. Ms C told her analyst about a difficult "intimate" conversation with her husband about disciplining her 13-year-old stepdaughter, who had come to live with them.

P: *I felt brave, I brought up hard things. It's sort of like progress. That's why I brought them up, told you about them. But as I was talking about them, they didn't feel good.*
A: *You thought they were going to bring you to a comfortable place, and they didn't.*
P: *No, I don't think so. . . . I brought them up thinking they were kind of "celebratory." I realized there was this hope, and it wasn't being realized, and then this desperation feeling came up. The hope disappeared. . . .*
A: *These things are kind of challenging, these interactions. And the break is there somewhere. Maybe you're struggling with, as you're saying, feeling kind of vulnerable. . . .*
A: *It does seem kind of exhausting having to fix things all the time. . . .*
A: *It's depressing, It's blah, not exciting. . . .*
P: *It is "unglamorous" and "not sexy."*
A: *It's a little depressing or a little empty.*

The analyst was helping her stay with "ordinary unhappiness." The analyst had shifted largely to an interpretive stance on transference, pointing out defensive shifts in the patient away from anxious affects and links to loss. But the concern with safety continued, as the interpretive process is very careful and done in small steps, staying close to the patient's material. The concern with containing had not disappeared, and the analyst still worked to help her patient verbalize her narratives and elaborate her bodily sensations as metaphors for internal states.

We can also see what the analyst did not do. For example, she did not interpret primal scene fantasies when the patient was curious, nor did she interpret rejection by the Oedipal couple, likely inferring that her patient was not ready.

The clinical material indicated a shift in therapeutic action between early and later sessions. At the beginning, the emphasis was on containing and holding. There was little or no interpretation of unconscious fantasy. Rather, the analyst focused on connection and breaks in connection, identifying states of closeness and states of loss. Relationship aspects of therapeutic action predominated. In the later sessions, there was a shift to interpretive efforts. The patient was now able to voice more complex fantasies about the analyst and much of the work is centred on transference and fears of loss of control, of being abandoned, and of being envied. The analyst had become a separate person in her mind, having a separate life, and there was a growing sense of object constancy, an enduring sense of being held in the analyst's mind. Yet the patient still could regress toward paranoia when faced with separations. Thirdness was hinted at but not yet ready for awareness and work. The work appears to have integrated many of the split-off fantasy states, and we see much less evidence of projection or denial.

Results and conclusions

We have presented the results of a long period of analysis (six years) through the "participant observation" of 40 analysts working in three different clinical observations groups. With the results of the questionnaires done before and after the experience, the reports done by the three groups, and the participation in the group discussion, the results reflect not only some illustrative material of one analyst but the views reached about this clinical material by a number of trained psychoanalysts and its resonances in the participants in a formal discussion group, using a setting and a specific method. The challenge has been to understand the clinical material as an insider and describe it for the psychoanalytic community.

We found that analysts with different theoretical frames and belongings (different societies and regions) had an empathic sensitivity and perceived changes in similar ways, as shown in reports and questionnaires.

With regard to the global changes of the patient, the reports describe that some groups underline more external changes, others more internal changes, and others privilege the lens of the different transferential positions that were taking place between analyst and patient. The three groups used these three criteria but with different emphases.

In the questionnaires filled before and after the group discussion we found that most group members report important global changes of the patient—important changes in the patient's use of her own mind and bodily resources for the analysis, and moderate changes in the patient's use of the analyst and her interpretations.

Regarding the 3-LM levels at the descriptive phenomenological level (clinical thinking), we found that the three groups underlined some of the same and some different anchor points, but they concurred in the lines of force: the stress on the analyst of her patient's acting out, her dissociative states, her disavowal. The groups also saw the same changes in Ms C's "use of the analyst and of her interventions," and the same changes in her old defensive strategies, allowing her more safety and continuity in relationships over the course of the analysis. The scenes we have selected, "the naked lunch," the "hide-and-seek," "the family party with abusing older cousin," "the earthquake and fungus fantasies," in response to separations from the analyst, show how the groups work at this level, where images and metaphors in the analysis are observed and others emerge from the clinical observation group. In the unconscious construction of meaning, metaphor plays a salient role. Arnold Modell (2005) suggests that metaphor functions unconsciously as a pattern detector and thus is pivotal to the organization and categorization of emotional memory.

We observe at the beginning of the treatment the intense needs of the patient, who was always looking for contact, which for her was a kind of rudimentary intimacy with mechanisms of dissociation, disavowal, and acting out. Six years later, all her pathology about sexuality was brought into the transferential relationship and into an inhibition with her husband. The analyst worked with the transference and the need of the patient to be in contact, to regulate contact with others, and to self-regulate.

Her story of hiding and being found did not resolve conflict; she wanted to be found but, at the same time, felt it would be humiliating to submit to her mother. In the first period of analysis the analyst reported the difficulties they had during breaks, when the patient would resort to action and boundaryless sexual goings-on, and there were unsuccessful efforts to connect the "acting out" with the breaks in the sessions, another version of hide-and-seek. The analytic process was full of "feelings of fear," loss, and abandonment.

The patient couldn't handle different affects, but she was able, as the analytic process advanced, to use the analyst to get to know that there was a missing affect in her experience of "hide-and-seek" and to know happiness at the reunion with the other. Years later we find a new meaning of hiding: being in the back of the car feels like being in her own world and doesn't feel like hiding, finding her own private space but without secrecy. We can observe the emergence of a different person, with a wider range of affects and remembering, wanting more contact, planning for the future.

In Level 2—Main Dimensions of Change—the group found improvement in all dimensions, changing from important disturbances and severe limitations in functioning to moderate disturbances, with some limitations in functioning in most dimensions. The group found a higher improvement in relational pattern with the analyst that got a higher score (from 2 to 3.5) and empathy that had a very low score at the beginning (1) and arrived to a 3 score.

Table 2.1 Level 2. Main dimensions of change. Mode scores in one group

Dimension	*Initial moment (mode)*	*Later moments (mode)*
1. Experience of illness: understanding of difficulties and hints of possible changes	2	3
2a. Relational patterns outside the analysis	2	3
2b. Relational patterns with the analyst	2	3.5
3. Defences and conflicts	2	3
4.1a. Self-perception, sense of identity, and integrity of the self	2	3
4.1b. Perception of the others. Empathy	1	3
4.2a. Regulation of impulses, affects, and self-esteem	2	3
4.2b. Regulation of the relationship with others (self-care and care of the other, reciprocity)	2	3
4.3a. Internal communication and symbolization (bodily and mental self)	2	3
4.3b. Communication with the others (depth and richness of affects and representations)	2	3
4.4a. Bonds with internal objects	2	3
4.4b. Bonds with others. Capacity to establish and end bonds, to face separation, and the existence of a third	2	3

Discussing the third level, Explanatory Hypotheses of Change, we see a shift from the early hours focused on clarifying and containing, to later hours where unconscious fears could now be explored—predominately fears of abandonment.

Alternative hypotheses that emerged in the group have to do with the personal involvement of the analyst in the process and in the relationship. Hence, questions arose in the group: Why is transgenerational transmission of trauma never brought to the analysis? Why was not the meaning of the different cultural backgrounds in the psyche of the patient worked on?

In the group discussion, ideas tended to lose their connection to their original theoretical framework and were used from a common clinical baseline. Hence, the concept of splitting, projective identification, continent function, and separation anxieties summarized clinical observations and were common, shared concepts closely linked to clinical observations in psychoanalysis. We could say that there was an integration and coherence centred in the patient, and, as the analytic process advanced and transformations took place, other hypotheses and implicit or explicit theories arose.

Clinical observation group members working with the 3-LM valued the fact that everyone talked in descriptive terms, even using metaphors from everyday life. This speech style helped participants develop a more clinical perspective and enabled them to get a better picture of the patient and her emotional functioning, while avoiding the risk of using more theoretically saturated approaches.

The 3-LM is another setting to see the psychoanalytic process, to detect psychoanalytic clinical facts, to make observations and inferences, and to communicate them. Within the group, we identified clinical facts and then we made inferences, trying to separate what was a fact, an observation, and a conceptualization.

Clinical experience and research evidence have confirmed that psychoanalytical treatments (among others) produce positive changes in patients. Our challenge was to answer the questions: How to improve the description of changes? (Level 1); What does exactly change? (Level 2); and How and why does it change? (Level 3).

Note

1 Internal object relations are the building blocks of psychological structures and organizers of motivation and behaviour. The building blocks of psychic structure are made up of a representation of the self, an affect related to or representing a drive, and a representation of the other (the object of the drive). This units of self and other, and the affect linking them are object relations dyads (Clarkin, Yeomans, & Kernberg, 2006, p. 2).

References

Bender, D. S., Morey, L. C., & Skodol, A. E. (2011). Toward a model for assessing level of personality functioning in DSM–5, part I: A review of theory and methods. *Journal of Personality Assessment, 93*(4), 332–346.

Bernardi, R. (2014). The Three-Level Model (3-LM) for observing patient transformations. In M. Altmann (Ed.), *Time for change: Tracking transformations in psychoanalysis—The Three-Level Model* (pp. 3–34). London: Karnac.

Clarkin, J. F., Yeomans, F. E., & Kernberg, O. F. (2006). *Psychotherapy for borderline personality: Focusing on object relations*. Arlington: American Psychiatric Association.

Green, A. (1996). *On private madness*. London: Karnac.

Modell, A. H. (2005). Emotional memory, metaphor, and meaning. *Psychoanalytic Inquiry, 25*(4), 555–568.

Nieto, M., Bernardi, R., Altmann, M., Bouza, G., Cárdenas, M., & de León, B. (1985). Investigando la experiencia analítica: una propuesta [Inquiring into the analytic experience: A proposal]. *Revista Uruguaya de Psicoanálisis, 83*, 117–135.

Chapter 3

Bodily metaphors as anchor points in facilitating change

Margaret Ann Fitzpatrick Hanly, Beatriz de León de Bernardi, and Marianne Leuzinger-Bohleber

Introduction

This chapter focuses on the nature and effectiveness of bodily metaphors to convey core presenting difficulties, which can act as landmarks for observations of change in later sessions. Bernardi presents key ideas on metaphor and psychoanalytic thinking:

> The emotional and cognitive processes in metaphor are especially relevant in psychoanalysis, since metaphoric polarities are part of the interpretative process established between patient and analyst facilitating emotional and conceptual transformations, also mediated by such elaborations and transformations in the analyst (see p. 63).

Leuzinger-Bohleber reflects on embodied metaphors and the unconscious:

> [T]he concept of the self is always based on unconscious embodied metaphors, so that a change in these metaphors is an indicator of transformations in the inner world of the self (see pp. 69–70).

This introduction sets the background for two discussions on metaphor, by briefly reviewing the history and three key metaphoric expressions in Ms C's early analytic sessions in the clinical narrative, which observes the nature of the difficulties, and the changes and absence of change in the patient and the process.

The patient, Ms C, was a 36-year-old single woman, half-Asian, half-Jewish, who worked in a senior position as a social worker. The analyst spoke vividly about having to contain the anxiety, during early years with Ms C, given the very risky behaviours she engaged in on weekends, involving dangerous sex and drugs. During Ms C's infancy and early childhood, her mother was depressed. The family had emigrated from Europe to the United States when she was 7, and moved within the country shortly afterwards. Her mother was hospitalized several times when Ms C was 10, as a result of medical problems (possibly following a hysterectomy). Some family members on the mother's side (not close) were probably killed in the Holocaust. The father and his extended family were from Asia; some still live there. Ms C said her parents were "distant" with her and often left her alone for weekends when she was a teenager, when she would have wild parties.

Three key metaphoric descriptors were used as landmarks or anchor points from which to assess change in her problems: "chill," "naked lunch," and verbatim passages in a session, which the group condensed as "hide-and-seek." When elements in the metaphors were elaborated by Ms C in later sessions, meanings that had been unconscious or split-off emerged into the light of the analysis, into new language, the setting, the relationship, the transferences, and counter-transferences.

Chill: In the first sessions Ms C said she liked to be "chill." She felt she was "above" normal needs and feelings; she liked to think of herself as self-sufficient, "on top." In this simple colloquial expression, "chill," Ms C conveyed a core problem, which Bernardi relates to her "emptiness of feeling" and which Leuzinger-Bohleber elucidates in relation to early bodily experiences with a depressed mother. The 3-LM group observed that through the years of analysis Ms C came to understand how she had used her body to avoid feeling psychic pain and vulnerable aspects of her female body, by setting up dangerous situations and trying to stay "chill." Two years into the analysis, Ms C was no longer engaging in dangerous sexual encounters, and in time she expressed much more about her bodily and mental states, and was able to say, "I am scared not to feel the fear." Later in the analysis, she spoke of "layers of non-contact" in herself.

Naked lunch: One morning at breakfast, after a "blissful" night with her boyfriend on Valentine's Day, Ms C told her boyfriend that she was thinking of having a second "naked lunch" with an older, married, male colleague. Her boyfriend became extremely angry. Ms C was still deeply distressed in her session, as she described to her analyst that she'd had a "hysterical reaction to M yelling" at her, that she'd felt "overwhelmed." She had "panicked." When she was "too opened up," "something went wrong." She could not recognize her part in provoking him as she set up a repetition and felt "overwhelmed."

By the seventh year of treatment, Ms C was married and had a 5-month-old baby. She said to her analyst (speaking of the session the day before), "It was very helpful. I just thought about it a lot. . . . When things make sense, [I have] more of a physical feeling of being in touch with a certain experience." In the session, Ms C spoke of her experience of observing her mother with her baby and expressed the lack of being held by the analyst: "In the morning I was thinking about you and me. Do we have a physical relationship? We don't have a physical relationship—being held or touched."

Hide-and-seek: In the first session of the analysis at four times a week, Ms C associated to the increased hours: "One feeling is like having nowhere to hide, and the other one was it feels really vulnerable. . . . I think of a field with low-cut grass. It's square and finite. You can see the whole thing and I'm on it somewhere and there's nowhere to hide."

Then Ms C remembered the day the family moved to a new house in a new city, when she was 6, and she ran across the street and hid from her mother.

P: *I don't remember what happened, but I was supposed to say "I'm sorry" to my mom and I wouldn't say I was sorry, and so I ran away. I went across the street. . . . I was hiding in some bushes and it felt scary. It felt scary, like I felt scared she wouldn't find me and that she would.*

The expression "hide-and-seek" captured for the 3-LM group both Ms C's vulnerability in hiding and not being found, and in being found and exposed. Later in the analysis, as Ms C felt more connected with, and afraid to separate from, the analyst, she recaptured a feeling of not being "tracked" by her mother, and unable to "track her":

P: *I feel very not thought of—like the opposite of feeling tracked. I don't have any clue if she understands or knows where I'm at, and I can't track her either.*

The following discussions by de León de Bernardi and by Leuzinger-Bohleber deepen our understanding of the crucial place of metaphor in understanding unconscious aspects of our patients' bodily minds, their simplest and most hidden experiences. Their discussions further elaborate ways to carry out an effective clinical thinking focused on the specific language of the patient, as her bodily metaphors develop over time.

Key embodied metaphors in the group work on Ms C's case—Beatriz de León de Bernardi

The clinical narrative of Ms. C's analysis, presented in Chapter 2 and reviewed in the introduction, prioritized certain expressions in the clinical material, which generated reflection on and discussion of central aspects of the patient's problems. These expressions in the session material were considered from the different points of view proposed by the 3-LM for group reflection: phenomenological observation of the clinical material, description of changes occurring in the analysis, and finally explanatory hypotheses on how these changes came about. The following perspectives converged in making judgments about meaning: the clinical material reported by the analyst, the analyst's interventions concerning the material, and finally the contributions of the analysts participating in the 3-LM group.

Selected verbatim passages, depicting Ms C's sense of self as "chill," a story of a "naked lunch," and an expression for a memory and transference, "hide-and-seek," clearly had a strong impact on the group's way of hearing the clinical material and were considered "anchor points" or "metaphors" that especially contributed to the reflections on change and no change in the psychic functioning, bodily experience, and life in Ms C's analysis. However, can these expressions be considered as metaphors? How could we characterize them? How can we position them within the field of analytical communication? What are their dynamics and clinical usefulness? How did they contribute to the group reflection?

Aristotle defines metaphor as an abbreviated comparison in which the meaning of a term is transferred to a second term, the latter losing its literal meaning to acquire a new figurative meaning. From this perspective, the notion of transmission of meaning from a source term to a second target term (goal) is central.

However, in contemporary developments, the idea of the metaphor has become more complex. Davidson (1978) has privileged the idea that the two terms of the metaphor retain their literal meaning and their conceptual weight. From his point of view, what is relevant is not the transmission of meaning but the relationship established between the terms of the metaphor, which generates associations and emotions in the reader or listener. For Lakoff and Johnson (1980), metaphors are part of our cognitive processes from the early stages of life, substantiated in our bodily and emotional experience, resulting in mental products rather than figures of speech. For Gibbs (2008), metaphors are part of the thinking process and contribute to the development of cultural expressions, whether artistic or scientific productions. Progressively the idea of metaphor has become independent of the classical views, which refer largely to literary works and forms of speech.

Metaphor can be considered a complex interactive unit, composed of polarities of meaning in which cognitive and emotional processes are put into play. The emotional and cognitive processes in metaphor are especially relevant in psychoanalysis, since metaphoric polarities are part of the interpretative process established between patient and analyst facilitating emotional and conceptual transformations, and mediated by these elaborations and transformations in the analyst. The emotional and embodied dimension of metaphor has been especially highlighted in psychoanalysis, such as in Susan Isaacs' ideas on unconscious fantasy. Caspi (2018) has highlighted how the unconscious emotionally charged ideas become determinants of metaphoric creation in psychoanalysis in the thinking of M. Klein, Winnicott, and Ogden.

The subject of metaphors in psychoanalytic communication has been important in the thinking of analytic authors such as Arlow (1979), Ogden (1997), and Rizzuto (2001, 2009). In a general sense, we can say that interpretation is metaphorical in seeking to establish relationships and analogies between the manifest sense of psychoanalytic interaction and its latent meaning (de León de Bernardi, 1999). However, in this chapter I will refer only to the key role, which certain expressions acquire in psychoanalytic communication, which I call "key metaphors."

The expression "key metaphor" was proposed by Siegelman (1990) to refer to metaphors that are used to conceptualize the theory of technique, to refer to the therapeutic space and frame. But in this commentary I will leave aside the subject of metaphors, which refer to theoretical and technical concepts in psychoanalysis. I will use the term "key metaphor" to refer to expressions that emerge in psychoanalytic communications that may be considered "key metaphors for the patient's self." Images referring to central aspects of the patient's subjectivity appear as key metaphors that embody corporal representations and emotions, and, in the course of the analysis, the shift in the metaphors shows transformations in the intrapsychic experience and patterns of relationship in the analytical process. In the analytic session, key metaphors may emerge in the communications of the patient, of the analyst, or in the exchange established between them. In work with the 3-LM, with certain cases, such as Ms C's, the 3-LM group working on the session material selects key metaphors as a starting point for the reflections developed in the group's work.

In Ms C's material, the group highlighted the expressions "chill," "naked lunch," and "hide-and-seek" in the patient's associations, in the analyst's intervention, and in the dialogue between them. These expressions were characterized by a strong figurative impact, evoking a variety of images of the patient, which seemed to refer centrally to the patient's subjectivity and condensed multiple senses. These expressions can be thought of as embodied, intrinsically linked to Ms C's emotional and bodily experience. Key metaphors can be considered embodied metaphors and are not determined by the logic of verbal language with a narrow aesthetic goal. They emerge and are transformed from the conscious, preconscious, or unconscious aspects of the analytical bond.

Key embodied metaphors are useful interpretive tools, keys that open doors or offer bridges in integration of emotional and bodily sub-symbolic experience, with the symbolic dimension of images and words facilitating the symbolization. This can be verified both in the clinical material presented by the case analyst and in the conceptualization of group work with the Three-Level Model.

It becomes necessary to discriminate the contribution of the patient, the contribution of the analyst, and the group work to the implicit and explicit significance acquired by the "key embodied metaphors." We see how Ms

C introduces the first of these expressions, "chill," with which she seeks to characterize herself to her analyst (Rizzuto, 2001).

Ms C's view of herself reveals the metaphorical and intrapsychic sense of the expression "chill," converting it into an embodied metaphor of herself. For Ms C this expression condenses her being empty of feelings and her experience of not needing another, as well as her narcissistic grandiosity: she felt that she was "above" "normal needs and feelings" (9–10). She liked to think of herself as self-sufficient, "on top" (62).

In the second metaphor she presents about herself, "naked lunch" condenses a relationship scene in which Ms C showed how she lived her sexuality: "Ms C has a 'risky' 'polymorphous' lifestyle involving 'sex and drugs', casual sex with heterosexual couples, with men, with women, with a stranger 'in the hood.'" Paradoxically, both "chill" and "naked lunch" are "embodied metaphors" that show the estrangement of the body and the emptiness of Ms C's feelings. Both metaphors are "anchor points" from which the group reflection on the unconscious aspects of Ms C's relational patterns enacted in her life.

After two years of analysis, transformations began in Ms C, who showed discomfort with, and concern about, her way of being "chill." Fear appeared as a central theme: "I was thinking about the word dissociation. I felt in my body that numb panic."

The expression "hide-and-seek" is about hiding and being afraid to be found and emerged in the material of the second year of analysis (hour 3, 2010) when the analysis began at a frequency of four times a week. "Hide-and-seek" also stood out as "key body metaphor" in the group reflection, and its meaning emerged from the dialogue established between Ms C and her analyst.

P: *One feeling is like having nowhere to hide, and the other one was it feels really vulnerable, and I guess it feels right now like it's revealing something about me.* (463–464)

A: *In these images it seems like there is a very ominous or scary feeling about being found. There isn't any sense of relief or something good coming out of it or being taken care of.*

P: *I was hiding in some bushes and it felt scary. It felt scary, like I felt scared she wouldn't find me and that she would. That all felt scary. . . . [T]he image I have of hiding somewhere—it feels totally scary. If someone finds you, it's going to be scary. If someone finds you, they're scared. It just seems clear to me now. I never thought it was fun to play hide-and-seek.* (488–494).

Hide-and-seek acquires new metaphorical meanings related to each other in the analytical field (Baranger & Baranger, 1961) by condensing feelings, sensations, and bodily representations embodied in a relational pattern. Ms C's fear of owning her feelings became the focus of the patient's and the analyst's expressions, as they finally integrated these fears into the transferential scene. At the end of the session, the analyst interpreted the patient's anger at not being protected (by friends, family, and analyst), which led her to turn to promiscuous behaviours with men: "It sounds like you feel unprotected by and angry at them [the friend and parents] and me also, and then you turn to men" (386–387).

During moments of the analysis "hide-and-seek" revealed the patient's central fears, but also her seeking transformation, which she expressed in the way she used the analyst from the beginning of the analysis. "Hide-and-seek" contrasts with the expressions "chill" and "naked lunch," which the group selected as anchor points in the initial period of group work. These metaphors of the self were dynamically and dialectically resignified (Pichon-Rivière, 1998) in a "retrospective and prospective" way in relation to each other, both in their intrapsychic significance and in relation to the bond with the analyst and bonds in the patient's life. Thus, defensive unconscious aspects expressed in "chill" and "naked lunch" can be understood retroactively as representations of a mental space, empty of feelings, in which the patient took refuge from the fear of emotional contact with herself and the others.

Based on the material presented, the group reflection considered that the transferential–counter-transferential relationship centrally contributed to the changes of the patient. It is only when the analyst brings up wanting to be found that she can label her feelings hide and seek. From this anchor point, we see a clear transformation: The ability to name and identify discrete emotions, the ability to describe frightening experiences, the beginning of identifying needs and wishes, wanting to be found and held. She no longer needs the defense of projection and paranoia.

To synthesize, Ms C's narrative about hide-and-seek showed relational patterns that led her to hide and, at the same time, to seek contact in her life connections and in the transferential relationship with her analyst. Group work allowed participants to infer implicit unconscious fantasies in this patient's relational pattern. The fantasy of hiding implied a flight from contact with the maternal figure and from the feminine in herself, which had a very terrifying meaning. The group's reflections on these fantasies suggested that they were associated with repeated traumatic childhood experiences of distance from the parental figures and especially from the mother, resonating with Green's conceptualization of the dead mother, reflected on in Level 3 of the 3-LM. The group commented, "Her core conflictual relationship seems to be with the depressive mother, the 'dead mother' (in Green's sense). If she depends on this dead mother, she imagines she will die. She has to have control and omnipotence." "She needs to be self-sufficient—her mother cannot supply reassurance or meet her needs."

Key embodied metaphors had a key role in the psychoanalytical conceptualization of Ms C's material, enabling bridges (Modell, 2009; de León de Bernardi, in press) among the group experience of contacting and hearing the clinical material and with the group's theorization about it.

In the first stage of the group's work, each analyst presented a subjective position in which the psychoanalytic theory was regressively integrated with the analyst's activity of free association. This inferential process is similar to Freud's oneiric model in the mechanism of dreaming. The analysts participating in the group discussion, resonating emotionally (Bernardi, 2017), listened to the clinical material with free-floating attention to their own preconscious and unconscious reactions, but at the same time observing their reactions to the presented material, reflecting, selecting, highlighting, and spontaneously assigning implicit metaphorical meaning to certain expressions (de León de Bernardi, 2018).

Leibovich de Duarte (2010), taking up the notion of abduction formulated by Charles S. Peirce (1903), has shown how our clinical inferences are based on prior internalized knowledge whose relationship gives rise to new hypotheses. These abductive processes are especially evident in the allocation of metaphorical meaning to expressions of the self that, as in the case of Ms C, acquired a specific sense at each moment of the analysis, but at the same time could be related to each other differently as the analysis progressed.

Abductive processes implicit in the selection of the key embodied metaphor imply the analyst's previous internalization of aspects of general psychoanalytical theories, the analyst's clinical experience and, in the case of the group work, the actual experience of listening to the clinical material. In this sense it involved implicit (Bleger, 1969; Sandler, 1983) theoretical deductive processes. But, at the same time, metaphors create bridges towards inductive processes that allow articulation of different clinical problems and explanatory theoretical hypotheses regarding the phenomena described.

In Levels 2 and 3 of the 3-LM, the analysts step back from the empathic contact with the clinical material to take a "second look" (Baranger, Baranger, & Mom, 1983), and in a reflective-critical inferential process ask questions about the dimensions and theoretical and technical hypotheses concerning mechanisms of change. In the case of Ms C, key embodied metaphors were the basis for the critical-reflective–critical-inferential process of the group work. The discussion group created a common flexibly operative reference space (ECRO, in Pichon-Rivière's vision, 1998), which allows a rich, deep, and vivid understanding of the clinical material.

The transformations and the deepening in the meanings of the key metaphor "hide-and-seek" contribute to understanding the patient's conceptual and emotional changes in relation to her central fears and her defences against them. Group members observed important changes in the patient and in the analytic process, but noted areas of work still to be done: "There are still problems to be resolved, with intimacy and sexuality, with fears of not being connected, with her identification with her mother's depression, with the intergenerational transmission of trauma."

The discussion about whether depression was an important risk for the patient or if her intense phobia was a consequence of unexplored Oedipal aspects and considered in the problems referred to Ms C's sexuality was left open, highlighting the absence of the fatherly figure in the material presented. It is necessary to keep in mind that specific theoretical contexts of a specific work group and psychoanalytic community can condition the formulation of explanatory hypotheses on a certain clinical material, a subject that can be considered in relation to future experiences.

Discussion—Marianne Leuzinger-Bohleber

In Chapter 2, Altmann de Litvan, White, and Fitzpatrick Hanly have summarized the results of 3-LM groups with 40 analysts on this psychoanalysis. They impressively illustrate that the 3-LM is suitable for systematically clinically investigating and documenting the transformations of patients at three different levels of the model in psychoanalytic groups (see Bernardi, 2014).

This is one of the most important objectives that our committee has pursued since the European Psychoanalytical Federation Congress in Copenhagen. We have tried to take up the experiences of 10 years with the clinical working parties in the EPF. These groups have been involved with different ways psychoanalysts work with their patients, their specific techniques, models in the back of their minds, identifications with certain psychoanalytic groups, concepts, etc. The clinical working parties in the EPF had created a new culture of mutual listening to each other, to psychoanalysts coming from different psychoanalytical cultures and different theoretical orientations. Instead of the infertile "faith wars," which psychoanalytical theory was "best," "the true and only one," etc., it was now a matter of looking at the opportunities, but also the risks, of the theoretical pluralism in contemporary psychoanalysis.

At the EPF Congress in Copenhagen (2011), I postulated that it was time to return to our real task of psychoanalytic treatments and their outcome: the changes patients make during such treatments due to different psychoanalytical techniques (Leuzinger-Bohleber, 2014). Since then, our clinical observation group has developed the 3-LM to study the patient's transformations in groups clinically.

In my discussion I can pick out only a few aspects and refer to the interdisciplinary exchange on embodiment and embodied memories, which I have been involved with, together with Rolf Pfeifer, an internationally leading expert in embodied cognitive science.

I am referring to the description of the analyst's first session with her patient:

> *Initially Ms C presented only a vague interest in growth and referred to herself as "chill"; she liked to think of herself as self-sufficient and "above" normal needs and feelings. In her first session,* ***I said something about how under her "chill" exterior, I sensed that there was a lot of pain*** *[emphasis added]. This seemed to touch her and she started crying. I was also left with the feeling, though, that somehow this was too quick or that it had been too easy to get in or have access to her.*

The analyst took up the metaphor of the patient's being "chill" and spoke of a "chill exterior," behind which she felt a lot of pain. This metaphor seemed to reach the patient right away: she began to cry: "[T]he analyst was also left with the feeling, though, that somehow this was too quick or that it had been too easy to get in or have access to her." As I will discuss below, these self-doubts speak on the one hand to the professional self-critical attitude of the analyst. On the other hand, I suspect that these verbalizations also hint at the analyst's own defence. She unconsciously perceived that she had hit the mark with her metaphor and unconsciously immediately empathized with the patient's severe traumatization. Probably she was not able to endure the patient's despair, panic, fear of death, and distress contained in it and to keep all this psychic and bodily sufferings in her consciousness. Instead she had to keep it away from herself, with the help of defence mechanisms.

The analyst might have adhered to the central, embodied meaning of metaphors as a "direct path to the unconscious" and thus placed more trust in the patient's spontaneously created metaphor capturing unconscious meanings of her sufferings, which she had understood intuitively right away.

Lakoff and Johnson (2008, p. 3) characterize metaphors:

> The mind is inherently embodied. Thought is mostly unconscious. Abstract concepts are largely metaphorical. There are three major findings of cognitive science. More than two millennia of a part of these discoveries, philosophy can never be the same again.

The authors argue that metaphors are universal and indispensable. For example, the concept of the self is always based on unconscious embodied metaphors, so that a change in these metaphors indicates transformations in the inner world of the self (and objects). "We have found . . . that metaphors permeate our everyday lives, not only our language, but also our thinking and acting. Our everyday conceptual system, according to which we both think and act, is at its core and fundamentally metaphorical" (Lakoff & Johnson, 2008, p. 11).

For our context here, what is crucial is that Lakoff and Johnson illustrate the close connection between people's original, embodied experiences mostly with their primary objects, sensomotoric experiences and subjective assessments. For example,

> "Affection is warmth."
> Subjective judgment: Affection
> Sensorimotor domain: Temperature
> Example: "They greeted me warmly."
> Primary experience: Feeling warm while being held affectionately.
> (Lakoff & Johnson, 1980, pp. 49ff)

When this patient described herself as "chill," she unconsciously and accurately used a bodily metaphor that indicated that she perceived herself as cold because, as a child of a depressed mother, she experienced too little warmth in her earliest bodily experience during times of an emergent self and identified herself with a "cold object" in the sense of a primary identification. It was a great empathic achievement of the analyst when she simultaneously felt what an unbearable suffering this had entailed for the patient, for her as a helpless infant totally dependent on the love of the primary object.

Eight years later, when the patient herself had a baby, she observed her mother holding the baby and could say about her,

P: *[A]nd my mom's not a comfortable physical person. I mean she's pretty athletic—she plays tennis, and my parents are competent hikers—but she's not physically comfortable in her own skin, and when she holds R she seems so uncomfortable. When I got there he was awake and he was happy—it was really cute when he saw me—it was pronounced—he had eventually fallen asleep on my mom, she had gotten him to eat, etc. Then she goes to kiss him—like, do things she's seen me or my dad do. It felt so awkward, there was this whole feeling of awkwardness.*

It doesn't feel like she's ever taken care of a baby before, it just seems so unnatural—even just holding him. He's still a little floppy sometimes—there are many ways to hold him. She's figured out one way to hold him, and that's the only way. It's all awkward—it's all a big to-do. Then in the morning I was thinking about you and me. Do we have a physical relationship? We don't have a physical relationship—being held or touched. The feeling is everyone I've ever had contact with, there was the possibility of sexual contact.

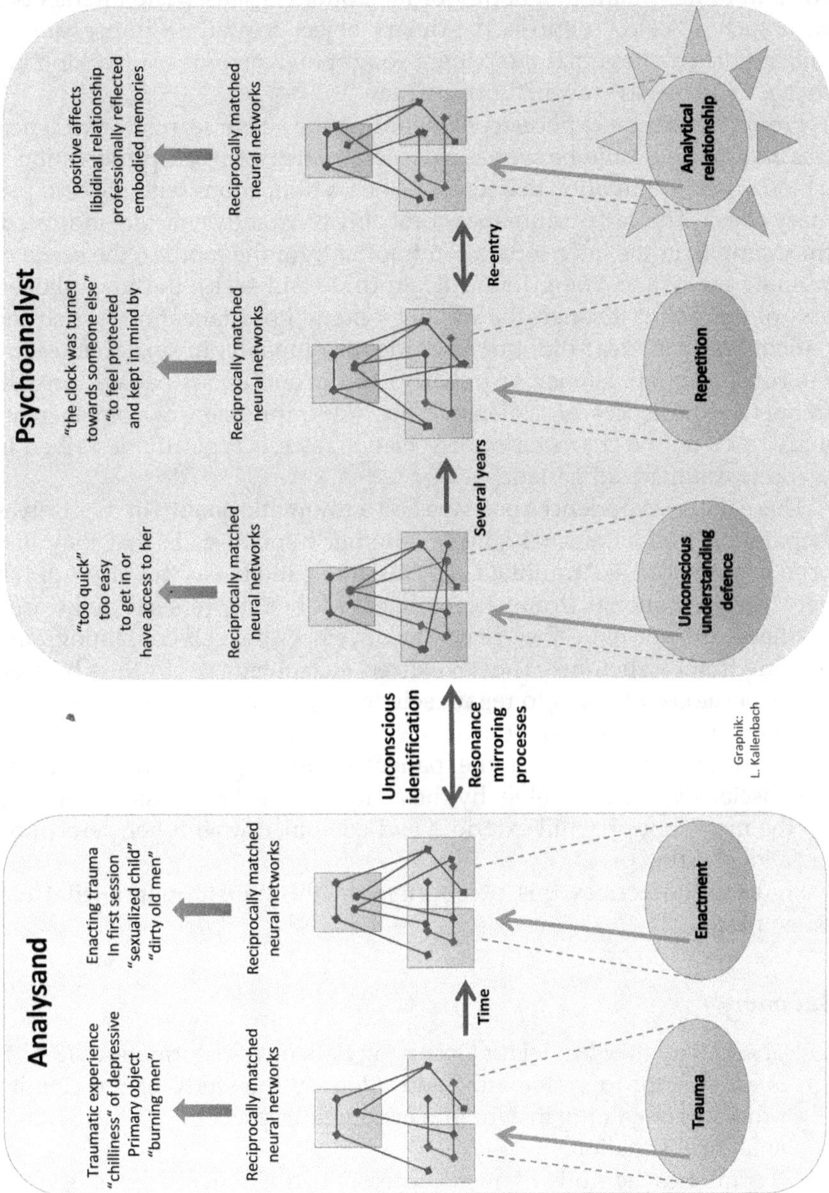
Analysand
Traumatic experience
"chilliness" of depressive
Primary object
"burning men"
Reciprocally matched
neural networks
Time
Trauma
Enacting trauma
In first session
"sexualized child"
"dirty old men"
Reciprocally matched
neural networks
Enactment
Unconscious
identification
Resonance
mirroring
processes
Graphik:
L. Kallenbach
Psychoanalyst
"too quick"
too easy
to get in or
have access to her
Reciprocally matched
neural networks
Several years
Unconscious
understanding
defence
"the clock was turned
towards someone else"
"to feel protected
and kept in mind by
Reciprocally matched
neural networks
Re-entry
Repetition
positive affects
libidinal relationship
professionally reflected
embodied memories
Reciprocally matched
neural networks
Analytical
relationship

Only through long psychoanalysis was the patient now able to observe how "awkward" her mother was when she held her baby son and how she felt strange in her own body. Such a mother could not convey enough warmth to her infant in a bodily or metaphorical sense. The interactions with such a "cold," depressed primary object created an impression of unbearable coldness that the patient sought to overcome by "seeking hot sexual experiences" (even "Burning Men").

From "hot sexual experiences" including the active search for violence, this background could be seen as a desperate attempt at self-preservation—a kind of self-stimulation to overcome the identifications with the cold primary object. The early trauma was probably constantly enacted, indicated, for example, in the later separation trauma from the mother, the scene of running away and being found again (hide-and-seek), the unexplained loss of the object through the mother's many hospitalizations when the patient was a 10-year-old, but also due, presumably, to sexual abuse by the cousin (in late latency or puberty) and promiscuous behaviour with frequent experiences of violence. Thus the impression of cold increasingly takes on the character of dissociation, as it is typically described in severely traumatized patients.

These (later) experiences perhaps had a traumatic quality in themselves (separation trauma, sexual abuse). Another hypothesis is that they had been experienced as "traumata" because the patient—as the result of her very early emotional (traumatic) neglect by her depressed "awkward" mother—did not have the chance to develop safe, self-containing, and holding inner structures. The sexualized enactments could thus be seen as unconscious attempts to regain self-agency, "emotional warmth," and excitement in intimate relationships with an object.

The traumatic quality of the patient's suffering was also captured unconsciously and accurately by the analyst in the first session. She took up the metaphor of "chill exterior" and combined it with her perception of "a lot of pain."

Figure 3.1 describes this perspective on the transformation that has taken place.

Summary

1 The Three-Level Model for Observing Patient Transformations (3-LM) is an attempt to systematize and intensify the study of the circular processes of gaining insight into unconscious processes in the psychoanalytical situation.
2 It combines the study of microprocesses in different phases of psychoanalyses with summaries of the "macro-processes," the transformation in the inside and outside world of our patients.

3 It focuses the transformation of the patient which can best be studied in the relationship with his or her analyst (in the transference/counter-transference, etc.) One example is the transformation of the metaphors created by the analytic couple.
4 It is a method with great similarities to the ones used in supervisions and intervisions—and thus close to the clinical and institutional practice of psychoanalysts.
5 The 3-LM can be applied in different settings (clinical study groups, training, clinical and extra-clinical research, interdisciplinary projects).
6 Thus it can be considered a first step in *clinical research in psychoanalysis*, e.g., to improve case reports or detailed case narratives (by systematic application of the psychoanalytical expert validation, particularly on the third level of the 3-LM) or by systematic use of clinical (expert validated) material to illustrate "clinically evaluated" conceptual ideas in psychoanalysis (*conceptual research in psychoanalysis*).
7 The 3-LM can also be used in *extra-clinical psychoanalytical research* if it is combined with non-psychoanalytical methods in diagnostics and evaluation of outcome.
8 Analysts from different parts of the IPA are fascinated and inspired by the 3-LM, offering an innovative new tool to share clinical observations, conceptual and technical ideas, as well as doubts and concerns with psychoanalytical colleagues.
9 Finally the 3-LM could be used in outreach projects, e.g., having students and interns participate in 3-LM groups with experienced analysts and thus offering them a possibility to get to know transformation processes in psychoanalyses in detail. Many of the interns and students who participated in 3-LM and the clinical conferences of the LAC study (Studie LAngzeittherapie bei Chronischen Depressionen, LAC-Depressionsstudie) have decided to apply for full psychoanalytic treatment: one of the best unexpected side effects of our study! Therefore, clinical as well as extra-clinical research in psychoanalysis is always a transgenerational endeavour and thus saves the future of psychoanalysis!

References

Arlow, J. A. (1979). Metaphor and the psychoanalytic situation. *Psychoanalytic Quarterly, 48*, 363–385.

Baranger, M., & Baranger, W. (1961). La situación analítica como campo dinámico. *Revista Uruguaya de Psicoanálisis, 4*(1), 3–54. Published also as Baranger, M., & Baranger, W. (2008). The analytic situation as a dynamic field. *International Journal of Psychoanalysis, 89*(4), 795–826.

Baranger, M, & Baranger, W., & Mom, J. (1983). Process and non-process in analytic work. *International Journal of Psychoanalysis, 64*, 1–15.

Bernardi, R. (2014). The Three-Level Model (3-LM) for observing patient transformations. In M. Altman de Litvan (Ed.), *Time for change: Tracking transformations in psychoanalysis—The Three-Level Model* (pp. 3–35). London: Karnac.

Bernardi, R. (2017). A common ground in clinical discussion groups: Intersubjective resonance and implicit operational theories. *International Journal of Psychoanalysis, 98*(5), 1291–1309.

Bleger, J. (1969). Teoría y práctica en psicoanálisis. La praxis psicoanalítica [Theory and practice in psychoanalysis: Psychoanalytic praxis]. *Revista Uruguaya de Psicoanálisis, 11*, 287–303.

Caspi, T. (2018). Towards psychoanalytical contribution to linguistic metaphor theory. *International Journal of Psychoanalysis, 99*(5), 1186–1211.

Davidson, D. (1978). What metaphors mean. *Critical Inquiry, 5*(1), 31–47.

de León de Bernardi, B. (1999). Attualità di una polemica: le due dimensioni dell'interazione analitica. *Revista Uruguaya de Psicoanálisis, 45*(1), 131–152.

de León de Bernardi, B. (2018). Teoría del campo, segunda mirada y procesos inferenciales en el analista [Field theory, the second look and inferential processes in the analyst]. In M. Gómez & J. M. Tauszik (Eds), *Psicoanálisis contemporáneo* (pp. 475–495). Buenos Aires: Asociación Psicoanalítica Argentina.

de León de Bernardi, B. (in press). Key metaphors as a multiple bridge for clinical research. In M. Altmann de Litvan (Ed.), *Clinical research in psychoanalysis. Theoretical basis and experiences through working parties*. Abingdon: Routledge.

Gibbs, W. J. (2008). *The Cambridge handbook of metaphor and thought*. New York: Cambridge University Press.

Lakoff, G., & Johnson, M. (1980). *Metáforas de la vida cotidiana* [*The metaphors we live by*]. Madrid: Ediciones Cátedra, 1991.

Lakoff, G., & Johnson, M. (2008) *Metaphors we live by*. Chicago: The University of Chicago Press.

Leibovich de Duarte, A. (2010). Psychotherapists at work: Exploring the construction of clinical inferences. In R. S. Frensch & A. Peter (Eds), *Personality, human development, and culture: International perspectives on psychological science* (Vol. 2, pp. 29–43). New York .

Leuzinger-Bohleber, M. (2014). Depression and trauma: The psychoanalysis of a patient suffering from chronic depression. In M. Altmann de Litvan (Ed.), *Time for change: Tracking transformations in psychoanalysis—The Three-Level Model* (pp. 122–163). London: Karnac.

Modell, A. H. (2009). Metaphor: The bridge between feelings and knowledge. *Psychoanalytic Inquiry, 29*, 6–11.

Ogden, T. (1997). Reverie and metaphor: Some thoughts on how I work as a psychoanalyst. *International Journal of Psychoanalysis, 78*, 719–732.

Peirce, C. S. (1903). Lectures on pragmatism: Three types of reasoning. In *Collected papers of Charles Sanders Peirce, Volumes V and VI: Pragmatism and Pragmaticism and scientific metaphysics (1935)*. Boston: Harvard University Press.

Pichon-Rivière, E. (1998) *Teoría del vínculo* (Vol. 19). Buenos Aires: Nueva Visión.

Rizzuto, A. (2001). Metaphors of a bodily mind. *Journal of the American Psychoanalytic Association, 49*(2), 535–568.

Rizzuto, A. (2009). Metaphoric process and metaphor: The dialectics of shared analytic experience. *Psychoanalytic Inquiry, 29,* 18–29.
Sandler, J. (1983). Reflections on some relations between psychoanalytic concepts and psychoanalytic practice. *International Journal of Psychoanalysis, 64,* 35–45.
Siegelman, E. Y. (1990). Metaphors of the therapeutic encounter. *Journal of Analytic Psychology, 35*(2), 175–191.

Part II

Change in metaphors and dreams

Chapter 4

Changes and no changes in the representation of self and others through images and metaphors

Marina Altmann de Litvan, with a discussion by Ricardo Bernardi

Introduction

The purpose of this chapter is to observe changes in the representation of self and others in an analytical process through metaphors, showing the usefulness and limitations of metaphors and images to observe patient transformations, in the study of a case discussed using the 3-LM (17 analysts from Argentina, Brazil, Peru, and Uruguay[1]).

A metaphor is a rhetorical figure or trope in which the meaning is transferred from one concept to another, establishing a relationship of similarity or analogy between the two terms (Gelo & Mergenthaler, 2012). Metaphors are images, concepts, or ideas that have a subtle relationship between them that is summoned or suggested when they are associated in a text, and that produces impressive relationships that give new significance to the literal meaning of words (Kopp & Craw, 1998).

Metaphors in the analytic setting appear as bridges between clinical practice and theory, which reveal themselves through preconscious and unconscious fantasies and construction and deconstruction during the analysis. Exploring them enables psychic change and leads the patient to the creation of new metaphoric versions of themselves (Rizzuto, 2009; de León de Bernardi, 2013).

In this chapter, we emphasize the importance of observing the emergence of metaphors in the first sessions and regarding them as core anchor points, from which to observe subsequent changes. These metaphors, which have to be disassembled through analytical procedures, represent deep dynamics, resistances, and splitting experiences.

This chapter will focus on an anchor point that arises at Level 1, when the group makes a phenomenological observation of the material, separately from theories (Bernardi, 2014). These observations are then contrasted with analysis of the change of the patient in Level 2 discussions about the patient's mental capacities.

Clinical observation with the 3-LM[2] considers different dimensions of mental functioning: relationship of self with others, relational patterns with the analyst and outside the analysis, self-perception, sense of identity and integrity of the self, perception of others and empathy, regulation of impulses, affects and self-esteem, regulation regarding others (care of self and of others, reciprocity), communication with others (depth and richness of affects and representations), bonds with internal objects and bonds with others, possibility of separation and of establishing and ending bonds.

Reflecting on the group work, we asked ourselves about the scope and limits of the metaphors that were displayed. What do the metaphors account for in the process? What changes or no changes are observed through them? How is it possible to triangulate Level 1 with some dimensions of Level 2 to observe the same phenomenon from a different angle, to broaden the diversity of observation?

Clinical case: Helena

Helena was a professional woman who began analysis at 53 and was now 60 years old. She was a single daughter, married, with three adult sons. She was in the process of retirement. She was in her eighth year of analysis, with a frequency of three times a week and had already had two previous analyses.

She consulted for panic attacks that were accentuated in the two months before treatment began. These crises included physical symptoms like dizziness and tachycardia, accompanied by a fear that she "cannot cope."

Despite talking about her intense anxiety, her facial expression was neutral, as if she wore a "mask," and her appearance was not feminine. She felt imprisoned, afraid of getting sick and suffering from serious illnesses. The analyst described her posture and gait as somewhat rigid, with a strange way of walking. She was "as if in a state of perplexity, suspension and disconnection." During the group discussion, the analyst revealed, "I felt that she was feeling puzzled, like someone facing an abyss." According to the analyst, it became difficult to have a clear idea of what she felt, as if the linguistic means were missing to express her emotions, but the patient was "not depressed."

Helena described her mother as little sensitive to her needs, and her mother's motto was "You have to endure." Despite all this, and at an advanced age, she now sought her third analysis. Her life was emotionally impoverished, and she was very distressed.

Metaphors that emerged in the dreams: First level of analysis

Significant clinical patterns can be expressed in metaphors (Modell, 2005) that emerge in the dreams, they "transmit in a vivid and

> unsaturated form some of the core of the patient's problems. Some of them appear from the beginning and become the focus of therapeutic work and can be considered as "anchor points" that serve as a background on which it is possible to identify subsequent changes.
>
> (Bernardi, 2016, p. 373)

Metaphors represented the more revealing anchor points, parts of the clinical material that had great resonance during Level 1 and that can be used as clues of patients' transformations through the analysis. Listening to the material, a strong figurative anchor point was selected by the group: houses and hotels. Conceptually, we hypothesized that these were representations of the self, rooted in the body.

Metaphor 1: A hotel with no walls (1 year, 3 months of analysis)

In the first year of analysis, Helena remembered a dream:

P: *I arrive at a place, something like a hotel. There are a few cottages and chalets. The numbers were hidden. Finally, I found mine, but to my surprise, there were no walls. The furniture was a kind of sleeping bag hanging like a suitcase, and I tried to sleep in it. I was outraged at being put in a room like that.*

The hotel without walls was a representation of how the patient experienced herself, giving an account of her structural problems. The dream showed aspects of herself: precarity, non-discrimination: "no walls" and difficulty in finding her place. At the same time, the hotel, cottages, and chalets represented a search for containment. The dream was communicated to the analyst, the patient made no associations. There was a figurative process of symbolization in the dream but not an internal communication with what it meant for Helena.

The analyst interpreted:

A: *It is as if you were looking for a place to sleep, to live and dream, and what you find is this paradoxical house without walls, with a suffocating bed without space. . . .*

P: *The part of not having walls did not bother me. I was able to see the others . . . and they saw me.*

A: *Then, it is as if you need to escape from the hard, rigid part inside in which you feel trapped, to find a comfortable bed, feel at ease. . . . In a certain way, it is what you are trying to build here when you lie down and dream.*

The analyst expected a dreaming attitude. For the analyst, the patient had a conflict between her tightness and rigidity (the suffocating bed) and the difficulty of expressing her emotions (the rigid body posture). This conflict prevented her from relating to herself more freely (associated with the hotel with no walls). Helena had no ears for her wishes and needs, an indication of instability and vulnerability with scarce integration. The analyst was providing her patient with latent content that the patient could not accept. There was no conflict for her, only "her need to see and be observed, without walls." It is in immediate relation with the sensory-motor aspects and lacks reference to an alive inner object.

The analyst interpreted the dream as the patient wished and desired (a conflict) and not as the self-representation concerns (a structural problem). There were no walls, no differentiation between the self and the other.

Metaphor 2: No furniture and the walls are peeling (3 years of analysis)

At the third year of analysis, Helena brought a transference dream. In one scenario, she felt uncomfortable because someone else was with her analyst. "I was watching you and that person; it was as if you weren't paying attention to me."

In another scene, she went inside the analyst's house: "Fire and smoke are coming out of the house," and she felt afraid to be discovered invading and felt scared that someone would think she were intruding. "There is no furniture, and the walls are peeling."

The dream continued: she got into the closet, and she saw different clothes. We saw now a different representation of her body looking for different outfits. Transference was facilitating the processing of these emotional and bodily sub-symbolic experiences through the relationship patterns with the analyst. Very regressive moments were recreated in the transference that alluded to what the patient did not have in her primary bonds. But again the dream was brought without associations or comments.

In this new context, there were walls, a differentiation between the analyst and herself. She felt the desire to get into the analyst's life, but she was concerned about the effects of her actions on the other, and different feelings of exclusion and invasion appeared.

Metaphor 3: Trying to rob my house (3 years, 2 months)

A few sessions later, she brought another dream:

P: *I went to a family lunch in a restaurant, where we used to go. I entered. There was a big table where everyone was sitting, but I had to stay at another table*

> *nearby, with my father and another person. I got very angry and decided to leave. My husband followed me, but I got lost, couldn't find the car and got very irritated. Some horses passed by and I was afraid that one of them would trample on me. Then I was at home, but outside, with my children, my family. Suddenly, at the gate, some people appeared, who apparently wanted to get in. Then I saw they were police officers, who said that other people were trying to rob my house.*

Now she was not alone; she was with her family and people "wanted to come in" (not invading), but there was the presence of the other (police officers) who tried to defend her from robbery.

Persecutory anxieties were now the content of her dream and not acted out, as was observed at the beginning of the analysis. In her dreams, she could express her hostility, her irritation. Her emotions began to be processed. There was a pattern of relationship: she felt excluded, then very angry, and she escaped.

Although we observed these emotions in the recollection of the patient's dream, we did not find evidence in the clinical material of the analytic work done in the transference about these emotions. Regarding this matter, Fain and David (1963) state the importance of the capacity to dream and remember the dreams as an important clinical fact, because of their capacity to link tensions and traumatic situations. As Marty states (1984), dreaming in itself has an elaborative capacity.

Metaphor 4: Large, spacious, bright, white house (6 years, 10 months)

The analyst interpreted her feelings of exclusion and immediately Helena reported this dream:

> I was in a large, spacious, bright, white house. The house was on top of the mountain. Outside, there are people around a hole in the ground. I go out and get scared with the hole; I have the feeling that I am falling into it. I grab my husband's arm. He is not afraid, and that does not reassure me. I am afraid of falling.

She became scared, needed the support and reassurance of her husband because she perceived herself as unstable. Now there was a bright, spacious white house, herself, but challenging to reach: at the top of the mountain. The analyst's interpretation tried to link the mind and body, but the patient rejected it. Instead, she brought the suicidal falling: she saw a person falling from her window. She was still perceiving herself as fragile and unstable, and the fear of falling was still present.

Helena also associates the white house with their beach house, which she inherited from her mother.

P: *I want to have it renovated so that the children can frequent it and have it full, but I fear that in the end, they will not go.*

A: *Are you afraid that the house is not as full as it was in your mother's time?*

Associations appeared that linked the beach house with the mother's house and her current beach house, with her sons and granddaughter: the milestones of her life. The analyst interpreted that she was the girl who fell into the hole out of envy for her mother. It was the analyst who brought up unconscious feelings and there was a strong emotional connection between them. The analyst tried to establish a link between her childhood and the present, to weave the associations that the patient did not make. And in this dream, the houses were associated with representations of different periods of her life, as well as her feminine identity concerning her maternal figure.

For the unconscious—as we see in dreams and literature—the house can represent the maternal body and our own body. Our life is deposited within their walls, in their corners, and we go to them every time we need to locate ourselves in time or the place of dream or fantasy (Maberino de Prego, 1977).

The analyst tried to link dizziness (physical aspects) with dreams, but the patient did not respond to her interpretation.

The observation group still perceived that her self-representation had not been totally stabilized yet, for she could become unsettled or incapacitated by some aspects of her daily life. Although the house had changed and was larger, brighter, and more comfortable now, the intensity of her negative emotions, such as fear, still prevented her from overcoming this instability.

Metaphor 5: A house under construction (8 years, 2 months)

Helena brought a dream of a house:

P: *I was going alone, to L.'s new house. I know he has people working, but I come in. The room is long, has a barbecue outside. I walk to the back, and I perceive my cousin Leo behind me. I didn't expect to find him, he's happy. I go on until I find a space, in the background, big, it impresses me. Many people are working in the garden, and then I see a river, with a waterfall. I find it beautiful, but strange. When I woke up, I discussed it with Ruy and he says it's the sum of L's two houses (the beach and the new one). At first, it's similar, but then most of it's unexpected.*

She was silent.

P: *I never had the opportunity to do this, to talk about a dream at breakfast.*

In this moment the house was the representation of a differentiated body, with walls, and different places and functions. The husband was there to secure her, to talk, but we know nothing of what he felt and thought. It was presented as an object at the service of Helena's needs. The affects were more positive: there was no fear or irritation, no feeling of rejection or indifference.

Metaphor 6: The hotel starts to look bigger and nicer (8 years, 2 months)

P: *I had a different dream. It was a hotel in Z; I was there on business. I get the key and bring my suitcase to my room, which was very small. It is a see-through suitcase and I see a mannequin inside it, but only from the waist up. The hotel lobby is modest, and a man I don't know offers me a room upgrade, for a little extra money. I accept it and go look for my room, but I can't find it. The hotel starts to look bigger and nicer.*

She perceived herself in a more active way, giving agency to her things and revealing a more integrated representation of herself, although there was still a representation of her body as a mannequin, from only the waist up. Her physical cohesion was disrupted, and she experienced her body as fragmented.

Now there were associations with experiences of her daily life: she associated them with an episode with her granddaughter, whose hair was dishevelled, and she combed it very delicately. She told her that she didn't know how to comb because she had short hair, and her husband told the girl that Helena used to have long hair.

A: *And we recently talked about long hair in the last session. . . .*
P: *Yeah, I told you I was delighted with my granddaughter's hair.*
A: *You also remembered your artificially curled hair in the photo where you were little.*
[The analyst introduces the tyrannical mother.]
P: *That's right. . . . what did she do to curl my hair? I was almost a baby. . . .*
A: *It looks like we're weaving a story together: you bring all kinds of feelings and even envy. It's a fabric, it's not just waste. [The analyst refers in metaphorical terms to the analytical work showing a historicization.]*

Representations of the self and the others: Second level

The second level of analysis allows a focalized observation in different dimensions. In this case, I will focus on the changes or no changes in mental functioning.

At the beginning of treatment, Helena failed to perceive herself and others (she did not trust others because she found their responses unpredictable). She had experiences, but she could not represent them in a way that remained inscribed in herself. She played many roles, but with no affective depth. Helena was not able to integrate body and mind; she presented flaws in her self-perception, as she was unable to integrate her achievements with a self-assessment of her self-experience. She perceived herself as an outsider, and she felt less valuable.

A variation was observed in her sense of identity and integration, but she still appeared troubled.

Helena had little thickness in her representations, and she needed to work from the body, to find and repair basic aspects of her feminine narcissism and self-esteem. She needed to invest her body, see her body, libidinally, for her body was experienced as cut off.

At the beginning of treatment, she showed difficulties in regulating her impulses and her affects, which compromised everything related to self-esteem. She had dysfunctional defences and excessive idealization of others.

As for interpersonal relationships, the group noted that the patient had serious relationship difficulties with others. In the beginning, the patient excluded herself, and when invited she did not accept the invitation. She had no close friends and she called the professionals who attended her "friends." There was a subjectivity deficit, because of her lack of confidence and the unpredictability of the other's response, so she fell into isolation and subjective loneliness. Then she began to look for interactions; there were modifications of affects, her fears diminished, and there were scenes of pleasure linked to sensorial, sub-symbolic contents, which could not yet be adequately represented.

As for links with internal and external objects, the patient improved but still had disturbances. At the eighth year of analysis, in a dream, "a handsome young man appears and asks me if I remember him. . . . When he goes away I felt bad because his presence was reassuring." She needed an object to give her reassurance, look at her, to receive pleasure.

She could talk more with her husband after eight years of analysis, and the link with her mother image improved. A change was noted regarding her children: she was more able to enjoy their company and to enjoy her granddaughter.

Table 4.1 Dimensional analysis of change and no change

Dimension	*Beginning*	*Change*	*No change*	*Group evaluation**
Self-perception	She plays many roles, without affective depth, that have not been integrated. No ears for her own wishes and needs.	*Metaphor 5: A house under construction* *Metaphor 6: The hotel starts to look bigger and nicer* Brings changes and her conflicts between the mannequin and the integrated body that dives into the sea.		From 1 to 2
Sense of identity and integrity of the self	Difficulties in perceiving herself in an integrated way. *Metaphor 1: A hotel with no walls* Perceives herself as not stable *Metaphor 2: No furniture and the walls are peeling*	*Metaphor 5: A house under construction* The *real* house. Contact with feminine aspects of herself		From 1 to 2
Perception of others and empathy	*Metaphor 2: No furniture and the walls are peeling*		Not worried about the other. Her significant others are poor and function at her service, not as independent selves.	From 2 to 3
Regulation of impulses, affects, and self-esteem	She has fears of being excluded, of being trampled upon, getting sick and dying, falling, losing ground, being watched, being invaded, afraid that the house is not as crowded as in the time of her mother. *Metaphor 3: At home they are trying to rob my house*	*Metaphor 5: A house under construction* More pleasure and enjoyment: water, sea. Better self-esteem as mother and grandmother. Less fears, better regulation of her impulses, which appear in the dreams and not in real life.		From 2 to 3

(*Continued*)

Table 4.1 (Continued)

Dimension	*Beginning*	*Change*	*No change*	*Group evaluation**
Regulation regarding others (self-care, care of others, reciprocity)	*Metaphor 4: Large, spacious, bright, white house* Others appear as threatening or at the service of her self-regulation. Feelings of exclusion, being ignored.	*Metaphor 5: A house under construction* The other (her cousin) appears less threatening and with positive affects.	Scarce reciprocity. No evidence of care of others.	From 2 to 3
Communication with others (depth and richness of affects and symbolic internal representations, fantasies, bodily self, sexuality)	*Metaphor 1: A hotel with no walls* *Metaphor 2: No furniture and the walls are peeling* There are few people in her universe. She calls people "friends" who are not really her friends.	*Metaphor 5: A house under construction* A change was noted regarding her children: she is more able to enjoy their company and to enjoy her granddaughter. She is able to talk more with her husband after eight years of analysis. A little more confident in her relationships. Less persecutory.	No deep communication with others. More positive but not richness of affects. *Metaphor 6: The hotel starts to look bigger and nicer* Communication with her sexuality is very limited. Improved (more discriminated parts) but still conflictive relations with body self.	From 1 to 2

Bonds with internal objects and with others	She had no close friends. She excludes herself.	In the transferential bond the capacity to have intimacy and reciprocity with the analyst is evidenced. With her husband it improves a little, and with her children and granddaughter. The link with her mother image improved.	There is no evidence that it has been established with bonds outside the analysis.	From 2 to 3
Possibility of separation and of establishing and ending bonds	She shows difficulties in establishing significant bonds.		She shows difficulties in ending bonds, no grief scenes about her mother or father. In the clinical material the process of separation with the analyst or the grief of her mother are not described.	From 2 to 3

**Scale:* 1: Extreme disturbances. Non-integrated functioning; 2: Important disturbances. Severe limitations in functioning; 3: Moderate disturbances, with some limitations in functioning; 4: Minimum or imperceptible disturbances and limitations.

Note: Intermediate values can be marked with half a point (for example 1.5, 2.5, etc.).

She showed difficulties integrating her mind and body. After eight years of analysis the change presented as part of a conflict between two aspects of herself, from the mannequin to a figure of herself with a full body facing the sea. The analyst said that in the dream she could leave the body that was severed at the genitals and devitalized in the small room to look for other things, and reminds her that the final scene, in the sea, could be a photo of a wider relationship with her whole body.

The patient was able to link her mind and body, and from there, in the eighth year, she began to recover her relationship with her mother. A new house emerged, her son's house, a house that had different parts and functions. It almost became a discriminated body with different roles, which was being repaired, fixed. The patient began to discover the different places she had within herself.

She showed difficulties in regulating her impulses and her affects. Fears were a version of the initial panic that brought her to analysis. The analyst perceived her fears and panic, but in the clinical material, these fears did not appear to be the analyst's focus.

At the beginning of analysis, there was no internalization of her problems. She brought dreams but she could not learn from them. We can observe a fear of feeling emotions. She did not analyze what happened in her relationships, and her desires and goals focused on avoiding facing conflict instead of ruling them.

At the beginning and middle of analysis, she also showed difficulties in giving continuity to her experiences and her history. In the eighth year of the analytic process, there were more memories and she went on "weaving the story," bringing memories and now linking them with her granddaughter.

Conclusions

Reflecting on the work of clinical observation groups using the 3-LM, I used a clinical case to show the possibilities and limits of metaphors to observe changes in the representation of the self and others in a psychoanalytic process.

This is relevant because, in the unconscious construction of meaning, metaphor plays an important role. Modell (2005, 2009) suggests that metaphor functions unconsciously as a pattern detector and thus is pivotal to the organization and categorization of emotional memory. We could assume, therefore, that the metaphors the patient brings are a representation of the patient's inner world, and the changes accomplished or not during the analytic process would be reflected in the metaphors.

The images condense aspects of life experiences and the construction of the patient's identity, that open in multiple senses, which are still unknown to the analyst (de León de Bernardi, in press). The different images of the self represent polarities, retrospective and prospective layers of the internal world of the patient, which are a dialectic spiral circuit of senses that acquire progressive experiential density (Pichon-Rivière, 1998). Metaphors "provide a mode of apperception of otherwise disparate aspects of self-experience, and it creates a private mode of objectification of ineffable experience" (Rizzuto, 2001, p. 557).

Houses are metaphors identified by the clinical observation group in this clinical case as a result of an intuitive clinical observation that captures emotional, bodily, and cognitive states of the patient—partially unconscious—that effectively communicate the patient's experiences. They are bridges between the unconscious processes of the patient and the preconscious representations that arise from the analysts in the group work.

At Level 1, metaphors give us an account of the patient's structural problems and her difficulty in perceiving her mental states and those of others, her representations of the self and the others, and their changes and no changes:

- *A hotel with no walls*: precarity, non-discrimination, difficulty in finding her place, difficulties in differentiating her representations of herself from the representation of the others.
- *No furniture, and the walls are peeling*: the place of the other, the body.
- *Clothes*: the feminine aspects of herself; she is beginning to explore her interior and recognize her different sides.
- *"Trying to rob my house"*: her fears and difficulties in the relationship between the self and the other, how close to others or separated from them she can be. She can express her hostility, her irritation. Some of her emotions begin to be processed.
- *Large, spacious, bright, white house*: more positive feelings, fear of falling, need of the other for reassurance.
- *A house under construction, the hotel starts to look bigger and nicer*: The other is not seen as a threat. Hotels and houses also represent a search for containment.
- We can also observe her different patterns of interactions, her worries and fears regarding relationships: to see others and to be seen by others if they pay attention to her or not.

When we compare our observations at Level 1 with some dimensions of Level 2 to observe the same phenomenon from a different angle (triangulation), we have an account of the patient's problems and some of her advances in treatment.

To what extent do the dimensions of Level 2 overlap, broaden, or question the changes observed at Level 1 with the metaphors? The second level allowed us to observe and extend certain observations that were raised:

- We find with the 3-LM that the categories of mental functioning at the second level confirm some trends and expand our knowledge of the analytic process.
- However, metaphors alone are not enough to see the full scope of Helena's difficulties. Here moderate changes and those difficulties that still require transferential work are underlined.
- Metaphors showed changes in mental structure and functioning, but the metaphors of the houses are less accurate in describing the patient's conflicts.
- The group found a difference between the written presentation of the clinical material and the personal expressions of the analyst, when she was present in the group discussion, that helped greatly in understanding other dimensions of the patient that the analyst neither explored nor asked. Among group observations, it was noted that Helena "is a box of surprises." She wrote several books, worked, had a family, a pragmatic side that allowed her to study, to practise a profession. These were not mentioned in the material the analyst selected and made us reflect on the analyst's selection of the clinical material.

Regarding these observations, we can also mention what different authors point out regarding changes in the manifest dreams and the work with dreams in the psychoanalytical situation: Andrade (2007); Marty (1984); and Altmann de Litvan (2002, 2014, 2018). They are key to understanding unconscious conflicts and fantasies and possible transformations of psychic functioning (Leuzinger-Bohleber, 2012).

Nevertheless, the clinical material shows few of the patient's associations. These failures in associative capacity were explained by Rizzuto (2001) as linked to numerous preverbal representations of the self (visceral, sensory, iconic, motor) that organize internal and external experiences so that the analyst has to focus on the development of verbal communication. They are signs that remain at the preverbal level.

Dreams, metaphors, and images are very powerful. However, we found some limits:

- There is no evidence in dreams of the patient's regulation regarding others (self-care, care of others, reciprocity), or empathy, because the analyst did not include real-life episodes of the patient. The patient's relational episodes with her closest relatives do not appear clearly, except in the dreams. What we observe are inferences from dreams with internal objects and not real interactions with people. We can ask ourselves if the intersubjective problems improve as an effect of intrapsychic analytic work or whether analysts should work on them specifically.

- The analyst doesn't inquire about the patient's sexuality with her husband. She focuses on preconscious content, and the questions she introduces aim to enhance the associative process. The areas of sexuality are related to getting in touch with her bodily sensations, but not directly to adult, genital sexuality.

In short, we were able to go through some of the ups and downs in the representation of the self and the others in these eight years of analysis with the sessions selected by the analyst, especially through the patient's dreams. Metaphors are a powerful clinical tool but were not enough to know how the external world of the patient changed and to assess the perdurability of the changes achieved.

An enriching polemic was held with the discussant regarding whether it is accurate to consider the images that emerge from the manifest content as metaphors. Metaphor is a very broad term. What is a metaphor in the analytical field? First, we define it as "a vivid and unsaturated pathway to the patients' problems" (Bernardi, 2015, p. 14).

If metaphors are images, concepts or ideas that have a subtle relationship between them that are associated and related (Rizzuto, 2009), the patient scarcely reached that association, because she could not give the transferred meaning to them, even though the analyst showed her possible meanings.

We also find there are "key metaphors" (de León de Bernardi, in press). This concept entails a metaphoric process between the patient and the analyst that allows access to different layers—conscious and unconscious—in the patient–analyst interaction. In this clinical case, we observe that this last process began in the sixth year of analysis.

Nevertheless, I believe the houses can be considered as metaphors for the clinical observation group, because they served as anchor points and showed us the patient's problems as well as her evolution throughout the analytic process, and served as bridges to reveal her preconscious and unconscious fantasies during the analysis.

References

Altmann de Litvan, M. (2002, September). *La capacidad de soñar como indicio de la salud psique-somática* [*Dreams and the capacity to dream as evidence of the functioning of the psyche-soma*]. Paper presentation, XXIV Congreso Latinoamericano de Psicoanálisis, Montevideo. www.fepal.org/images/congreso2002/adultos/altmann_m___la_cap.pdf.

Altmann de Litvan, M. (2014). *Time for change: Tracking transformations in psychoanalysis—The Three-Level Model*. London: Karnac.

Altmann de Litvan, M. (2015). Panel report, IPA Congress Boston 2015: Metaphors and the use of analyst as tools to improve our clinical practice panel and small discussion group organized by IPA project committee on clinical observation. *International Journal of Psychoanalysis, 96*(6), 1651–1654.

Altmann de Litvan, M. (2018). Escuchando la voz consciente e inconsciente del paciente y el analista en un encuadre grupal. El Modelo de los Tres Niveles para la Observación de las Transformaciones del Paciente, 3-LM [Listening to the conscious and unconscious voice of the patient and the analyst in a group setting. The Three-Level Model for Observing Patient Transformations, 3-LM]. In *Latin American psychoanalytic thinking*. Buenos Aires: APA FEPAL.

Andrade, V. M. (2007). Dreaming as a primordial state of the mind. *International Journal of Psychoanalysis, 88*(1), 55–74.

Bernardi, R. (2014). The Three-Level Model (3-LM) for observing patient transformations. In Altmann M. (Ed.), *Time for change: Tracking transformations in psychoanalysis—The Three-Level Model* (pp. 3–34). London: Karnac.

Bernardi, R. (2015). What kind of discipline is psychoanalysis? *International Journal of Psychoanalysis, 96*, 731–754.

Bernardi, R. (2016). La evaluación de los cambios del paciente. El modelo de los tres niveles (3-LM) [The evaluation of changes in the patient: The Three-Level Model (3-LM)]. In R. Bernardi, B.Varela, D. Miller, R. Zytner, L. de Souza, & R. Oyenard. *La formulación psicodinámica de caso. Su valor para la práctica clínica [The psychodynamic formulation of a case: Its value for clinical practice]* (pp. 369–383). Montevideo: Grupo Magro Editores.

de León de Bernardi, B. (2013). Field theory as a metaphor and metaphors in the analytic field and process. *Psychoanalytic Inquiry, 33*, 247–266.

de León de Bernardi, B. (in press). Key metaphors as a multiple bridge for clinical research. In M. Altmann de Litvan (Ed.), *Clinical research in psychoanalysis. Theoretical basis and experiences through working parties*. Abingdon: Routledge.

Fain, M., & David, C. (1963). Aspects fonctionnels de la vue onirique [Functional aspects of dreamlike view]. *Revue française de psychanalyse, 27*, 241–399.

Gelo, O. C. G., & Mergenthaler, E. (2012). Unconventional metaphors and emotional-cognitive regulation in a metacognitive interpersonal therapy. *Psychotherapy Research, 22*(2), 159–175.

Kopp, R., & Craw, M. (1998). Metaphoric language, metaphoric cognition, and cognitive therapy. *Psychotherapy: Theory, Research and Practice, 35*, 306–311.

Leuzinger-Bohleber, M. (2012). Changes in dreams: From a psychoanalysis with a traumatised, chronic depressed patient. In P. Fonagy, H. Kaechele, M. Leuzinger-Bohleber, & D. Taylor (Eds), *The significance of dreams: Bridging clinical and extra-clinical research in psychoanalysis* (pp. 49–85). London: Karnac.

Maberino de Prego, V. (1977). La casa: escena de la fantasía [The house as fantasy scene]. *Revista Uruguaya de Psicoanálisis, 56*, 105–118.

Marty, P. (1984). A propos des rêves chez les malades somatiques [About dreams in somatic patients]. *Revue française de psychanalyse, 48*(5), 1143–1161.

Modell, A. H. (2005). Emotional memory, metaphor, and meaning. *Psychoanalytic Inquiry, 25*(4), 555–568.

Modell, A. H. (2009). Metaphor: The bridge between feelings and knowledge. *Psychoanalytic Inquiry*, *29*(1), 6–11.
Pichon-Rivière, E. (1998). *Teoría del vínculo* [*Theory of binding*] (Vol. 19). Buenos Aires: Nueva Visión.
Rizzuto, A. M. (2001). Metaphors of a bodily mind. *Journal of the American Psychoanalytic Association*, *49*(2), 535–568.
Rizzuto, A. (2009). Metaphoric process and metaphor: The dialectics of shared analytic experience. *Psychoanalytic Inquiry*, *29*, 18–29.

Discussion—Ricardo Bernardi

In her challenging paper, M. Altmann de Litvan examines "the usefulness and limitations of metaphors and images to observe patient transformations, in the study of a case discussed using the 3-LM." For this purpose, she uses the first two levels of analysis, with reference to the comments made in the group discussion and by the analyst. Her work highlights the new questions that arise when considering extended periods of analysis. Altmann de Litvan specifically proposes combining the phenomenological understanding of Helena's changes acquired in the analytic listening at Level 1 with the conceptualization of these transformations using the psychopathological categories described by the second level of the model (Bernardi, 2014).

The study of the metaphors from the 3-LM discussion groups has been the subject of several communications, as Altmann de Litvan points out. In metaphors, says Altmann de Litvan, "meaning is transferred from one concept to another, establishing a relationship of similarity or analogy between the two terms." I would like to add that this transfer of meaning does not cancel out the meaning of the original terms, but creates a tension between them that generates a creative effect. Arieti (1964) pointed out that the poetic metaphor combines two classes of phenomena in such a way that we can see one class in the other, but, unlike schizophrenic thought, this does not imply merging them, but rather suggests a third class that brings them together. Similarly, Arieti points out, creativity arises when we are able to combine the primary and secondary processes without confusing them, giving rise to what he called "tertiary processes" (p. 61), an idea that was later taken up by other authors. This double view is also present, to a certain extent, in Altmann de Litvan 's attempt to combine analytical listening at the first level with descriptive categories at the second level.

Altmann de Litvan's interest is in the dreams which were an important part of Helena's communication with her analyst. Having participated in the clinical discussion group to which Altmann de Litvan refers, I too was surprised by some lack of consistency between the abundance of dream images and the restricted nature of other types of communication. The analyst made multiple interpretations in a subtle and non-intrusive way for Helena to consider, at transferential and extra-transferential levels. Helena responded to them with few associations, using a literal, non-figurative language, referring to external events rather than to emotions or fantasies. However, Helena and her analyst agreed that the analysis was helpful for her. This situation certainly opens up a series of questions. I am interested in examining them and at the same time in discussing problems concerning clinical evidence in psychoanalysis and asking to what extent it is useful to add information from extra-clinical research. In that sense, this commentary can be seen as the application of the criteria discussed in Chapter 14 of this volume, dedicated to the problem of evaluating clinical evidence.

The first metaphor we find in the material does not come from Helena but from the analyst. Commenting on Helena's lack of facial expression and her bodily rigidity she says, "I felt that she was feeling puzzled, like someone facing an abyss." And she adds, "as if the linguistic means were missing to express her emotions." The expression "facing an abyss" suggests the persistence of the annihilation anxiety experienced by Helena during her panic attacks. Helena is paralyzed before an abyss and lacks words to express what is happening to her. I believe that the question of the relationship between panic and lack of words is central to this analysis. I will return to this point.

For the analyst and for the group, as for Altmann de Litvan, dreams were a source of free associations and metaphorical processes, but not for Helena. Dream images in themselves are not metaphors, at least according to classical dream theory. The processes of meaning transfer between the source domain of a metaphor and its target domain (Lakoff & Johnson, 1980) are very different from the processes that transform the latent content of a dream into its manifest content. Dream work is not a creative process of metaphorizing, but of distortion. Purely symbolic interpretation of dreams plays at most a secondary role in Freudian theory, while the patient's associations have the essential role (Freud, 1900, p. 360). Helena's few associations allow us to identify some residues of the day, such as memories of houses and fragments of scenes from her family life. However, they offer us less access to the dynamic aspects of her dream-thoughts, without which it is not possible to understand the context of the dream.

Taking into account only the manifest content of dreams exposes us to multiple biases. Although biases are inevitable, we can reduce them when the patient's associations provide evidence from different sources: transference, recovered memories, unexpected affects, enactments, etc. Without these references, we lack valid criteria that allow us to choose between possible meanings. Take, for example, the fourth dream referred to by Altmann de Litvan, which she calls "Large, spacious, bright, white house (6 years, 10 months)." As Altmann de Litvan says, in the manifest dream we find the spacious, bright, and white image that Altmann de Litvan highlights but also negative emotions and the fear of falling into a hole, despite being held by the husband's hand. There are also references to a suicidal falling. Which of these aspects should be privileged? How do we know that "bright, white house" does not mean the opposite, as the result of the oneiric distortion? The same doubt arises with the following dreams, in which we also find images of antithetical meaning. If we are looking for repressed meanings, we need the associations of the patient and the context of the analysis.

Altmann de Litvan intends to move in another direction. In her comparison with the second level of the 3-LM, she does not take into account the unconscious conflicts, about which the material gives us little information, but rather the integration of the basic functions of the personality.

I agree with Altmann de Litvan that structural vulnerabilities in Helena make it difficult for her to cope with stressful external situations. They are probably related to how much she uses denial, repression, and conscious suppression of affects, which suggest that she flees from external as well as internal conflicts. Her strong inhibition probably includes problems of structural integration and defences against fears of any kind of conflict. Structural vulnerabilities increase the need for strong defences, which in turn make inhibitions and vulnerabilities more evident. It is difficult for me to determine the contribution of each of these factors on the basis of the available data.

To advance the discussion of the role of dreams in this analysis, I would like to discuss the relationship between two clinical facts that occupy a prominent place: panic attacks and the difficulty in expressing her emotions. In what follows I must rely on hypotheses that have a significant speculative component. Despite this limitation, the type of "thought experiment" that I will present points out directions, which we should explore more deeply. It also leads to a more precise formulation of the operational models that can guide the analyst and facilitate discussion of their similarities and differences.

Helena's difficulty in expressing feelings is similar to what Marty called operative thought (*pensée opératoire*) and Sifneos called alexithymia. From Marty's (1968) perspective, panic attacks would correspond to the type of diffuse anxiety that precedes or accompanies the psychosomatic disorganization. This leads to states in which life becomes mechanical and devoid of fantasy, and may lead, in his view, to somatic diseases. The analysis could offer Helena the possibility of stopping the progression of these movements of disorganization, helping her to regulate the stimuli that overwhelmed her protective mechanisms. Through her dreams and the analyst's commentary on the day's residues, Helena could make attenuated contact with aspects of her life without feeling threatened. Altmann de Litvan also mentions the importance of the dream's sensory images, which coincides with the importance that Marty (1976) gave to reorganization that took place through what he called lateral chains or parallel mechanisms of a sensory nature. As far as the interpretative strategy is concerned, likely Marty would have advised pointing more directly to the paralyzed aspects of Helena's libidinal life. Marty (personal communication) called these interventions "scraping," that is, trying to remove the inert and non-reactive parts in order to reach deeper layers, reactivating libidinal movements. How would Helena have responded to an intervention of this type that investigated, for example, her sexual or aggressive fantasies? Probably it depends on how safe she feels in the analysis. The advantage of this type of thought experiment is that it puts into play not only conceptual models but also helps to put empathic understanding into action. In the case of Helena, for the reasons I will show later, I would be extremely cautious with this type of intervention.

The concept of alexithymia proposed by Sifneos (1973) is similar to that of Marty's "operative life." Sifneos makes a distinction between primary alexithymia, related to neurobiological factors, and secondary alexithymia, of traumatic origin. His descriptions served as a basis for constructing scales of alexithymia, such as the TAS-26 (Taylor, Ryan, & Bagby, 1985), which study diverse facets: difficulty in identifying feelings and in describing feelings; reduced daydreaming and fantasies; and externally oriented thinking. Helena would very probably score high on these types of scales. It would be interesting to see if this score changed during the analysis. Often this kind of research tool is considered, as opposed to psychoanalytic clinical research. Of course, it is important not to disturb the therapeutic process, but in principle it is possible to find research designs that combine clinical and extra-clinical methods.

Several studies have drawn attention to the relationship between panic attacks and alexithymia. Sometimes it is not easy to decide in which cases alexithymia should be considered as a previous trait or as a defensive state against anxieties (Fukunishi et al., 1997; Hemming et al., 2019). It has also been pointed out that from a methodological point of view there is an overlap of variables between both phenomena (Marchesi, Brusamonti, & Maggini, 2000; Cox et al., 1995). Neurobiological studies also show the relationship, since patients with panic disorder and difficulty in identifying and managing emotional experience present a dysfunction of fronto-temporal-lympic circuits (Galderisi et al., 2008). It would be important to investigate if alexithymia appeared only during or after Helena's panic attacks, or if it were a permanent feature in her, which seems more likely.

It is also possible that symptoms of agoraphobia and perhaps social phobia persisted after the panic attacks. Patients often minimize these disorders and they may go unnoticed when there is a restricted lifestyle, with little social contact and early retirement, as with Helena. If this were the case, we should ask ourselves how far the image of the house is both the representation of the self and others and also represents, perhaps primarily, the refuge that Helena needs to feel protected.

She invites her analyst to her house-refuge, where they go through the different images of her dreams, but the condition is that she should not go outside it, where she feels that the abyss and annihilation anxiety are lurking.

We thus arrive at the central point: the role of manifest dreams as an indicator of structural changes. At this point, it is useful to review some studies on this subject.

Unlike in Helena, it is common for alexythmic patients to have difficulty in remembering or relating their dreams (De Gennaro et al., 2003; Parker, Bauermann, & Smith, 2000). When dreams do exist, patients who have difficulty identifying and describing feelings tend to have more disturbing, bizarre, and aggressive dreams, while in those who have a predominantly outward orientation, dreams tend to be unremembered or short, boring, and not vivid (Lumley & Bazydlo, 2000). In alexithymic patients in treatment, the traumatic content decreases as affective regulation improves (Trijsburg, 1989). Alexithymic people have difficulty recognizing the personal meaning of sleep images because of the disconnection between cognitive, affective, and memory processes. As a result of this flaw in mentalization, and more specifically, of affective mentalization (Jurist, 2005), traumatic contents remain unlinked to personal memories, fantasies, or situations. Helena probably does not clearly perceive these difficulties in mentalization, although she does see the consequences and feels that she lacks the resources to face internal or external stressful situations, which leads her to the restrictions and the search for a refuge that I have already mentioned.

Individuals with high degrees of alexithymia exhibit deficits in mentalization and do not respond well to traditional interpretive therapies (Taylor & Bagby, 2013). From this perspective, clinical dream investigation should be directed towards mentalization and the functions of structural integration. Let us take as an example the presence of antithetical contents in some dreams (e.g., bright and white house vs. falling into a hole). A key point is Helena's willingness to actively explore the connection of these contradictory feelings in the dream scene with her memories, her affects, her current significant relational episodes, etc. Helena appreciates the analyst's capacities in containing and holding her, which help her to feel comfortable within certain limits. But, returning to the dream, she does not know how far the hand that holds her will be able to do so if they try to go beyond this protective circle (I am aware that this metaphorical allusion is mine and I do not know how far Helena would recognize it as hers). All of this leads me to the question of how far Helena is willing to take the risk of exploring new challenges that will test her resources and those of her analyst to face her fears. In any case, I would be careful not to try to go beyond where Helena desires to go.

Notes

1 Presented in Montevideo, Uruguay in 2016.
Reporter: Luisa Pérez (Uruguay)
Moderator: Beatriz de León de Bernardi (Uruguay)
Group: Adela Leibovich de Duarte (Argentina), Liliana Fudin (Argentina), Haydée Zac (Argentina), Mayela Falvy (Peru), Bruno Salesio (Brazil), Nancy Delpréstito (Uruguay), Luis Villalba (Uruguay), Mercedes Gallinal (Uruguay), Mónica Eidlin (Uruguay), Nahir Bonifacino (Uruguay), Silvia Sapriza (Uruguay), Fernanda Cubría (Uruguay), Adriana Gandolfi (Uruguay), Sylvia Braun (Uruguay), Griselda Revello (Uruguay), Vera Regina Fonseca (Brazil), Liana Pinto Chaves (Brazil), and Vanessa Ems (Uruguay).

2 The IPA Clinical Observation Committee and Research Committee have been working on metaphors since 2015, presenting the panel "Metaphors and the use of analyst as tools to improve our clinical practice" (Altmann de Litvan, 2015) at the International Psychoanalytic Congress in Boston, July 22–25, 2015, and leading the International Conference "Working from the clinic. Metaphor and interpretation," Montevideo, October 20–21, 2017.

References

Arieti, S. (1964). The rise of creativity: From primary to tertiary process. *Contemporary Psychoanalysis, 1*(1), 51–68.

Bernardi, R. (2014). The Three-Level Model (3-LM) for Observing Patient Transformations. In M. Altmann de Litvan (Ed.), *Time for change: Tracking transformations in psychoanalysis—The Three-Level Model* (pp. 3–34). London: Karnac.

Cox, B. J., Swinson, R. P., Shulman, I. D., & Bourdeau, D. (1995). Alexithymia in panic disorder and social phobia. *Comprehensive Psychiatry, 36*(3), 195–198.

De Gennaro, L., Ferrara, M., Cristiani, R., Curcio, G., Martiradonna, V., & Bertini, M. (2003). Alexithymia and dream recall upon spontaneous morning awakening. *Psychosomatic Medicine, 65*(2), 301–306.

Freud, S. (1900). The interpretation of dreams. *S.E. 4/5* (pp. 1–625).

Fukunishi, I., Kikuchi, M., Wogan, J., & Takubo, M. (1997). Secondary alexithymia as a state reaction in panic disorder and social phobia. *Comprehensive Psychiatry, 38*, 166–170.

Galderisi, S., Mancuso, F., Mucci, A., Garramone, S., Zamboli, R., & Maj, M. (2008). Alexithymia and cognitive dysfunctions in patients with panic disorder. *Psychotherapy and Psychosomatics, 77*(3), 182–188.

Hemming, L., Haddock, G., Shaw, J., & Pratt, D. (2019). Alexithymia and its associations with depression, suicidality, and aggression: An overview of the literature. *Frontiers in Psychiatry, 10*, 203.

Jurist, E. (2005). Mentalized affectivity. *Psychoanalytic Psychology, 22*(3), 426–444.

Lakoff, G., & Johnson, M. (1980). *Metaphors we live by*. Chicago: The University of Chicago Press.

Lumley, M. A., & Bazydlo, R. A. (2000). The relationship of alexithymia characteristics to dreaming. *Journal of Psychosomatic Research, 48*(6), 561–567.

Marchesi, C., Brusamonti, E., & Maggini, C. (2000). Are alexithymia, depression, and anxiety distinct constructs in affective disorders? *Journal of Psychosomatic Research, 49*, 43–49.

Marty, P. (1968). A major process of somatization: The progressive disorganization. *International Journal of Psychoanalysis, 49*, 246–249.

Marty, P. (1976). *Les mouvements individuels de vie et de mort.* Paris: Payot.

Parker, J., Bauermann, T. M., & Smith, C. (2000). Alexithymia and impoverished dream content: Evidence from rapid eye movement sleep awakenings. *Psychosomatic Medicine, 62*(4), 486–491.

Sifneos, P. E. (1973). The prevalence of "alexithymic" characteristics in psychosomatic patients. *Psychotherapy and Psychosomatics, 22*, 255–262.

Taylor, G. J., & Bagby, R. M. (2013). Psychoanalysis and empirical research: The example of alexithymia. *Journal of the American Psychoanalytic Association, 61*(1), 99–133.

Taylor, G. J., Ryan, D., & Bagby, R. M. (1985). Towards the development of a new self-report alexithymia scale. *Psychotherapy and Psychosomatics, 44*, 191–199.

Trijsburg, R. W. (1985). Dreams as a sign of change in alexithymia in psychosomatic patients. *Psychotherapy, Psychosomatik, Medizinische Psychologie, 39*(12), 471–475.

Chapter 5

Changes in dreams in the psychoanalysis of traumatized, chronically depressed patients in the frame of the LAC Depression Study[1] applying the 3-LM

Marianne Leuzinger-Bohleber, with a discussion by Carolyn S. Ellman

Introduction

The question of how patients change in the course of psychoanalysis touches on the complex and difficult question of their outcome. In Germany and other Western countries it is closely connected to outcome research. To "prove" the outcomes of psychoanalyses and psychoanalytic therapies has become a major issue in Germany in order to save the still very generous support of psychoanalyses and psychoanalytic long-term treatments (300 sessions are paid for by the insurance companies) (see, e.g., Leichsenring, 2008; Leuzinger-Bohleber & Arnold, 2020). I was responsible for two endeavours in this context: a large follow-up study by the German Psychoanalytical Association in the 1990s (see Leuzinger-Bohleber et al., 2003) and—since 2005—the large multicentric LAC Depression Study comparing short-term and long-term outcomes of psychoanalyses and psychoanalytic long-term therapies of chronically depressed patients on the one hand and cognitive-behavioural therapies on the other hand (see Leuzinger-Bohleber, Hautzinger et al., 2019).

A bitter pill that psychoanalytic researchers have to swallow is that in these comparative studies, which must follow the criteria of evidence-based medicine in order to be taken seriously in the non-psychoanalytic world, the focus is mainly on symptom reduction (see also, e.g., Fonagy et al., 2015). Psychoanalysts certainly also want psychopathological symptoms to be alleviated in their treatments, but their aim in psychoanalyses and long-term psychoanalytic treatments is on transformation of patients' inner object world and the associated unconscious fantasies and conflicts, the "structural changes." Therefore, it was important in the LAC study that, using the elaborate and scientifically accepted method of *Operationalized Psychodynamic Diagnostics* (*OPD*), we showed that after three years of psychoanalytic treatments, structural changes were observed more frequently in chronically depressed patients than in the group who were treated by cognitive behavioural therapists (see Leuzinger-Bohleber, Kaufhold et al., 2019).

In this chapter I would like to discuss another "outcome criterion" for psychoanalysis and psychoanalytic long-term treatments: changes in dreams and in dealing with dreams, as one "via regia to the unconscious" (Freud, 1900). I have investigated such changes by using a theory-based, computer-supported content analysis (e.g., Leuzinger-Bohleber, 1989, 2012). The results were replicated by Kaechele et al. (2006). In the meantime, Moser and von Zeppelin (1997) have developed an elaborate coding method for reliable investigation of the manifest dream content. Fischmann and Leuzinger-Bohleber (2013) used this coding system to investigate the changes of manifest dreams in individual psychoanalyses in the LAC study. They were able to show that analogous changes can also be detected in dreams in the sleep laboratory, as well as with neurobiological methods (fMRI) in the same individuals. In the following sections I would like to illustrate such changes of dreams in a relatively detailed case study (see Chapter 3).

Within the limited scope of this chapter, I am unable to address the epistemological, philosophical, and methodological questions of psychoanalytical research that are always connected to research endeavours, such as the LAC study (see Leuzinger-Bohleber & Arnold, 2020). I also cannot summarize the conceptual and interdisciplinary discourses on psychoanalytical and empirical dream research here (see Bleichmar, 1996; Bohleber, 2010; Fonagy et al., 2012; Weinstein & Ellman, 2012).

Application of the 3-LM in the LAC study: One example

The case was studied with the Three-Level Model for Observing Patient Transformations (3-LM) in the frame of the LAC study. This model is discussed in other chapters of this volume. In weekly clinical conferences we discussed the treatment sessions that had been partially taped and systematically documented our discussion and applied the 3-LM. Based on this joint clinical research, narrative case reports that have been "expert-validated"[2] belong to the most important results of this study (see, e.g., Leuzinger-Bohleber, Negele, & Bahrke, 2020). These case studies convey psychoanalytic insights about the psychodynamics of chronic depression, its complex individual and cultural determinants, as well as details of treatment to the psychoanalytic and non-psychoanalytic community (see also Altmann de Litvan, 2014).

The psychoanalysis of Mr. W (see below) has been investigated with the help of the 3-LM. As anchor points I chose the changes of dreams, taking into account the manifest as well as latent meanings of dreams and their changes.

"As far as I can remember, I have always been depressed" (Mr. W)

Assessment interviews and short biography[3]

The patient came to the Outpatient Department of the Sigmund Freud Institute. He reported that he had always been depressive, but in the last two years his state had become steadily worse. He could hardly concentrate at work and suffered from severe sleep and eating disturbances: "I feel empty inside, like a dark hole: I can't imagine being important for anybody, not even for my wife." Before the interview the patient had not left his dark room for several weeks.

On enquiry he reported that his wife had had three miscarriages, the last one two years earlier. "This time she had been 3 months pregnant. Therefore we had already imagined a life with the baby. I was very sad." He reported that this event strengthened his depressive mood, but that it had always existed.

The patient was the younger one of two sons. His mother was a housewife and his father a natural scientist. During the assessment he did not have a single memory of the first years of his life, only of the time at primary school when his mother increasingly slipped into alcoholism.

> It was horrible. We had to hide alcoholic drinks from her or even had to take them away from her. She was angry, cross, uncontrolled, yelled at us or was just drunken. My father was very helpless and took refuge in work. The whole issue was up to me and my brother. It overshadowed my whole childhood and adolescence.

Fortunately the patient had a close and good relationship to his brother, who was two years older.

The patient described his social isolation and severe feelings of inferiority since his first years in school and particularly during adolescence. After his A-levels he completed basic military service. Also during this time he suffered because he hardly had any friendly contacts. Afterwards he studied in natural sciences (like his brother) and completed university time. When he was 30 years old he met his future wife, who was a natural scientist too.

The patient was highly motivated for treatment. During the assessment he showed a surprisingly differentiated capacity for self-reflection and was able to report dreams. He dreamed repeatedly of standing on a high object, such as a bookshelf, which suddenly started to quiver until he eventually fell down, and he woke up in a panic. These associations led to his mother's addiction, which made the "ground under him quiver" when he was a child and pushed the family into an abyss. The patient responded to the attempt to understand this dream in the first assessment interviews with another dream and his hopes connected with therapeutic treatment:

P: *I'm getting around by bicycle, wanting to reach any destination. . . . Then I suddenly stand in front of an abyss. I see my brother and a companion down in the valley. I take a big ladder and want to climb down to them in the abyss. But when I'm on the ladder, it starts to shake: it shakes and shakes so that I get scared that I might fall down. My brother's companion shouts to me that this would not work out and that I should ascend the ladder again and take the path down further right. . . . I follow his advice and really find my way down.*

The patient told me that this was the first dream in which he was not alone and from which he did not wake up in panic, and instead found a solution based on someone else's advice. Therein we saw his hope to find a way out of his loneliness and to leave behind the "shaking ladder" with the help of the professional relationship with his analyst, prognostically a positive indicator for the beginning treatment.

Summary of the psychoanalytic process with the focus on the changes in the manifest dream contents

Of course I can only summarize fragments of the psychoanalytical process (four sessions a week, for five years). As already mentioned, we discussed the material in the weekly clinical conferences of the LAC study, following the expert validation in the Three-Level Model (3-LM). My focus for systematically studying transformation processes in this psychoanalysis had been the changes in the manifest and latent dreams.

Nightmares and early enactments of the trauma in the transference

As discussed in other papers, central embodied memories of early trauma may be observable in the dreams of the initial phase in analysis (see Bohleber & Leuzinger-Bohleber, 2016). Often these embodied memories are enacted very early in the transference and evoke intensive affect in the counter-transference of the analyst. Often the meaning of the enactment cannot yet be understood during this early stage of treatment but only after years of psychoanalytic work. Here is just one example:

During the assessment interviews I had offered long-term psychotherapy in a vis-à-vis setting with one session a week, because, according to my clinical impression, Mr. W seemed too fragile for psychoanalysis. To my surprise Mr. W answered, "One session a week is not enough for me: you would never make it to reach me emotionally if you see me so seldom." I was very surprised but because I thought that analysands unconsciously are "always right." I agreed to take him into psychoanalysis. I managed to offer him four sessions a week.

At the beginning of our second week of psychoanalysis, Mr. W surprised me by not lying down at the beginning of the session. Sitting in the edge of the couch he turned his (frozen) face to me and said, "I have to ask you a question. If I should feel really bad and helpless during this treatment, can I contact your colleague, the medical doctor at your institute?" I was not only overwhelmed by this "action" but even more by my sudden, uncontrollable, intensive affects in my counter-transference. I was furious, felt devaluated and denigrated. Although I tried to control these intensive affects and did not say a single word, Mr. W. seemed to recognize them. He jumped up and said, "Sorry, I did something wrong—you probably don't want to work with me anymore. I will go then."

At that moment I did not have any idea about the unconscious sources of this enactment. Much later in psychoanalysis we understood that it had been an enactment of "embodied memories" of the traumatic experiences of Mr. W with his unreliable, affect-incontinent, alcoholic mother, which had been enacted immediately upon becoming involved in the psychoanalytical relationship. I will return to this central therapeutic experience.

To come back to the initial phase in psychoanalysis, for a long time it was difficult for Mr. W to freely associate. It was often hard to reach him emotionally. Many analytic sessions dealt with depressive self-accusations, massive inferiority feelings, and the unconscious belief that he was "a strange loner, who no one likes, much less isn't loved." One strategy to cope with his extreme anxieties about giving up control was working with dreams: the patient often remembered dreams, often nightmares, and filled whole sessions with them. The dream-subject in these narrations was often flooded by waves, stuck in narrow channels (see above-mentioned nightmare), tortured or persecuted. Here just one example:

P: *I was condemned to death and wanted to hang myself in the death cell. . . . I woke up in panic.*

Dreams like this one (and many others during this time) illustrate the enormous feelings of helplessness and archaic forms of guilt. These feelings were in the centre of Mr. W's depression: a feeling of being the passive victim of strokes of fate that he could do little to counter, as he was confronted during the 12 years of growing up with a severely ill mother. Besides, as the result of his pathological early object relationship in his first years of life (severely depressed mother, missing father) he probably had been hardly able to integrate his early sadistic and destructive impulses and phantasies or to regulate his unbearable affects.

Approaching aggression

After six months of psychoanalysis, the manifest dream contents started to change. As in the dream, mentioned above, which was told during the assessment interviews (with his brother), now the dreamer was not alone in the dream anymore. Other people were present. The dreamer also seemed to have at least some chance to decide "autonomously," as in the following example:

P: *It was a very short dream. I dreamt that I am in a room together with a friend. He explains to me that I will be executed. I can choose between two possibilities: either to have my head cut off or to be killed by a cord hanging around my neck in a fixed position which would be then strangulated by a running horse. . . . I awoke in panic.*

The process of regaining some control and activity in the dreams continued. In the eighth month of psychoanalysis, after Mr. W had spent one night in the sleeping laboratory in the context of his severe sleep disturbances, he reported the following dream:

P: *I was in a party with my wife. I had to go to the toilet and found one in rooms in another floor. I could not close the door and had the feeling that someone was following me. There were two men—an older and a younger one. The first one had a strange look. He had thick glasses on his nose and stared at me continuously. This was threatening. I tried to chase him away with the toilet brush. And afterwards I woke up because I really was kicking with my foot.*

The associations led to experiences of helplessness—in the sleep laboratory where he felt unprotected, but also in the psychoanalytical sessions. Memories arose of scenes of complete loneliness during adolescence. We talked about his wish "to kick someone" instead of being "a good guy":

A: *In the dream you are defending yourself with a toilet brush in order to protect yourself. This seems to be an important, active step, in contrast to the situation in the laboratory last night or here on the couch—and probably also to many situations as an adolescent where you felt like a passive victim.*

This short example illustrates the importance of approaching one's own aggressive impulses, which until now could hardly be used by the patient as a source of activities of the self (in the sense of a self-agency) to get out of situations of extreme helplessness. These processes were possible thanks only to a reliable, sustaining, and containing psychoanalytic relationship.

Differentiation between self- and object representations

Then in a series of dreams his chronically ill brother appeared. Once he discovered that his brother was tortured and fled despite his feelings of guilt for not helping his brother.

After recognizing massive feelings of guilt as well as phantasies of envy and destructive rivalry in the analytical relationship, the motives changed in the manifest dream:

P: *In the dream I was with my brother. We both were sitting in the car. He was driving but drove faster and faster and did not control the car. I said, "I will now count 1, 2, 3 and then I will be taking over the wheel. And I really was able to prevent a catastrophe."*

This was an impressive example of the successive differentiation between the self-representation and object representation (the brother) as well as the struggling of the dream subject to gain activity and control (self-agency) in order "to prevent a catastrophe."

Working through this central topic in the transference influenced Mr. W's depression. At work he asserted himself in relationships with his colleagues as well as authorities but could feel triumph for only a brief moment. He immediately felt like a "bad person" and anticipated social disaster and exclusion from the team. Above all, he was increasingly able to feel his own aggressive-destructive fantasies and impulses in the transference relationship.

Mourning, revenge, self-destructiveness, and creativity

In the third year of psychoanalysis the patient felt able to work most of the time and was partially able to solve conflicts with colleagues openly and productively. He was able to reflect his tendency towards social withdrawal in order to work against it. He had partly regained his creativity and joy at work, although he still suffered from depressive breakdowns.

The massive fears that he would destroy his objects through his archaic revenge impulses and aggressive fantasies now became accessible in the transference and opened a window for psychoanalytical understanding. For a long time they still provoked massive fears and defences in Mr. W. It did not seem coincidental to me that a second relapse of the immune disease occurred in this difficult phase of psychoanalysis (he suffered from an illness of the autoimmune system). As a result of his autoimmune disease and still latent suicidal tendency, this dynamic in psychoanalysis thus had an existential dimension, which was shown in dreams.

In a dream people were destroyed by hurricanes. He was in a panic and did not dare watch how people were lifted up in the air by the hurricane and then smashed. This dream may illustrate his unconscious belief that his aggressive impulses could destroy his love objects and lead to an irrepressible catastrophe (like his mother's alcoholism). The psychoanalytic understanding of these archaic fears and omnipotent fantasies as well as the increased psychic integration of his aggressive and libidinal impulses often were in the centre of the psychoanalytical work in the transference during these months. Closely connected is the understanding of the psychic function of his rigid ego ideal and superego structures. It seemed favourable for the prognosis that the patient increasingly showed some signs of humour and partially revised his self-image as a "low-maintenance analysand." He partially endured intense conflicts in the analytic sessions, although they still threatened him. Thus there seemed to be some indicators that the psychoanalytic treatment of this severely traumatized patient led to a regaining of trust in a "helping internal and external object," connected with a felt reduction of his loneliness as well as an improvement of his narcissistic self-regulation.

After a session in which we are talking about his terrible loneliness as an adolescent again and that he constantly felt like an "odd bird" (*ein schräger Vogel*) he started the next session:

P: *Mrs. Bohleber, you will not believe it. I really dreamt of a* schräger Vogel *[an odd bird]:*

There was a large, black "odd bird" that was hopping on the street. It looked really interesting, original, and loveable. Then suddenly a sportscar stopped. Very fancy young people got out of the car and looked at the bird. They wanted to take the bird with them, but I protested and did not allow them to take it away: "The odd bird does belong to me," I said.

The associations led to the just-mentioned self-perception as an "odd bird" in his adolescence. In his adolescence he "always felt different from the other, strange, not loved. I felt I didn't belong" At that time he tried to make a virtue out of necessity: "I am just different from them, so what?"

As the manifest dream content as well as the associations illustrate, Mr. W had refound his sense of humour. In the dream this indicated a growing capability of the dreaming self to create a certain distance from feelings and thoughts and to create a sense of control and self-agency. Looking back to the transformation processes during psychoanalysis, the humorous creation of the "odd bird" in the dream was a turning point in the treatment: the analysand had refound his sense of humour. For me this was an indicator that he regained access to a good inner object. In the terminology of Moser and von Zeppelin (1997), the model of a depressed self and object no longer completely dominated the psychic reality of the analysand (the dream scene) and the generation of dreams but was replaced by "embodied memories" of more adequate, less traumatic early object relationship experiences (probably with his analyst, building on early embodied experiences with his mother before she became addicted as well as with his father and grandfather, in which positive affects as well as a "mobility of the self" (self-agency) had been present.

Thus during these months in psychoanalysis the patient dealt with his own part in his social isolation, such as his scorn for fun-loving colleagues during military service or his angry withdrawal from his colleagues at work. Working through this complex of problems led to a change of his position in the outside reality as well as in the transference.[4] In many dreams of the fourth and fifth year of psychoanalysis the dream self was supported by his love object, and thus able to fight against destructive violence as well as ask for help in this fight. The negative affects were integrated in the relationships. These changes may indicate that the traumatized self was no longer completely helpless and impotent, flooded by unbearable affects: there were helping "others" around, which could be seen as a sign that the destroyed basic trust in a helping object was partially restored.

Summary and discussion

Different contemporary interdisciplinary dream models that integrate knowledge from diverse scientific disciplines agree that patients' nightmares may be connected to analysands' (early) traumas. In analogy to the traumatic situation, the dream subject repeats being in a traumatic situation of extreme helplessness, impotence, and unbearable negative affects such as panic, despair, rage, and death anxiety again and again—also while dreaming. The dream-self has lost control of the situation and is confronted with annihilation anxiety and the threat of death. As Weinstein and Ellman (2012) discuss, nightmares are triggered not only by overflooding anxiety but also at the same time by the missing of a holding, containing object. As is well known, in trauma the basic trust in a helping "other" and in self-agency is destroyed—an experience with sustaining consequences (see

Cooper, 1986; Bohleber, 2010). Moser and von Zeppelin (1997) postulate that traumatic complexes can be characterized by the fact that extreme affects are not "bonded" (integrated) in a structure of human relationships. Finally, as illustrated in the case example, we can find indicators of "embodied memories"—bodily experiences in early relationships—in the manifest dreams, which can often be used as indicators for understanding the (unconscious) "history of the trauma" of the analysand in the psychoanalytical situation (see Leuzinger-Bohleber, 2015).[5]

These different conceptualizations of dreams agree that frequent nightmares, which are often told in the initial phases of psychoanalysis (also by patients in the LAC study), may hint at cumulative (early) traumas of the analysands, which may be considered as one unconscious source of chronic depression. As was illustrated in the clinical case, changes in the manifest dream contents as well as in the association of the dream (indicators for the latent dream content) thus can be used as signs for often hidden transformations during psychoanalyses. A dream subject who gains a more active stance and control over the dangerous situation and is no longer exclusively a passive, lonely victim but in the company of helping others often means that a turning point has been found in the psychoanalytical process. Another indicator is the systematic change of affects in the manifest dreams: the spectrum is enlarged. No single affect (like panic) dominates the dream plot anymore, as in the initial phase of the treatment. In the frame of this chapter I could only illustrate but not systematically show or theoretically discuss in detail that in "successful" psychoanalysis the analyst brings the (split-off) trauma with its unbearable affects and unconscious beliefs back into the transference relationship. This may lead to a modification of unconscious convictions that "no one—but no one—is interested in me when I am in an unbearable, life-threatening situation with complete helplessness and impotence, without self-agency." Of course, the traumatic experiences cannot be deleted by such experiences in the transference/counter-transference of the psychoanalytical relationship but they may lose their quality of unbearable horror as it manifests itself, such as in the psychic quality of nightmares.

Therefore changes of the manifest dreams as well as the working with dreams in the psychoanalytical situation still seem a "via regia to the unconscious" for me. They are key to understanding unconscious conflicts and fantasies and possible transformations of psychic functioning. Of course I don't want to simplify these processes: they are never unilinear but very complex. Often transformations take place in a very hidden way and are characterized by ups and downs (as in real life!). But, as I tried to show in this chapter, as well as in several extensive case summaries, a systematic clinical and extra-clinical investigation of the changes of dreams could be a more psychoanalytical way to study changes in psychoanalyses or psychoanalytic long-term treatments than an exclusive investigation of symptoms. The told dream in psychoanalysis is for me, as I tried to illustrate, a narrative that contains "truths" about the narrator's unconscious worlds that—beyond the patient's consciousness—may contain clues to possible changes in his or her unconscious fantasies and conflicts during psychoanalysis.

> Never trust the teller, trust the tale. The proper function of a critic is to save the tale from the artist who created it.
>
> (D.H. Lawrence)

References

Altmann de Litvan, M. (Ed.). (2014). *Time for change: Tracking transformations in psychoanalysis—The Three-Level Model*. London: Karnac.

Bleichmar, H. B. (1996). Some subtypes of depression and their implications for psychoanalytic treatment. *International Journal of Psychoanalysis, 77*, 935–961.

Bohleber, W. (2010). *Destructiveness, intersubjectivity, and trauma: The identity crisis of modern psychoanalysis*. London: Karnac.

Bohleber, W., & Leuzinger-Bohleber, M. (2016). The special problem of interpretation in the treatment of traumatized patients. *Psychoanalytic Inquiry, 36*(1), 60–76.

Cooper, A. (1986). Toward a limited definition of psychic trauma. In A. Rothstein (Ed.), *The reconstruction of trauma: Its significance in clinical work* (pp. 41–56). Madison: International Universities Press.

Fischmann, T., & Leuzinger-Bohleber, M. (2013). Trauma, dream, and psychic change in psychoanalyses: A dialog between psychoanalysis and the neurosciences. *Frontiers in Human Neuroscience, 7*, article 877.

Fonagy, P., Kächele, H., Leuzinger-Bohleber, M., & Taylor, D. (Eds). (2012). *The significance of dreams: Bridging clinical and extraclinical research in psychoanalysis*. London: Karnac Books.

Fonagy, P., Rost F., Carlyle J., McPherson S., Thomas R., Pasco Fearon R. et al. (2015). Pragmatic randomized controlled trial of long-term psychoanalytic psychotherapy for treatment-resistant depression: The Tavistock Adult Depression Study (TADS). *World Psychiatry, 14*(3), 312–321.

Freud, S. (1900): The interpretation of dreams. *S.E. 4/5* (pp. 1–625).

Kaechele, H., Leuzinger-Bohleber, M., Buchheim, A., & Thomö, H. (2006). Amalie X.: ein deutscher Musterfall [Amalie X: A German master case]. In H. Thomä & H. Kaechele (Eds), *Psychoanalytische Therapie* (pp. 121–174). Berlin: Springer.

Leichsenring F. (2008). Effectiveness of long-term psychodynamic psychotherapy. *JAMA, 300*(13), 1551–1565.

Leuzinger-Bohleber, M. (1989). *Veränderung kognitiver Prozesse in Psychoanalysen. Band 2: Fünf aggregierte Einzelfallstudien* [*Transformations of cognitive (affective) processes in psychoanalyses. Vol. 2: Five aggregated single case studies*]. Ulm: PSZ Verlag (Springer).

Leuzinger-Bohleber, M. (2012). Changes in dreams: From a psychoanalysis with a traumatised, chronic depressed patient. In P. Fonagy, H. Kächele, M. Leuzinger-Bohleber, & D. Taylor (Eds), *The significance of dreams: Bridging clinical and extra-clinical research in psychoanalysis* (pp. 49–85). London: Karnac Books.

Leuzinger-Bohleber, M. (2014). Depression and trauma: The psychoanalysis of a patient suffering from chronic depression. In M. Altmann de Litvan (Ed.), *Time for change: Tracking transformations in psychoanalysis—The Three-Level Model* (pp. 122–163). London: Karnac.

Leuzinger-Bohleber, M. (2015). *Finding the body in the mind: Embodied memories, trauma, and depression*. London: Karnac.

Leuzinger-Bohleber, A., & Arnold, S. (2020). Outcome research and the future of psychoanalysis: Clinicians and researchers in dialogue. In M. Leuzinger-Bohleber, S. Arnold, & M. Solms (Eds), *Outcome research and the future of psychoanalysis: Clinicians and researchers in dialogue* (pp. 26–35). Abingdon: Routledge.

Leuzinger-Bohleber, M., Arnold, S., & Kaechele, H. (Eds). (2015). *An open door review of outcome and process studies in psychoanalysis*. London: International Psychoanalytical Association.

Leuzinger-Bohleber, M., Hautzinger, M., Fiedler, G., Keller, W., Bahrke, U., Kallenbach, L., Kaufhold, J., Ernst, M., Negele, A., Schoett, M., Küchenhoff, H., Günter, F., Rüger, B., & Beutel, M. (2019). Outcome of psychoanalytic and cognitive-behavioural long-term therapy with chronically depressed patients: A controlled trial with preferential and randomized allocation. *The Canadian Journal of Psychiatry, 64*(1), 47–58.

Leuzinger-Bohleber, M., Kaufhold, J., Kallenbach, L., Negele, A., Ernst, M., Keller, W., Fiedler, G., Hautzinger, M., Bahrke, U., & Beutel, M. (2019). How to measure sustained psychic transformations in long-term treatments of chronically depressed patients: Symptomatic and structural changes in the LAC Depression Study of the outcome of cognitive-behavioural and psychoanalytic long-term treatments. *International Journal of Psychoanalysis, 100*(1), 99–127.

Leuzinger-Bohleber, M., Negele, A., & Bahrke, U. (Eds). (2020). Was nur erzählt und nicht gemessen werden kann Fallberichte aus der LAC Depressionsstudie [What only can be told but not measured: Case studies from the LAC Depression Study]. Giessen: Psychosozial Verlag.

Leuzinger-Bohleber, M., Stuhr, U., Rüger, B., & Beutel, M. (2003). How to study the "quality of psychoanalytic treatments" and their long-term effects on patients' well-being: A representative, multi-perspective follow-up study. *International Journal of Psychoanalysis, 84*(2), 263–290.

Moser, U., & v. Zeppelin, I. (1997). *Der geträumte Traum* [*The dreamt dream*]. Stuttgart: Kohlhammer.

Weinstein, L., & Ellman, S. (2012). Die Bedeutung der endogenen Stimulation für das Träumen und die Entwicklung: ein Versuch der Integration und Neuformulierung [The meaning of the endogene stimulation dreams and development: An attempt for integration and re-formulation]. *Psyche – Zeitschrift für Psychoanalyse, 66*, 833–861.

Discussion—Carolyn S. Ellman

Following Marianne's model, I would like to show that embodied memories can not only show themselves in the transference and dreams but that structural changes can also be seen in dreams over time. This will be the second case that I have written about in the past year (Ellman, 2017) in which I not only found the type of changes that Dr. Leuzinger-Bohleber found but I also attempted to show how one can trace a developmental sequence from more narcissistic primitive relating to structural, Oedipal content in dreams in order to show change in psychoanalytic treatment. I appreciate the changes that Marianne shows in the aggregated single case studies that were found in successful cases (Leuzinger-Bohleber, 2017):

1 The atmosphere of the manifest dream is more frequently positive and more successful in problem solving.
2 There is a broader spectrum of affects (in contrast to the domination of one single affect—most frequently panic) in early dreams.
3 The dreamer is in an active position and not just an observer.
4 There are more intensive and satisfying human relationships.
5 There are more human subjects, fewer animals.
6 I add that there is a more differentiated sense of self and a sign of triangular space, with the possibility of working through Oedipal conflicts.

The 3-LM groups I have participated in didn't focus on dreams, but they did help me to look at therapeutic change in a more sophisticated way in looking at clinical sessions over a number of years.

I would like to go over the dreams that Marianne presented in this case presentation to focus more on the sources of the patient's guilt and the desperate state of object-seeking that occurs in people that have been traumatized. Having treated a patient for a long time five times a week, I also was able to see the deep sense of helplessness, the horrible dreams of mutilation and terror, and the inability to function creatively in the world for many years, just as in this case. However, the tie to a deep pathological introject I believe is also important in why it takes so long for these patients to truly begin to separate, since they often cling to the past. In the patient whom Marianne presented, I would like to focus on his relationship to his brother, as represented in the dreams. Even though my interpretation of the dreams was somewhat different from hers, I felt the content of their sessions was very focused on the theme that I picked up quite early in the dreams.

Unlike most traumatized patients (where the trauma occurs early in life), Mr. W was not left totally alone with his alcoholic mother; rather, he had his elder brother, which I saw as an important part of this case and perhaps why he was so guilty and suicidal. He also in some ways lost his mother at the height of the Oedipal phase (which I also find important). In trying to separate from what I see as an almost symbiotic twinship with this brother, I think he couldn't let go of him for fear of damaging him further and blaming himself for his brother's disability. (Perhaps he was the cause of the mother's breakdown because of his birth. Why does the patient finally come for help when his wife loses the baby? Why is not having a baby so central to this man?)

In Ferenczi's view (1949) trauma often leads the child who is so abandoned to take on a role of a caretaker in order to feel attached to someone and the child often doesn't feel it has a right to life without having to sadistically kill off objects and endure object loss. The patient said during his consultation,

> I have a nightmare: I am in a narrow tunnel, kind of a tube. Behind me my brother is crawling. We cannot go backwards; behind us is the stormy sea. The tunnel turns out to be more and more narrow. I am waking up in panic.
>
> (Leuzinger-Bohleber, 2017)

I found this an unusual dream in that Mr. W's brother was with him (maybe in the womb) and I thought, Does he have to remain with his brother for life, or will he come out and leave his brother behind to drown? Then we were told he had dreams again and again of standing up on a high object that was very shaky. The analyst saw this as his family life that was so shaky he couldn't rely on anyone. The patient also associated to his mother's alcoholism. But I also see it as him wanting to stand on his own feet but he really couldn't (he had a great wish to be separate but he needed someone to be there for him in order to do that). Then we saw him getting around on a bicycle but again he was in front of an abyss. The mother's depression could swallow up both boys since his brother was down in the abyss with a companion and he had to go to him. Only the companion could show him another way. Was this the analyst? Why did the patient know he needed an analysis? Did the patient remember a time when he was held? Then we have the enactment of his surprising the analyst that he didn't trust her and wanted a name of someone in case he was in trouble. The analyst first got angry but then realized that the transference to the unreliable, depressed, and damaged mother had already taken place. The first few months of treatment were filled with horrible dreams of helplessness and pain (condemned to death and wanting to hang himself in the cell; in a room where he was told he would be executed—he could choose between his head being cut off or being hung to death with a rope that a horse pulled). Why his head? Why castration? Did he blame himself for his brother's depression, his wife's miscarriage? Would his success and desire to live cause irreparable pain to others? Did he wish he could have given his mother a baby to cure her depression?

He did seem to then have a series of dreams in which his ill brother appeared and he experienced guilt for not helping him (I think this is a turning point where they are separate people). Then he had a dream where he was letting his brother drive and realized how he shouldn't be putting his life in his brother's hands. It was at this point that he had a major setback where he got very depressed and had an autoimmune reaction. Taking the reins in his life really would make him alone and terrified in the world. It would destroy all his internal objects. Often people who are this traumatized can gain control only by not having anyone in their life or forming some sadomasochistic tie to someone whom they ultimately can escape from. This is truly a test of the treatment, whether the patient has let go of the past enough to internalize a good object through the analyst. In the next dream where he was watching this horrible hurricane, he seemed able to tolerate his destructive impulses without being hurt. It feels as if there was some beginning structure, since the impulses he experienced were being contained. He still "feels that he needs more analytic work in order not to be so afraid of his rivalries; and competitive situations and his massive inhibition of aggression. He is still upset that his marriage is childless." And if there was a psychological cause to the miscarriage (which of course I don't know), it could be because of his guilt about his birth or his incestuous wishes. I am struck by the degree of insight he had about what he needed as his self was growing through the treatment. He then had a dream about an odd bird, which he found amusing and a gift to the analyst, since it seems he realized some part of him was beginning to accept who he was. It is also important that there was humour here. There was pleasure. This was followed by the guitar dream in which there was ambition, a phallic representation, and a relationship with a man that wasn't filled with destruction, and again pleasure. The dream about going to the police seems like looking for a parental couple to care for him and deal with all the painful things that he had seen (even if the parents are not that adequate). In Britton's terms, it is as if he were trying to create "the capacity to envisage a benign parental relationship that influences the development of space outside the self capable of being observed and thought about which provides the basis for a belief in a secure and stable world" (1989, p. 87). I do believe that in looking at his own bodily representation and ability to own his phallus, we see a significant change in his capacity not to want to hurt himself, allowing himself to have some relationship with his wife (he is with her when the body is being dragged off in the last dream), and I believe there is hope for a baby—something creative and life-affirming that was destroyed by his mother's illness. I think the capacity to self-soothe is something that I find is very hard for most traumatized individuals that I have worked with. Trauma of any kind seems to bring up such archaic fears that one can destroy one's objects (and also a projection that someone else also wants to destroy the subject if they "live"). In this case and other cases that I have treated, patients who have been traumatized find it hard to tolerate their impulse life (including their sexuality). I believe in order to be in survival mode one may have to deaden all impulses, lest they lead one to danger. I felt this was represented in the dreams by his attacks on his head and all the dreams of destruction. One could also see this type of frozen state as the dangers of self-experience. I would also like to ask Dr. Leuzinger-Bohleber how often she has found conflicts over wishes for a baby in traumatized patients. For many of my patients who have been sexually abused, they seem terrified of having a baby, with some fear of repeating the trauma; for other patients, the wish for a baby seems to be the only thing that they can imagine will recapture their early loving feelings and bring reparation. Thus, I found it significant that his wife's miscarriages finally led to his wanting treatment. I thank everyone for the opportunity to go through these dreams and study once more how analytic work and the study of dreams is such a wonderful tool for understanding change.

Notes

1 LAC stands for *Psychoanalytische und kognitiv-behaviorale* **L**a*ngzeitbehandlungen von chronisch depressiven Patienten*. The short- and long-term results of psychoanalysis as compared to cognitive-behavioural long-term therapy among patients suffering from chronic depression: a prospective, multi-centric therapy effectiveness study, have been published in Leuzinger-Bohleber, Hautzinger et al. (2019) and Leuzinger-Bohleber, Kaufhold et al. (2019). Project directors: M. Leuzinger-Bohleber, M. Beutel, M. Hautzinger, and U. Stuhr. Supported by the Deutsche Gesellschaft für Psychoanalyse, Psychotherapie, Psychosomatik und Psychotherapie (DGPT), the Heidehofstiftung, and the Research Advisory Board of the International Psychoanalytical Association.

2 The method of expert-validation was developed in the DPV Follow-Up Study (see summary in the Open Door Review, IPA website (Leuzinger-Bohleber, Arnold, & Kächele, 2015). It is now integrated into the 3-LM (see Bernardi, in this volume; and Leuzinger-Bohleber, 2014). However, again the bitter pill is that publications based on these parts of the LAC study only convince psychoanalysts and interested friendly colleagues (mostly in the field of humanities), but not researchers from other therapeutic orientations, representatives of mental health institutions, or from the field of medicine and academic psychology. These groups accept the results only of the quantitative parts of the LAC study that strictly follow the criteria of evidence-based medicine (see Leuzinger-Bohleber, Hautzinger et al., 2019; Leuzinger-Bohleber, Kaufhold et al., 2019).

3 Mr. W agreed to publish material from his psychoanalysis as part of the LAC study. In order to protect confidentiality, some biographical and socioeconomical data are changed, although without destroying the "narrative truth."

4 In the limited frame of this chapter I can only mention that according to the clinical evaluation of the psychoanalytical experts, the dream sessions of that time illustrated transformations that the analyand already had gone through, but at the same time, the working through of his severe traumatizations was still in progress, which meant that psychoanalysis had to continue.

5 These changes also appeared in other dreams. Mr. W reported the following dream in the third year of psychoanalysis:

> P: *I had two dreams last night. One was quite funny: I played with the famous jazz guitarist Ralph Towner. I did quite well and had fun. I didn't fail and the neck of the guitar was also not soft [laughs]. The guitarist played along with my improvisations and held back. Of course I knew that he is better than me, but this did not play a role. It was just good fun.*

References

Ellman, C. S. (2017). Mirror, mirror on the wall: Who's the fairest of us all? Comments on Janice Lieberman's case: "Not quite a princess." In P. L. Ellman and N. R. Goodman (Eds), *Finding unconscious fantasy in narrative trauma, and body pain* (pp. 147–156). New York: Routledge.

Britton, R. (1989). *The Oedipus complex today: Clinical implications*. London: Karnac Books.

Ferenczi, S. (1949). Confusion of the tongues between the adults and the child (the language of tenderness and of passion). *International Journal of Psychoanalysis, 39*, 225–230.

Leuzinger-Bohleber, M. (2017). Embodied memories in dreams of severely traumatized, chronically depressed patients and changes during the course of psychoanalysis. Presented at the Toronto Psychoanalytic Society, April 22.

Part III

Foci of the analyst's interventions, mechanisms of change

Chapter 6

"I don't want to be like my mother"

Exploring change in identity using the analyst as model

Siri Erika Gullestad, Margaret Ann Fitzpatrick Hanly, and Mette Hvalstad

Introduction

In this chapter, we discuss gradual identity transformation in a 24-year-old woman—Kim—in an analysis lasting for three and a half years. Using the Three-Level Model (3-LM), exploring clinical material with analytic sessions from the beginning, middle, and late periods in the analysis, we examine how analytic process may create change. The 3-LM poses the question, How does the patient use the analyst, and does this change over the course of the analysis? Kim's analysis illustrates how attachment to unconscious identity-defining internal objects, revealed in metaphors, changed through use of the analyst as a new object (Loewald, 1960). In our discussion, we specifically emphasize the role of the analyst as a model (Gullestad & Killingmo, 2020), adding to the concept of the internalization of the analytic function (Rangell, 1987; Smith, 2007).

The case of Kim

Brief history

After having tried intensive cognitive therapy with little success, Kim was referred to analysis, diagnosed with depression and sleep problems caused by overthinking and excessive dreaming. Kim's parents and elder brother were in a group of boat refugees, picked up from the ocean by a Norwegian tanker before Kim was born. Together with the group of refugees, the family settled to form a Catholic minority society in a distant, rural part of Protestant Norway. Kim felt different, both from the Norwegians and from the refugees from the home country. Religion had a strong impact in keeping a closed community for the refugees, isolated from the Norwegians. While Kim's father became quite integrated, her mother held strongly onto her conservative and religious culture and traditions. In order not to bring disgrace to the family, Kim was expected by her mother to marry a husband chosen from their home country in an arranged marriage. In contrast, Kim's brother, mother's preferred child, was raised with a good deal of freedom, few responsibilities, and few expectations. The mother, who seems to have been seriously traumatized, was, according to Kim, unpredictable, attacking, unfair, selfish, and "the one who decided everything." Father was warm and caring, yet Kim was angry with him for being "weak and deceitful," always supporting mother in conflicts, thus letting the children down.

Kim's identity was torn by deep ambivalence in her affiliations, values, and faith. She experienced intense guilt and shame and a strong sense of the demands of duty. Wanting to be an ordinary Norwegian youth as a teenager, and describing herself as a "tomboy," she rebelled and broke with Catholicism. After high school, she was "thrown out" out of her home, because, according to mother, she brought shame on the family. At school Kim was an underperformer. Teachers and parents had low expectations of her academic performance, which hurt and offended her. In the opening phase of the analysis, she was proud of taking a master's degree in educational science, at the same time working as a leader in a kindergarten. Kim had been in short-term relationships, and one five-year relationship, all with Norwegian boyfriends. She had good friends and was close to her brother, his Norwegian wife, and their two small children. Most importantly, she had had one close early relationship with a neighbouring young housewife, J, with small children and a husband who later left his wife.

Presenting problems

Experiencing most things as unfair in life, Kim felt as if the whole world did not really want any good for her. She had to do everything herself and could not trust anyone. Talking about her life's problems, Kim told of breakdowns when she just wanted to die and had to lock herself up in her little bathroom and curl up in the darkness around the toilet, roaring loudly and crying. Rage, crying, and despair accompanied her descriptions in the sessions. Having no belief in future relationships, she often had the feeling that she did not want to live:

> *Relationships with boys, for example: I can't believe that I'll ever manage to be with anyone! . . . [A]nyone I can trust without feeling like I'm doing something wrong. I think I'm like Mom, and that gets me down so much.*

More particularly, Kim presented her reason for starting analysis as her anxiety about becoming like her mother. She did not want to have children, unable to bear the idea that she might put her children through all the "evil stuff" her mother had done to her:

> *Maybe having kids . . . will make my life meaningful. . . . But at the same time it's like, oh my God, I can't, I can't. I feel so broken, broken. So, first and foremost, I won't have a good relationship, and I won't be able to be a good mother . . . and I don't know if I can change now. I don't know if it's just the way I am.*
>
> *I don't want to lose control like Mom. I have no role model. Like a paedophile that doesn't know the difference between right and wrong because he has been assaulted himself. Someone must help to break out.*

The analyst thought that Kim wanted to "repair" her childhood and herself through education, work, and psychoanalysis, and, through that process, find out whether she should be a mother or not—a choice that seemed central to her identity.

First impression

Kim looked typically Asian, with an androgynous beauty, small, tender, slim, and very fit. Appearing vital and energetic, she came in training clothes and sneakers for the sessions, as if ready, noted the analyst, "to escape from me or fight against me." When the analyst arrived for the morning sessions, Kim was waiting outside the office building; she hurried up the stairs and into the office, turned on the light, and arranged the practical rituals, placed the serviette on the pillow. She spoke in her local dialect, sometimes using a rough language including provocative words in dialect, swearing a lot. The pace of her speech was so fast that the analyst rarely made a comment about what she was saying before it was too late or irrelevant. We learned as the analysis progressed that Kim's identity included images of herself as stupid and not belonging.

Yet Kim was easy to like—she could really "lighten up the room." A dominant counter-transference in the initial phase was a feeling of being reduced to an attentive audience, entertained and vitalized by an energetic actor. The analyst felt she was confronting a manic defence that protected Kim against entering into a relationship. Very early in the analysis Kim met a boy, E, and they quickly got into an intense and challenging cohabitation. A year later, the relationship ended and she spent a lot of time in the analysis trying to understand what had happened.

Early years

During the two first years of the analysis, Kim talked about things in a way that was often chaotic and fragmented. Her life from one session to the next was described chronologically and in detail. The analyst noted that she focused primarily on the concrete and material, especially on the body and sexuality. When talking about her relationship with E, she often talked about performing in their sexual life. Speaking about her earlier relationships, she compared them, especially focusing her own role as a sexual partner—as if being in constant competition. Later on, E experienced Kim as a demanding, controlling sexual partner and felt frustrated and inferior. Kim in this early period seemed rigid and constantly defensive, trying to take control in the analytic situation—there was little room for reflection. The analyst reported, "I often experience myself as an empty container, without any identity, position or role."

The unconscious material, in most sessions, expressed itself through the ways Kim acted, how she looked, or through her dreams. It was as if her physical appearance "spoke" about her mental states. In one period, Kim became depressed and gained weight. One time, when the analyst came to get Kim from the waiting room, for just a moment she thought it was Kim's mother sitting there waiting. In a later period, Kim unexpectedly came to the session with her black hair dyed totally blond, which matched the colour of her analyst's hair (but which is also, it should be noted, a common hair-colour in Norway), and wearing a dress the same colour and style as her analyst's. Failing to get a job she wanted, she considered changing her name to a Norwegian one (which she did not do). We learned that her Asian female identity was filled with ambivalence about female roles as well as demands for submission to her mother.

During the early part of the analysis, Kim's dreams did not mobilize thinking or affects in her associations—but only in the analyst's. By the end of this phase, the analyst interpreted Kim's fear that she would not be able to bear her rage: "You have said . . . that you cannot get into a rage (lose control) here with me." Kim now elaborated an important metaphor: "Yes, . . . I feel like 'the Hulk.'" "My rage . . . damages those I love. I have never shown these feelings to my parents . . . In my family, all difficult feelings appear as anger." The Hulk is a cartoon figure, who is an orphan wanting to be kind, but harbouring a destructive monster inside. Eventually, Kim could integrate the analyst's understanding of rage as human, working through her childhood identity as a monster.

Processes of transformation

Summary of the process

Kim began analysis as a deeply conflicted young woman. Torn between widely divergent cultural and religious values, she was furious with her parents and at the same time seriously depressed. The

Hulk—the unwanted, enraged monster—condensed an important aspect of her self-image. Appearing as a tomboy, Kim searched for an identity as a competent woman, different from her mother. Afraid of emotional intimacy—feeling that she could not trust anyone—sex was a preferred mode of relating. With her dominant, controlling way, she presented herself as quite masculine in her sexuality, seemingly a phallic mental position. An overriding relational scenario was one of being self-sufficient, managing rigidly on her own, not letting anyone come close.

Kim was in analysis for three and a half years, four times a week on the couch. By the end of the analysis, her relationship to her parents had changed quite radically. By then she could perceive that her father really did accept her. Moreover, she understood that he was in fact the one who also "carried" her mother—he was strong enough. Kim's thinking that they *have done as well as they have been able to* contributed to a reconciliation with her parents. While at the beginning of analysis she refused to accept anything from them, afraid of becoming dependent, she now allowed them to give her a deposit to buy her own apartment. Kim recognized and accepted her parents' relationship—the parental dyad—without feeling excluded. The analyst understood this as an expression of her having accepted both the parenting position and the generational difference.

By the end of the analysis Kim had opened up and resolved debilitating conflicts in her identity. She was now in the process of finding a job that matched what she considered her competence. Moreover, she clearly appeared more feminine, rarely coming to the analytic hours in sneakers, but rather wearing feminine outfits and with high heels. Proudly she told the analyst that her breasts were more beautiful than she had thought, and that she had bought her first bra. In this material, the analyst noticed an element of more robust competition with her, both in aggression and sexuality—as if Kim wanted the analyst to confirm her femininity, but also to affirm a connection between the two of them, as girlfriends.

Kim's way of being in the analysis changed visibly. In the ending phase, she appeared quite free, used humour and laughter, and worked confidently in the relationship with the analyst. The communication in the hours was characterized by free associations, wonder, and reflection.

Observing dynamics of change

What can account for the observed changes in Kim's inner states, psychodynamics, and ways of relating in her life after three and a half years of analysis? We cannot know to what extent the observed changes were due to the treatment alone. As with all therapies, there were interactions with real-life events. Nevertheless, through detailed analysis of session material we can articulate hypotheses about formative treatment processes. In particular, we focus how key dynamics related to presenting problems with conflicts in identity, self-image, and identifications were expressed in Kim's dreams and how these dynamics changed.

Initial dreams: Session 4

Although at the beginning of the analysis Kim appeared self-sufficient and controlling, she nevertheless expressed desire and hope in various ways. The analyst had the sense that Kim was very motivated to get help and to change. Coming to the fourth session, Kim started by saying,

P: *You're just waiting for me, are you?*
A: *Yes, it's not* just. *You are the main person here. It's as if it's hard to think out loud.*
P: *It's unfamiliar, still; it's different.*

Struck by the fact that someone was waiting for her—being there for her—Kim seemed touched, becoming aware that the analyst created a new space. In this same session, she said that she had a dream the night before—actually a recurring dream—about J in the house next door to her parents' house:

> *There is a large garden, with a small dollhouse and with a garage. The house has an ugly orange colour, and where you go in, there is a fairly steep hill down, if you want to enter the main door. Opposite there is the garage. Inside it's a staircase up to the living room and kitchen, and then there's a bathroom and two bedrooms and a master bedroom. . . . The colours are not so good in the dream. . . . In the dream it's not bright and nice, the colours are a bit dark and cold, blue. It's cold to stay there. I see her there in the dream with the three kids. Sometimes her ex-husband is in the dream too.*

Talking about the dream, Kim said that the relationship with J ended quite abruptly, which was very hard on her. Kim was left with a feeling of being utterly alone, suggesting that her sense of self, basic identity, was lost with the loss of the regard of this important m/other. Thus the dream seemed to actualize a theme of loss and sadness. The analyst commented,

A: *I get a feeling that you are a bit sad or maybe longing for something there where you stand and look.*
P: *Yes, I have such a sad feeling. Feeling so heavy, yes.*

This interpretation of her longing for a warm maternal relationship created an early moment of meeting—a break into Kim's self-sufficient pattern.

Kim continued, saying that before this dream she had another dream—also a recurrent dream—which created a strong feeling:

P: *There have been two, three times, maybe four, that I'm very pregnant, that I have a baby in my womb. That feeling is so strong, such a kind feeling. It's such a real love, like . . . Well, when I wake up, it's really strong. It's not mine, it's just a kid, a baby. . . . It's a feeling I've had for many years then. A really strong and good feeling, a strong love as well. It's almost that I really will not wake up because it's such a good feeling.*

We do not have Kim's associations to this dream. The analyst commented that perhaps the dream was about the analysis and the possibility of getting in touch with the child within—maybe a child they could love together? Kim responded with silence, but not defensively, and for the first time in the analysis she seemed to take in what the analyst communicated. Looking back, it seems likely that the baby represented an idea of being "born" again through the analytic treatment. The analyst interpreted that Kim's love for the baby was like her "strong feeling" for the mother/neighbour whom she "could not hold onto." Then Kim associated to the food and music they shared: "We could just relax and just enjoy a good lunch. Made lots of rolls (baked goods), put on music and drank tea and had a cosy time. That time, I remember it, it was so good. I miss it." This use of the analyst's interpretation of longing for maternal nurturance allows an important regression on the way to the formation of a new identity.

Dream of the doll: Session 26 (two months into analysis)

Two months into analysis Kim presented the following dream:

> *I had an interesting dream tonight. I don't quite remember how it started, but I remember going to the doctor. And my doctor, he's very kind, he's from my hometown. . . . He's very decent so I feel pretty safe with him. . . .*
>
> *Then I looked around and then I saw that there was a doll there, who had a face, who had eyes like black buttons. She had blonde hair . . . which was made of fabric—a blue dress. They lay on the table and on the couch. There were several of them [dolls] in different sizes. It was creepy. What was this then?*

As Kim had no thoughts about the dream, the analyst shared her associations to the dream with the 3-LM group. To this first part of the dream she associated:

> I was touched by the content of the dream. Could it be that the vulnerable and feminine in her was "laid dead" and that the mother's

interior as she experienced it was dead and that she had not reached her mother in the early stages of life, but met lifeless, black, and judging eyes? It was as if she placed maternal objects in "lifeless" positions while she got the man (libidinal-object), triumphing over the maternal object. She described one of the women in the dream as "blonde and with a blue dress." I thought it was me.

The dream continued:

P: *Then I suddenly saw a picture. Then I saw that the doll was in the picture. Then he saw that I noticed it. He said, "It's my mother—I do not have a good relationship with her." And suddenly he was gone with the other scientist. . . . Then I got such a bad feeling that it was really heavy for him . . . with his mother and that he had experienced lots, lots of heavy things. And then I got to know the feeling he had. And like he should try to explain what happened to his family . . . and then I turned away. And when I turned back, suddenly there was this artist LidoLido. Do you know who that is?*

A: *No.*

P: *Well I like his music quite a bit. He is a Norwegian artist then. Suddenly it was he who was there instead [laughing a little bit]. Then we sat holding hands and were very passionate, unable to keep our eyes apart. We just looked at each other to see each other deeply in the eyes. We were kissing and kissing, really deep kisses. And he filled the whole room, and the dolls had something to do with him. . . . Yes, I do not think I remember anything else. There was something more about the doctors and the dolls but I do not remember completely.*

The analyst's associations:

> The situation with the intense "deep kiss" made me think of the little child who sucks her mother's breast and holds her mom's eyes—where I was the mother she wanted contact with by looking deep into my eyes. And I noticed both a social and a sexual component both in her and in the mother (me). I resisted a strong urge to act, to interpret the dream for her and to show that I understood her.

Working with this dream, the group asked whether it might express an Oedipal sexuality, introduced by the counter-transference jealousy. LidoLido—his name easily associates with *libido* and the Norwegian term *lidenskap* (= *desire*), as well as with the cabaret scene *Lido* in Paris—seems to be a metaphor for sexual desire. Or did the deep gaze and kissing rather present a maternal infant scene? Or both? Concluding, the group resonated with the LidoLido as an anchor point for Kim's use of sexual experiences to deal with depression and the "dead mother."

Looking at the dream from a dynamics-of-change perspective, we notice how the person of the analyst was introduced in the dream—blonde hair and blue dress, as she was in reality. The analyst, associating to the dream, said that one of the women had blonde hair and a blue dress, while it actually was the *doll* with the black button eyes. Thus, it would seem that the doll conflated two female figures—the dead mother as well as the new analyst-object. It may be that Kim's unconscious here provided her with an embodiment of a transformational object, a hope for change.

Dream of the polar bears: Session 91 (eight months into analysis)

Coming to the session, Kim stated, "Today I can start with several dreams":

> *One dream: We are partying out on the town. There are not any familiar faces. I knew them anyway. One was E, but not him, in a way. We had to drive over a river, and there were polar bears under the water. We got over. The polar bears started chasing us at full speed. We were split. I and one other person could not hide—the polar bears were so clever—but they were unable to reach us. We managed to get over a 2-metre-high fence.*
>
> *The second dream: We were in café—a group of friends. One of the girls I am closest with at school was with E and me. She started intimate kissing and stuff with E, who did not seem to think much about it. He gave her many compliments (also intimate). And that was enough for me. E gave me a friendly kiss. He explained he did not mean to hurt me—just take care of my friend (ours?). But I just walked away.*

At this point in the analysis, Kim could associate more fully to the dreams: "I was in the middle in dream number two. I was not accepted or respected." The analyst, commenting on the clever polar bears, asked whether they expressed something about being smarter than people think. Kim responded, "It's familiar for me to feel tiny and stupid . . . I'm not as stupid as people think." In this session, Kim was in contact with deep feelings of having been hurt by people devaluing and underestimating her (teachers in school). The analyst commented, "When you get hurt, you can get angry." And later:

A. *You . . . cannot get into a rage [lose control] here with me, because you think I will not tolerate it very well.*

P: *Yes, but you know I feel like "the Hulk."*

A: *So those who think you are nice and cute, they should only have known what's inside you?*

P: *Yes, it damages those I love. I did not even dare to show E how angry I can be. I have never shown these feelings to my parents. I was not even allowed to pretend. I was so sorry that I was crying. . . . In my family, all difficult feelings appear like anger. . . .*

A: *Maybe there was a relationship between the dreams, two ways to show aggression.*

P: *Yes, and when will I use either way? It will be so embarrassing.*

A: *Embarrassing? . . .*

P: *I do not want to lose control like Mom—I have no role model. Like a paedophile that doesn't know the difference between right and wrong because he has been assaulted himself. Someone must help me to break out.*

In this session, difficult feelings of jealousy, hate, and the intense, inhibited rage were brought into the therapeutic dialogue. Importantly, the analyst commented on how the fear of destructive aggression was actualized in the transference, thereby conveying that she *could* tolerate Kim's internal world.

Embodiments

The middle phase, about one and a half years into the analysis, was difficult. Kim became increasingly gloomy and depressed and made almost no eye contact. She wanted the frustrating relationship with her boyfriend E to end, but at the same time she was afraid of losing him. Full of doubt, she did not know whether she wanted to live or die. During this period she gained a lot of weight, wore loose, dark, formless clothes, and looked increasingly older. One day, meeting Kim in the dark corridor outside her office, the analyst thought she saw Kim's mother standing there, which provoked catastrophic feelings that Kim was dead or that Kim's mother was furious with her for having destroyed her daughter. Kim now seemed to look like her mother, as Kim perceived her—another embodied enactment expressing what was happening in her inner states in the analysis. The analyst thought that Kim probably felt increasingly vulnerable, and that the masculine, phallic defence was no longer working or useful.

A new shift, in embodied form, occurred one year later. After the third summer holiday Kim came to the session, slim, beautiful, and full of energy. She had probably lost 10 kilograms in three months and looked more feminine and agile. At the same time, having stopped living with E, she was struggling with heartbreak, suicidal thoughts, and, with loss of E's "regard," she regressed to an identification with the mother who loses control:

P: *I started to get stupid thoughts. "Nothing can be worse than this life. I can quit it and die . . ."*

The analyst tells us, "I'm feeling here that she's pretty scared and wishes that I'll do something," but she contains the anxiety and urge to act.

P: *I've gone all the way down—I want to die. I think I'm losing control. I need something really there, to help me. . . .*
A: *Then you come here and I just sit here.*
P: *That's important . . . that you just sit there. . . . It takes time to find my way back. I lost my identity when I lost E. . . . He does not answer me.*
A: *It hurts you. . . .*
P: *Yes, "Hello, can you answer me!"*
A: *A feeling you have here in the analysis too—that I do not answer.*

The analyst here gave space for Kim to bring the "impatient" internal object that could not put up with her into consciousness, and to differentiate this object from the analyst, a new "patient" object.

P: *Yes, you are putting up with me. But I often find it difficult. I'm incredibly glad you're putting up with me.*
A: *You're glad I've been putting up with you.*
P: *You must be incredibly patient. You know the answers a year before I do. I do not think I would have managed to wait a year for you to figure it out.*

Kim projects her own inability to put up with her feelings, thoughts, and impulses (in part, an identification with her critical, traumatized mother) onto the analyst, using the analyst to digest and elaborate her fears.

A: *I get the impression that you think you can be replaced at any time. Here in the analysis too.*
P: *Yes, I'm so scared that you cannot put up with me. That I'm wearing you out. [She starts to cry.]*
A: *And you might think it's difficult to give me a really hard time—to criticize me.*
P: *Yes, it is.*

Here we witness a crisis of identity (with loss of the object), resulting in suicidal thoughts. Here-and-now transference interpretations addressed Kim's fear of being replaced and fear of aggressively criticizing the analyst. At the same time there seemed to be a movement in Kim towards increased openness and gratitude to the analyst, who apparently was now experienced as an admired, benign parental figure—the one who "knows."

Termination

Approaching termination, after three years of analysis, Kim met with her dearly loved friend J with whom she lost contact a long time ago.

P: *I got so calm. I got back my life—the meaning. . . . It's good not to be lonely anymore—and allowed to be angry. . . . I was very angry. I spoke up.*
A: *As if it was safer to say what you meant after last weekend with J.*
P: *I was inspired by her. She is so vulnerable—but strong.*

It would seem that Kim was now more able to contain and express her anger. A new psychological "position" now seemed possible, that of being strong and vulnerable at the same time.

Just a couple of months before the end of analysis Kim dreamed that she and the analyst formed a lesbian couple who were having a child together, a girl. Kim thought the child might symbolize her, and that she was getting to know the child in her through the analytic process. In the transference the analyst also felt a wish for something creative in their relationship—a feeling of strong love from Kim, which she believed was mixed with erotic feelings. In this period, Kim started to copy the analyst's feminine style. One session she came with blond hair, blue dress, and blue eye makeup just like the analyst's—apparently an external, embodied expression of Kim's identifying with the analyst's ways of being emotionally present and in control. Gradually, the analyst noted that Kim found her own style, different from that of the analyst.

Discussion

What accounts for the changes obtained in Kim's treatment? What were the curative factors? While the state-of-the-art of psychotherapy research is that therapy helps people, to identify mechanisms of change, now framed as question of mediators, remains a challenge. Examining the course of Kim's analysis on a phenomenological level, bottom up, through detailed verbatim session reports, allows us to establish hypotheses about processes of transformation in her treatment.

First, let us summarize the structure of Kim's problems. Starting analysis, Kim was in search for an identity, first some aspects of a "personal identity" (McDougall, 1992), and then more specifically an identity as a woman. Was she Asian or Norwegian, or neither—or both? Was she able to be a university student and become a strong, competent woman, or was she destined to work in a shop, as her teachers as well as her mother thought? How was she to live her sexuality? Kim's identity seemed to be that of a rebelling tomboy in training clothes and sneakers, controlling and with manic activity—and deeply afraid of emotional intimacy. Theoretically, we may speak of a phallic-narcissistic mental position characterized by self-sufficiency and omnipotence developed as a defence against the feeling of being rejected by a non-affirming mother and deceived by the father. This self-sufficient position seemed to shield an underlying lack of coherent self—the "heart" of personal identity (McDougall, 1992)—related to deficits in self-other differentiation. Due to lack of separation/differentiation between self and object representations, primitive aggression against a destructive mother-introject also became directed towards Kim herself, resulting in devastating feelings of being a monster that did not deserve to live. At the same time, the phallic-narcissistic position protected against a traditional female role, as defined in her family and culture. Such a mental position would seem to imply a fantasy of the phallus (Birksted-Breen, 1996) denying the Oedipal triangulation—a distorted version of the paternal function, with no room for capacities traditionally associated with the feminine/maternal function, such as receptivity, reverie, bearing children.

What were the curative factors? Certainly, the containing function of the analyst experienced by Kim as "You are putting up with me" was essential. Transference expectations of being rejected, as well as fear of the raging internal monster able to destroy the analyst, were not met in ways Kim's psyche expected. The analyst, not responding with the expected strictness and reproaches, thereby became an "auxiliary superego" (Strachey, 1969), which manages more realistic and current ideas than those stored in archaic superego introjects. In Kim's analysis we have seen how here-and-now transference interpretations (e.g. "I get the impression that you think you can be replaced at any time—here in the analysis too") enabled Kim to "take back the projections" (Gullestad & Killingmo, 2020).

Another factor that we think should be particularly emphasized in Kim's analysis is model learning (Gullestad & Killingmo, 2020). In a long analysis, changes in the ego's organization are made possible through dialogue with an object that has a more nuanced and differentiated ego-repertoire than the patient herself. Identification is an essential mechanism in this process, usually discussed, within different theoretical traditions, as the identification with the analytic function of the analyst (Rangell, 1987; Lander, 2007; Smith, 2007). Central to this process is that the patient "takes in" more adaptive ways of thinking, such as the therapist's reflective mode (Fonagy et al., 2002). The patient may also identify with the analyst's attitudinal patterns, ways of being, and alternatives for action (Gullestad & Killingmo, 2020). Identification with the analytic function of the analyst as a curative factor implies that emphasis is put on what the analyst does (as opposed to discussing the therapeutic action of analysis without referring to the analyst's activity; see Smith, 2007)—thus indirectly focusing on the person of the analyst. This is in line with contemporary psychotherapy research, which in recent years has increasingly emphasized the importance of the qualities of the person of the therapist—therapist effects—for therapeutic outcome (Baldwin & Imel, 2013; Nissen-Lie et al., 2017; Heinonen & Nissen-Lie, 2019; Johns et al., 2019).

For the therapist to be "a model," of course, does not mean that the patient becomes like the therapist. To be like the other means that otherness is lost, as well as the capacity to discriminate, and the asymmetrical relationship with the analyst (Lander, 2007). In this context, it is relevant to distinguish between identification with persons as opposed to identification with modes of functioning. The wish to "resemble"—to imitate—as well as the need to admire and idealize the therapist, and in this sense to identify with the therapist as a person, should be subject to therapeutic working through. Rangell (1987) here speaks of identification as defence. Identification with modes of functioning, on the other hand, refers to "taking in" specific ways of functioning—such as more nuanced treatment of problems, a more realistic attitude, a greater tolerance in interpersonal ways of being and more independent self-representation (Meissner, 1973; Gullestad & Killingmo, 2020). In the analysis of Kim, however, we observed that, at least for a period, there was a process of actually trying to be, very concretely, like the analyst. How shall we understand this imitation?

Two aspects seem relevant. First, in the beginning of the analysis Kim had little capacity for reflective functioning—she was a woman of few words and much action. Entry into her internal world was not primarily through associations. Rather, dreams expressed Kim's unconscious dynamics—and, not least, her ways of being, carrying implicit relational messages. With Kim, the analyst captured how non-verbal affects and unsymbolized experiences manifested in bodily action language—the analyst was sensitive to find the mind in the body (Gullestad, 2015; Leuzinger-Bohleber, 2015). Importantly, the analyst addressed Kim's lack of self-other differentiation and her primitive conflicts over aggression, threatening her basic self-identity. It was striking when, after a year of analysis, Kim brought her guilt and shame about not taking care of her mother into the analysis: "I'm tired–no, not sad—I'm guilty of everything that has happened to Mom and Dad. I blame myself constantly and feel a lot responsibility for them. It will never be enough for them, they will never get enough."

Two years into the analysis, the analyst took on being the unresponsive, dutiful maternal object in a questioning way:

A: *A feeling you have here in the analysis too—that I do not answer.*

P: *Yes, you are putting up with me. . . . I'm incredibly glad you're putting up with me.*

Working through the negative transference, the analyst allowed Kim to find her as a new object, integrated in functions by Kim by ending the analysis. Kim worked through guilt and shame about her mother, sufficiently to go back and find a loving object in the neighbour/mother/friend. It would seem that the analytic work on personal self-identity later allowed Kim's feminine identity to emerge, and her use of the analyst as model, a strong female professional (McDougall, 1992)

Second, being the child of immigrants, rejected and with a sense of belonging nowhere, it seems that there was in Kim a hunger to find someone to accept her identity as a monster and as an aggressive polar bear, and then to act as a female, Norwegian role model. She was in need of what Lacan (1966) calls the *sujet supposé savoir* (subject supposed to know). As it turns out, her analyst became a model, not only as concerns containment of affects and ability to reflect instead of acting, but also for being female. It would seem that Kim, in searching for a more secure identity, needed to incorporate the feminine qualities of the analyst quite concretely. Wille (2008) also points out that sometimes imitation cannot be avoided and might sometimes even function as an intermediate stage towards identification (p. 1201). It should be underscored that in Kim's analysis, the physical imitation was a passing process. In the end, she found her own style.

What about having a child, a central theme in Kim's presentation of her life's problems? At the termination of the analysis, Kim said this was no longer a pressing problem—the idea of having a child (or not having a child) did not frighten her anymore. It would seem that in Kim's analysis, the analyst had been especially receptive to and welcoming of the erotic dimension of Kim's transference. The analyst noted that in the transference relationship she could feel Kim's wish for getting "into my femininity, to my womb" (Chasseguet-Smirgel, 1984), to identify with me and my maternal care (fusion), but also to create life together with me—to make me pregnant—thereby binding us together." The early dream about LidoLido seems to represent identification with the analyst/doctor's capacity to bear difficult feelings involving the mother. An odd phrasing in the dream—"I got to know the feeling he had"—suggests a magical use of the doctor's "experience" as her own: "Then I got such a bad feeling that it was really heavy for him, like . . . with his mother and that he had experienced lots, lots of heavy things. And then I got to know the feeling he had." The dream about the lesbian couple being creative and having a child expressed identification with the analyst's creativity and capacity to love in a transference fantasy (a reimagining of a mother/daughter love?).

In conclusion, the analyst let herself be taken in as an introjected or fusional model and then used as a role model with whom to identify in Kim's search for identity. We remember Kim's words starting analysis: "I do not want to lose control like Mom—I have no role model." She conveyed a self-image as a "paedophile that does not know the difference between right and wrong because he has been assaulted himself." "Someone must help me to break out." Kim found somebody who helped her to break out.

References

Baldwin, S. A., & Imel, Z. E. (2013). Therapist effects: Findings and methods. In M. Lambert (Ed.), *Bergin and Garfield's handbook of psychotherapy and behavior change*, 6th edn (pp. 239–258). Hoboken: Wiley.

Birksted-Breen, D. (1996). Phallus, penis and mental space. *International Journal of Psychoanalysis, 77*, 649–657.

Chasseguet-Smirgel, J. (1984). The femininity of the analyst in professional practice. *International Journal of Psychoanalysis, 65*, 169–178.

Fonagy, P., Gergely, G., Jurist, E. L., & Target, M. (2002). *Affect regulation, mentalization and the development of the self.* New York: Other.

Gullestad, S. E. (2015). How to capture character through the patient's language? *Scandinavian Psychoanalytic Review, 38*(1), 31–37.

Gullestad, S. E., & Killingmo, B. (2020). *The theory and practice of psychoanalytic therapy: Listening for the subtext*. Abingdon: Routledge.

Heinonen, E., & Nissen-Lie, H. (2019). The professional and personal characteristics of effective therapists: A systematic review. *Psychotherapy Research*, May, 1–16.

Johns, R. G., Barkham, M., Kellett, S., & Saxon, D. (2019). A systematic review of therapist effects: A critical narrative update and refinement to Baldwin and Imel's (2013) review. *Clinical Psychology Review, 67*, 78–93.

Lacan, J. (1966). *Écrits*. Paris: Éditions du seuil.

Lander, R. (2007). The mechanisms of cure in psychoanalysis [Supplement]. *Psychoanalytic Quarterly, 76S*, 1499–1512.

Leuzinger-Bohleber, M. (2015). *Finding the body in the mind: Embodied memories, trauma and depression*. London: Karnac.

Loewald, H. W. (1960). On the therapeutic action of psycho-analysis. *International Journal of Psychoanalysis, 41*, 16–33.

McDougall, J. (1992). *"The psychosoma and the analytic process": A plea for a measure of abnormality*. New York: Brunner-Mazel.

Meissner, W. W. (1973). Identification and learning. *Journal of the American Psychoanalytic Association, 21*, 788–816.

Nissen-Lie, H. A., Rønnestad, M. H., Høglend. P. A., Havik, O. E., Stiles, T. C., Solbakken, O. A., & Monsen, J. T. (2017). Love yourself as a person, doubt yourself as a therapist? *Clinical Psychology & Psychotherapy, 24*(1), 48–60.

Rangell, L. (1987). A core process in psychoanalytic treatment. *Psychoanalytic Quarterly, 56*, 222–249.

Smith, H. F. (2007). In search of a theory of therapeutic action [Supplement]. *Psychoanalytic Quarterly, 76S*, 1735–1761.

Strachey, J. (1969). The nature of the therapeutic action of psychoanalysis. *International Journal of Psychoanalysis, 50*, 275–292.

Wille, R. S. G. (2008). Psychoanalytic identity: Psychoanalysis as an internal object. *Psychoanalytic Quarterly, 77*(4), 1193–1229.

Chapter 7

Sequence of changes and interventions in the analysis of a violent patient

Bruno Salesio, with discussions by Ricardo Bernardi and Juan Pablo Jiménez

The case of John

John was a man around 40, very talkative, of Spanish and German origin.

His father did not recognize him much as a son, and his mother was his father's lover. His mother was a vain and beautiful woman, a source of conflict between the social and the sexual, for his rough, impulsive, and elusive father.

The father was an entrepreneur providing public utility services, with a primary level of education, and he accumulated goods and money throughout his life. He had three children from his first marriage (two boys and a girl). His sons worked in the company with their father; the daughter was divorced and became a chronic alcoholic showing early symptoms of dementia.

John was the eldest child, along with a sister. Among his friends, he was discriminated against for being the son of a man with his mistress. Among his friends' parents, John was the son of an illegal couple. Due to his comfortable economic situation, he was also the target of envy. He lived in this environmental crossfire: "I was ashamed to be my mother's son because it represented something dirty and wrong."

John's family life followed a torturous routine for him: the father would come home every night at around 8 o'clock, sat for a short while in the living room, with his mother and the two children, both of which were to be bathed and cleaned prior to his father's arrival. Each visit was an uneasy experience. Anything could happen, from fights and arguments between father and mother, to complaints from mother to father about the children's behaviour. There was always tension, either because the mother would ask the father for money for the upkeep of the house, or because she would ask him to spend more time with them. Or simply because she just wanted him to accept the key to the house, although this never happened.

The mother's complaints about John's misbehaviour led his father to beat him. In the most serious situations, the father would physically assault the mother as well. The two of them would go into a room and John would hear the slaps and pleas of the mother begging to be spared from the father's aggression. "That was when I wanted my father to die."

John feared that the father would separate from his mother because of the complaints regarding his behaviour. He had to be as careful as possible, silencing everything, keeping everything inside himself in the form of thoughts so as to prevent his deepest imagination from becoming true.

In these visits, in front of the children, still in the living room, his mother would begin to touch the father, opening the fly of his pants. Everything was done as if John and his sister did not notice. After some time of masturbation, his father and mother would then retreat to the bedroom, never for an extended time. The children could hear groanings and the noise of the bed shaking. His father "would then leave the room, wash his hands, and then immediately leave." John would then go into the room to confirm his suspicions of his parents' sexual intercourse, discovering little wipes on the floor, which held a smell that he couldn't yet identify.

His feelings were always those of apprehension and anguish. When he came to understand the sexual meaning behind his mother's touching his father and their flee to the bedroom, he "was very angry with them both." The mother was seen as a whore; the father, as an impostor. During the nights he "was controlled by these memories," devising ideas and feelings, "unable to sleep."

Reason for treatment

John sought treatment to decide whether or not to continue in his marriage, since "my wife and I haven't had sexual relations in more than two years." His wife was about two years younger than him. "Before getting married, our sexual life was intense. It began to decrease as soon as we got married and gradually diminished until it was completely over." John mentioned being interested in another woman whom he had dated a few years earlier, and who had worked in the same newspaper as his mother, "but I didn't go on with this relationship because I wasn't really that excited about it."

Other general complaints: "I have always needed organization. If when I got home some object was out of place, I had to put it back in its place right away." John would wash his hands quite frequently, driven by feelings of dirtiness, not knowing exactly why and in daily relationships, when some sort of aggression was needed or likely to happen, he would withdraw and turn to an intense and habitual internal soliloquy of struggles, arguments, and violence.

Addiction to drugs

John started to use varied and excessive drugs in the beginning of his adolescence (marijuana, cocaine, and alcohol) with a group of friends. "I was 8 years old when I first got drunk." He used marijuana to ease some states related to his social origin, or to alleviate his solitude. Alcohol was a releaser of inhibitions within relationships and group integration. He "found a climate of intimacy, value, acceptance, and affection, which he had neither at home nor when he went out." Drug use allowed him to feel powerful and wield his identity card, to tell the world (and the police, in his delinquent hours), that he was "so-and-so," the businessman's son: "I wouldn't order just a shot of whiskey, but the full bottle." He snorted cocaine because it was an expensive drug and he wanted to show off.

P: *I didn't know who the real me was: the one who got drunk, used drugs, felt loose and talkative, or the one who got reclusive, suspicious, and uneasy. When I used a lot of drugs one day, the next day was devoted to "discrediting" the day before, because of the shame it held.*

He would later refer to this experience as "today, each day is added to the other, because there is no longer any shame." When I interpreted that both the drug and the drink held aggression to some family member, and thus the shame, John added,

P: *Yes, it had to do with my father. The more euphoric I got, the more I felt like a man. Through violent attitudes and acts I felt like I was identifying with him.*
A: *It was a way of having your father.*
P: *It was, but the very things I used to get closer to him also prevented me from becoming close to him: the shame it involved.*

Our beginning

Initially John spent many sessions talking nonsense: he reported his daily activities, avoiding any revealing or compromising information. He would arrive in a cheeky fashion, well rested and apparently not committed to me or to our work. These sessions felt as if I had accomplished very little. One day he told me,

P: *My wife hides things from me and I pretend that I don't notice.*
A: *This is related to what you pretended not to see when your mother touched your father's penis; this used to happen because it aroused you, just like it does now in our relationship. You are not always willing to come, but when you do, it "arouses" you, you become happy.*

He came drunk to many sessions. He spoke slowly, slurring his words. I smelled the odour of alcohol in his breath. Following my intuition, as part of the more complex field that guided me, I was comfortable with not mentioning my observation, as I realized that doing so could cause him to walk away from our sessions. Another reason was a feeling that one day there would be an opportunity to talk about it without the risk of turning him away. It was merely an approach taken before someone who presented an attitude distinguished from his verbalization. John was never silent during our sessions, nor did he ever cancel appointments. My listening to him was very important to him. From an initial feeling of unproductiveness, an interest of carrying on grew within me, both of us driven by the increase in his participation. One day,

P: *I want to tell you something, I feel ashamed and guilty, I've been drunk for a few sessions.*

A: *I had already realized this.*

He was very surprised I had not told him about it before. There were associations of how much my attitude touched him, and how it presented him with the novelty of not needing to hide in a relationship. This first experience between us was impactful.

John was always surprised by my position of seeking in him some kind of understanding rather than criticizing him. In his previous therapeutic experiences, he sought to deliberately deceive his therapist, followed by a sense of triumph over him, and at the same time made John feel protected. I came to understand that the relationship with his former therapist was very denigrating.

Our relationship became more and more transparent and the sessions were vivid: I was excited to meet him and, for my part, the sessions were pleasant, light, and productive.

The wife

The greater transparency in our relationship lead him to talk about his sexual difficulty with his wife.

P: *I married my wife because she decided that we should; she was offended at being called a concubine. . . .*

A: *You also told me that your wife made you look for treatment.*

John commented that he could not decide between not drinking and having sex. When I interpreted the opposition between drug and sex inside him, he added: "I have already given up many hot pussies to keep snorting cocaine."

His associations relied on old ideas of dirtiness, when he had seen a photo album of his mother performing erotic positions. He used to become aroused at the sight of his mother's legs, with "that body." One day he saw his mother with a driver who fucked her and he became so angry, he nearly lost his self-control. When he called her a whore and threatened to beat her, she replied that she would have him admitted to a mental hospital.

P: *I figured out how a man would penetrate my mother and I even thought about doing the same with her [Later this appeared in a dream, along with the wonder of why it could not actually happen.] I often looked at my mother's hands and remembered that they had touched someone's penis; looked at her mouth and imagined that her mouth had given some guy a blow job. When I was 3, I saw the driver touching my mother's butt.*

A: *Many fantasies and disapprovals linked to ideas of touching things that are dirty.*

Drugs and sexual life

His daily involvement with marijuana replaced sexual activity. "When I used marijuana, I felt more free, I masturbated, looked at magazines, but had no one." One day John's wife decided that he should leave home because of their devoid sexual life. She had him go to a hotel for a weekend so that she could think. John was very distressed and asked me for an extra session on a Sunday. Besides the shock he experienced, he spoke of having suicidal ideas. They sounded unlikely to me, but I imagined that feeling abandoned when you have such an impulsive personality could eventually lead to suicide. The patient had a gun and took it to the hotel. Professionally, I decided to offer to keep his gun myself, stressing that this could go for as long as he felt this help was needed, so that he wouldn't feel completely alone. Visibly moved, the patient refused my offer and said, in a voice of complicity, that he would not attempt to take his life. This represented a trustworthy alliance to me, given everything we had been sharing and experiencing together.

He let me know that he had not been using cocaine in a long time. It was like a ritual: at the end of the day he would arrive home a little bit drunk, have dinner, shower, and smoke his joint. Then he would go to sleep, usually without any sexual interest in his wife. The understanding emerged that this schedule of consuming marijuana coincided with the exact time his father would visit them daily in their house to have sexual relations with John's mother, when John was a child.

The Nazi

John had two half-brothers who called him a Nazi. This nickname made him proud. His victims were humiliated and physically assaulted after well-planned ambushes, followed by feelings of triumph and superiority, without remorse. He was aggressively repeating what he had suffered passively with his father (both in the physical assaults and in his story of illegitimacy). When he succeeded, such an aggressive discharge gave him a sense of satisfaction, of restored balance, of victory: he was affirmed. On the day following these episodes he would sleep late and recover from his drunkenness, restarting the cycle of aggressiveness again the next time he went out. When telling me of these events, John became very talkative, spoke in a loud voice, and sounded excited, as if telling me about an achievement that asserted him before me. He certainly expected my compliment and perhaps I would tell him, "Like father, like son!" At this time, by associating that drug and drinking would be related to the father, he added: "Yes, it had to do with my father. The more euphoric I got, the more I felt like a man." I realized that John had no affective experience that could connect the author of these barbarisms to himself. I interpreted that at the same time that he complained of a father who beat him, he himself was overjoyed, proud of his own violence. When he drank too much, "I would take stock of the shit he was doing: if they noticed it, I would slow it down; if they didn't, I would intensify it." I resolved to transform my feelings of nauseating transferential repetition into interpretations that brought us closer, and that brought John closer to his split personal traits.

A: *You expect me to see you so that you can see yourself in full. If I do not see you, you increase the violence.*

Over time John became aware of his destructiveness (to self and other). Faced with an answer to my first interpretations, I found out that instead of moving away from me, he continued our transferential dialogue, able to talk about such unconscious patterns of conduct. In the transference, John forced me to watch and participate in his atrocities, repeatedly reporting his violent adventures. After we connected these attitudes to himself, he began to share tender reports about his first, very young daughter: he liked to take care of her at night to give his wife a break and discovered the pleasure of being in an affectionate relationship. This closeness towards the daughter was followed by sexual feelings for her. It was confusing for John. Seeing her daughter's body, her skin, he felt pleasure, but unavoidably he would torture himself between the feeling of caressing her and the feeling that he was abusing her. He referred to this as "a whirlwind that tortured him."

Twenty months after the beginning

In the last session of the year, we made our appointment at a time different from the usual one, to accommodate an impediment of mine. He arrived a few minutes late. He soon went on commenting that he thought about what we had discussed in our last session:

P: *I set my thoughts, defined some idea, and at the same time had a certain pleasure in defining threats.*

A: *How did you set these thoughts and how do you feel differently today?*

P: *[Hesitates] My sister appeared in the newspaper as one of the celebrities to be present on New Year's Eve, scheduled to take place at a nautical club in the city. At one time, I would think of the danger it could involve: there will be cocaine, people will fall into the water, there will be death. I had to move away from this idea. Today I think there could be cocaine, that people will find a way to defend themselves and that there will not be such a big disaster.*

A: *[At this moment I think how much his fear of me has changed, to the extent that he can share with me these contents of his inner world, which in the past had kept him so isolated from other people, his own thoughts burning within him.] A more comfortable condition for your thoughts is arising inside of you. Disasters and sinister outcomes are now imagined, but mitigated. They are no longer mortal or deadly. This relieves you.*
[At this moment his cell phone rings. In his conversation, I learn that public prosecutors want to remove one of his company's vehicles from circulation because it has no licence plate or identification.]

P: *The documentation has been submitted and the licence plate will be there by the end of this morning.*

A: *You are feeling threatened by an officer in your feelings of illegality/illegitimacy regarding your filiation. You are charged to provide documentary evidence as proof that you are a legitimate son and owner of yourself [I thought about the fight between him, his father and his mother].*

P: *[Suddenly] I'm remembering the relationship of my father and mother. It was a constant threat: whether or not the father would come that day; if he did come, a riot might befall them; if there were no riot that day, there could be one tomorrow; if I gave a gift to my father, he could not take it home, because his wife would know that it had come from the* other *family. My thoughts were all about torturing and threatening. If I thought about solving a conflict, another problem came up into in my mind immediately. And so on.*

A: *[I felt him very loose and happy, even making free associations by himself, which were aligned to the very thoughts I had had: an experience to be reckoned with, for this was lacking in his primitive relations. I preferred to say nothing in order to make room for his own sayings. His association had confirmed what I had imagined. Feeling him loose and satisfied, I also thought of the premeditatedly avoidant relationship that he established with his previous therapist.]*

P: *One day, when I was going to a session with my former therapist, I stopped by a bar and took two shots of whiskey just to have courage to tell him I was not having sex with my wife. Besides, I used to arrive 10 to 15 minutes earlier to think of a subject that could divert the therapist from talking about my issues.*

A: *[He had exceptionally arrived 10 minutes late. I did not feel uncomfortable and did not signal anything to him, though. I thought of the delay as internal loosening and freedom.] I see you talking more about yourself.*

P: *In the beginning, I tried to be like that here too, but that didn't work because you kept bringing things up.*

A: *Our relationship is serving for an experience you hadn't yet had.*

P: *[After some silence] For a long time, I used only my money and my wallet to relate to others.*

A: *Like the officer who requires the licence and is not satisfied with the vehicle ownership document. You are able to experience the difference between one situation and another, trying to own more the bonds of your origin from here on.*

P: *Yes.*

A: *You have acquired a mental certificate of your parentage and your legitimation.*

P: *You have just put into words what I had been meaning to say.*

Fifth year

P: *That bloodstain in the office hall just outside the elevator disturbed me, and reminded me of Isabella's murder [a 5-year-old girl who was thrown through the window by her father, a tragedy that was all over the media]. I'm heartbroken about it [silence]. At my father-in-law's place last weekend, where we went for lunch, I felt sleepy after eating and wanted to go to home, but my wife objected. . . . Before leaving I saw a police movie that moved me. In the plot, the policeman risked his own life to save the president's. I turned off the television so I wouldn't see the news about Isabella anymore [silence]. My oldest daughter is dying ever since the birth of the youngest. My wife's family asks my eldest daughter to do a lot of things. Yesterday she reacted and said that her uncle "sucked." She can already defend herself, you see! Yesterday morning, I hugged my oldest daughter and was moved by feelings of tenderness towards her.*

A: *The sight of the spot in the hall, coupled with fantasies about violence and mistreatment of children, points to a murderous father that I might eventually be, somewhere inside of you.*

P: *I do not know if that would be you. I would say it's my analyst dismantling my father. You and I are the same as my eldest daughter's affection for me. There is something that triggers this that goes beyond merely my liking it.*

A: *Based on the experience of our relationship, you are reaching new understandings between violence and intimacy.*

P: *Here I can figure out and unravel what I didn't have and what I can have. If it were not for our relationship, I would never be able to bring out the other side that I'm able to talk about here.*

A: *A separate side, unspoken, that the two of us are able to put together.*

P: *Yes. It is possible to undo this unpleasant discomfort connected to my father. We have to dig deeper, talk more, to get things fixed, you and I. But it has become a pleasure, though an ironic one, because it still hurts. We've talked about my birth. . . . M [psychoanalyst] said that today young people are the ones who look for the analytical couch because they don't know what they want. I arrived here without knowing what I wanted, and today I find myself wanting. It's laborious, it's complicated, it's painful, but it's also good. I remember Isabella's father giving an interview: he had a wry smile that seemed fake, showing his teeth and saying he loves her. Is there some murderous part within myself? [He was referring to anger toward his younger daughter, who as a newborn did not let him and his wife sleep.] When I said it here, it relieved me. Between fantasizing and actually committing an act, there is a way out.*

Here I can let loose. I no longer have the violent and aggressive load I used to carry. Today I like myself, I take care of myself. But I was a victim of violence.

A: *The stain in the hall connects me to a possibility of violence and not to the likelihood of increasing the violence between us.*

P: *I didn't go fight with the junkie who fled from the Army (the one who used to show up at the company gate to beg). With my father, I wouldn't have missed an opportunity to attack him. I also brought violence within myself, from inside of me, which ended up in a glass of alcohol or in drug use.*

A: *The violence of the father and the violence of John/father.*

P: *Yes, yes, now I can make sense of it. What I understand at the moment is the sexual relationship between my father and mother. I did not have to see that. The father is now 83 years old, he is an old and fragile man, quite dependent. Today when he saw me he asked, "How are the girls?" He walks past me and I find myself staring at him: this man clashes with the version of my father that exists inside of me.*

A: *The old man/analyst from here causes many other impressions too.*

P: *He would come home, slap my mother, and wouldn't even look at the table set with a gift for him. Today I need my daughter and my daughter needs me. When my wife curses my eldest daughter, I see it as my wife disregarding our eldest daughter's love for her, driven by emotions that run high.*

A: *The spot in the hall connects me to a killer inside of you.*

P: *I thought, holy shit, my analyst is out for blood. It was fast. I catch myself thinking about the face of my eldest daughter and I get very emotional [he speaks in a trembling voice]. These are crises of love. M referred to Prozac, and how young people use it as a virtual/chemical means of increasing the mental pleasure of sexuality, to the detriment of a more real relationship with a person.*

A: *For a long time you have interacted with the world in a virtual/aggressive/pleasure-seeking way. You are aware that some time ago your world was lived only virtually, leading to the reality of violence with your father. Today your world can be less virtual and less aggressive, and within a better reality.*

Vignette

P: *My father told me these days, "John, you are the driving force of this company."*
A: *"John, I'm proud you are my son."*
P: *I wanted a father. It still hurts me to this day.*
A: *It touches you.*
P: *I just wanted my father's attention. When he didn't want me, I decided to pull away from my feelings, as a kind of self-defence.*

Postscript

John came back to me a few years later.

August 2012: Three years after treatment termination

John was having difficulties with his sister, sharing the assets left by the death of their mother. Apparently he had not realized the deep and primitive meaning of losing his mother. The quarrel between him and his sister over his "betrayal" for taking the father's family side arose again. By going to work with the siblings of his father's first marriage, he broke the loyalty to their family group: the mother (father's lover) and the children (John and his sister) that resulted in a second family. His sister accused him of abandoning his family, and in the property division process she sought financial compensation for his betrayal. Our relationship allowed John to acquire understanding and ways to talk with his sister, and the conflicts eventually ceased.

Speaking in the transferential sense, I felt that I had been sought out as a father who was still alive within him, and with whom he had created a more loving and positive relationship.

We worked once a week, face-to-face, for six months.

October 2015: Six years after treatment termination

John came to see me because he was worried about taking up drinking again. He had noticed that the quantity and frequency of his drinking had increased. He also started to use marijuana again, though not so often. We worked together for five months. On the basis of his description, I revived the reports in which he would get home to drink so as to defend himself against possible sexual interactions with his wife. She lived under the constant stress of her father's illness.

I was surprised that immediately after our first sessions at once a week, he felt strong, his need to drink decreased, and he stopped using marijuana. Since these changes did not seem to come about through verbal interventions, I wondered how the changes in his psychodynamic functioning had come about. What was the use of the analyst as a transformational object? Did the simple presence of the analyst as a non-verbal transference object restore an internal situation that had existed through the previous analytic experience? Did this restoration result in the quick change in his mental functioning (outside conscious awareness) and thus reduce his need to use alcohol and marijuana?

He also reported having a poor sexual life.

Discussion—Ricardo Bernardi

John's case offers us the opportunity to reflect on the degree and sequence of the changes that occur in an analysis. I participated in the 3-LM discussion group that discussed this case, and I remember that the group and I were impressed by the way in which the analysis helped John to overcome his suffering. The frank and transparent narration of Bruno Salesio helped us to have a more vivid understanding of his change.

I will rely on criteria and evaluation instruments used not only in psychoanalysis but also in the whole field of health studies. This strengthens the dialogue with neighbouring disciplines and allows the triangulation of our perspective with that of other approaches. I will also point out the limitations of my analysis, indicating where the information and therefore the available evidence is not enough for drawing firm conclusions and another type of methodological approach would be necessary.

To answer the question about the nature and degree of change, I will use the International Classification of Diseases (ICD-11) of the World Health Organization (WHO) (World Health Organization, 2019). The ICD is the diagnostic classification standard for all clinical and research purposes. The ICD-11 was submitted to the 2019 World Health Assembly, and member states will start reporting using it on January 1, 2022. The ICD-11 description of personality disorders is closer to the psychoanalytic perspective than the previous one. The core criterion for personality disorders assessment is the relationship with oneself and with others. In this respect, it coincides with current psychoanalysis and with some parts of the alternative model of the *DSM-5*, Section III. It is important for us psychoanalysts to be aware of the meaning of this shift in international criteria of psychopathology and to contribute to its development.

When John comes to analysis, he clearly suffers from a personality disorder. His condition meets the ICD-11 criteria:

> Personality disorder is characterized by problems in functioning of aspects of the self, and/or interpersonal dysfunction that have persisted over an extended period of time. . . . They are associated with substantial distress or significant impairment in personal, family, social, educational, occupational or other important areas of functioning.

John's clinical material shows his identity and self-esteem problems, his difficulties as a couple, his self- and hetero-aggressive behaviours and his inner stress that he sought to calm with alcohol and drugs.

It is more controversial to assess the level of severity of his personality disorder. The ICD-11 establishes three levels (mild, moderate, severe), according to (1) the degree of disturbances in the functioning of the self and (2) of interpersonal dysfunction; (3) the pervasiveness, severity, and chronicity of personality dysfunction; and (4) the degree of distress or psychosocial impairment. In my opinion, John's case suggests a disorder of personality of moderate severity. I am taking into account that his disturbances affect multiple areas of personality functioning (e.g., sense of self, ability to form intimate relationships, ability to control impulses and modulate behaviour, etc.), while other areas of personality functioning are relatively less affected. There are marked problems in interpersonal relationships (family, friends), and many relationships are likely to be characterized by conflict associated with harm to self or others (the "Nazi" attitude, drug abuse, etc.). In moderate disorders, circumscribed areas may be maintained unscathed.

Perhaps a more systematic exploration of the extent of these healthy aspects might lead one to consider John's personality disorder as of mild severity. This question could be considered interesting for psychiatrists but irrelevant for psychoanalysis. I do not agree with this viewpoint. First, the ICD-11 is for all health-related professionals, not only psychiatrists. There is an even more important reason: psychoanalysis cannot remain outside the study and treatment of the disturbances that affect the functioning of the self and the relationship with others. Psychoanalytic work requires a clear understanding of the resources and the vulnerabilities of the patient (Bernardi, 2014, 2015, 2016). Otherwise, the analyst can lead the treatment to an impasse or produce iatrogenesis. Emphasis on self and other functioning is also the perspective developed by current manuals such as *OPD-2* (OPD Task Force, 2008) and *PDM* (PDM Task Force, 2006). Comparing the conceptual content, the diagnosis of a moderate disorder according to the ICD-11 is equivalent to a level of disturbance of severe neurotic or high borderline level, according to the *PDM*. From the *OPD-2* perspective, after an appropriate interview, John's diagnosis would probably be of a limited integration at the structural level with destructive conflicts that affect identity and relationships.

Has John's condition changed during the analysis, using the same ICD-11 criteria?

At the end of John's analysis, his functioning regarding the relationship with himself and with others no longer corresponds to a personality disorder. I believe that this achievement of the analysis should be highlighted. This does not mean that all the consequences of the traumatic situations experienced by John or vulnerabilities from other origins have disappeared. The ICD-11 includes trait domains that range from the normal to the pathological, that imply fragilities that may become evident in situations of stress. At the beginning John exhibited traits of dissociality (disregard for the rights and feelings of others), and disinhibition (tendency to act impulsively). When these traits are accentuated, they can constitute a special diagnostic category: Personality Difficulties. This category does not constitute a personality disorder but it is included in the ICD-11 because it may affect treatments or health services. As the clinical material points out, John needed to consult his analyst again years later. However, this need was not due to the type of traits indicated in the ICD-11 but to vulnerabilities of a different kind that the analysis revealed and to which I will refer later. This is an aspect where psychoanalysis can contribute to the international effort for reaching a better understanding of personality vulnerabilities.

In plain language, psychoanalysis helped John heal from his personality disorder and its predictable consequences. I mean the consequences of persistent substance abuse and from impulsive aggressive behaviours. Do we have evidence that the analysis was the key factor of the improvement? Sometimes personality disorders spontaneously evolve in a favourable way. However, clinical evidence suggests that in John's case, analysis is the best causal hypothesis, because the clinical material permits relating John's changes with the therapeutic process without other factors that could explain the changes. I will focus on the process of change. To do so, I will use the categories of two widely used scales that allow us to observe the sequence in which the changes occur in a psychotherapeutic treatment: the Assimilation of Problematic Experiences Scale (APES) by Stiles (Stiles, 2001) and the Heidelberg Structural Change Scale (HSCS), taken from the *OPD-2*. The assimilation model states that, in successful psychotherapy, patients follow a sequence of recognizing, reformulating, understanding, and eventually resolving the problematic experiences that brought them into treatment (such as painful memories, threatening feelings, or destructive relationships). The HSCS is a modification of the APES that seeks to reflect structural change in psychoanalytic treatments (e.g., of depressed patients; see Leuzinger-Bohleber et al., 2019). Both scales identify several levels (APES: 0 to 7, HSCS: 1 to 7) that describe the changes from the initial non-acceptance of the problems, towards their progressive assimilation. The use of the HSCS as a research instrument requires an independent researcher and a diagnostic process according to *OPD-2* criteria. Regarding APES, there is no strict formula for how to do assimilation analysis in qualitative research. In the selected transcribed or audiotaped sessions, the aim is to identify the passages related to the assimilation of problematic experiences and observe how they change across sessions. The goal, more than to reach a set of falsifiable statements, is to reach a better understanding of the transformations of the patient (Stiles & Angus, 2001). Fluctuations among levels and setbacks are usual, and these fluctuations have been researched using dynamic system analysis (Basto et al., 2018). I will use the levels of the two scales as a clinical guide. The 3-LM relies in the analyst's observation, and the group members are participant-observers of the group process.

John begins psychoanalysis under pressure from his wife for his lack of sexual interest and for his substance abuse. The way he expresses his presenting problem corresponds from my point of view to what the second level of HCSC calls "2. Unwanted preoccupation with the problem (reluctance. disconnection)."

At a deeper level, some key problems are at a lower level of the assimilation scale and can be better consider under the heading: "1. Problem area is warded off" ("no problem"). At the beginning, John's aim was to repeat his previous analytical experience, in which he "sought to deliberately deceive his therapist followed by a sense of triumph over him." The analyst tolerated this attitude for a long time, while seeking to integrate the split aspects of the patient and to relate them to the traumatic situations of childhood.

The analytical field progressively changed. The analyst's interest in his patient increased, and John began to admit his psychic pain. There is a greater acceptance of painful difficulties: "3. Defensive/aversive attitude. Negative affects." Perhaps acknowledgment of the shame about of his origin and the pain for the traumatic episodes of his childhood is the first manifestation of this progress.

We can observe the next level of the HSCS: "4. Incipient active preoccupation. Sporadic destructive or rejection responses" in the following dialogue:

P: *I want to tell you something, I feel ashamed and guilty, I've been drunk for a few sessions.*

A: *I had already realized this.*

This is a very interesting analytical dialogue. The analyst simply tells John that he had been aware of his destructive attitudes towards the analysis, but the analyst's attitude also recognizes that John is now able to communicate this. APES points out that in this level the patient can acknowledge the existence of a painful problematic experience but is not able yet to formulate the problem adequately.

The impressive episode, in which the analyst offers to take over John's gun, but also expresses that he is confident that John will not use it, also describes this level very well. The analyst adds, "This represented a trustworthy alliance to me, given everything we had been sharing and experiencing together." It is interesting to note the relationship of mutual understanding between patient and analyst during this episode with the idea of "epistemic trust" pointed out by Fonagy and Allison (2014) as a key factor in the treatment of personality disorders.

John begins to speak with greater acceptance of the thoughts that he cannot tolerate in his mind: "I often looked at my mother's hands and remembered that they had touched someone's penis." Other example: "With my father, I wouldn't have missed an opportunity to attack him. I also brought violence within myself, from inside of me, which ended up in a glass of alcohol or in drug use."

This prepares the passage to the next level, which is key to patient changes. The HSCS calls it: "5. Deconstruction in the problem area. Disintegration of accustomed coping modes. Uncertainty. Perception of limitations. Resignation alternates with reparation. Old modes are lost, new ones are not yet accessible." This definition does not exactly match John's process of change. I cannot identify, at least in the available material, clear moments of crises of the defence or the identificatory systems. It seems rather that there are non-integrated or split-off aspects, some of which are occasionally dominant but do not constitute a consolidated defensive organization. Nor was the identification with "the Nazi" permanent or a core aspect of his identity. For that reason, in my opinion, it is better to describe this level as APES does "Understanding/insight. Mixed feelings." There is an increasing insight and new patterns of relationship, while the old ones are only slowly abandoned.

The following description shows this coexistence of non-integrated heterogeneous aspects. At the beginning, the analyst tells us that John forced him

> to watch and participate in his atrocities, repeatedly reporting his violent adventures. After we connected these attitudes to himself, he began to share tender reports about his first, very young daughter: he liked to take care of her at night to give his wife a break and discovered the pleasure of being in an affectionate relationship.

The analyst tells us that these mixed feelings also occur in the transferential situation, and took place inside John's mind:

> This closeness towards the daughter was followed by sexual feelings for her. It was confusing for John. Seeing her daughter's body, her skin, he felt pleasure, but unavoidably he would torture himself between the feeling of caressing her and the feeling that he was abusing her. I have referred to this as "a whirlwind" that tortured him.

This "whirlwind" of feelings does not have the characteristics of obsessive ambivalent ideas, but of the coexistence of non-integrated emotions. Old and new modes coexist in John. This is probably due to his structural vulnerabilities, which presumably are the consequence of his infantile trauma and suggest probably a limit to the transformations that the analysis can reach regarding his capacity for intimacy.

The HSCS describes the next level in the following way: "6. Reorganization in the problem area. Increasing self-reliance. Responsible in the problem area. Spontaneous and unexpected integrative solutions." The first advances in this direction can be seen at 20 months of analysis when the analyst says to John, "A more comfortable condition for your thoughts is arising inside of you. Disasters and sinister outcomes are now imagined, but mitigated. They are no longer mortal or deadly. This relieves you." APES underlines that in this level the working-through has already begun and the patient can put into play new resources to solve the problems.

The working-trough is more clearly marked in the fifth year of analysis. John says,

> It is possible to undo this unpleasant discomfort connected to my father. We have to dig deeper, talk more, to get things fixed, you and I. But it has become a pleasure, although an ironic one, because it still hurts. We've talked about my birth.

Also when he says, "I arrived here without knowing what I wanted, and today I find myself wanting. It's laborious, it's complicated, it's painful, but it's also good." The analyst has a similar view of the situation:

> I felt him very loose and happy, even making free associations by himself and that were aligned to the very thoughts I had had: an experience to be reckoned with, for this was lacking in his primitive relations. I preferred to say nothing in order to make room for his own sayings.

The HSCS describes the last level in the following way: "7. Integration of the problem. Dealing with the problem is natural, it belongs to the past as a memory." The words that APES uses for the last two levels are similar: "Problem solution" and "Mastery."

The follow-up of the case shows that at the end of the analysis John acquired an adequate sense of self-direction, affect regulation, and well-being. However, 3 and 6 years after the end of the analysis he twice needed to consult his analyst when stressful life events joined with old vulnerabilities. The vulnerabilities at stake were in his first consultation related with anxieties about his identity as a family member and in the last one, to the deep difficulty of integrating sex and intimacy. This integration is probably in the core of his traumatic experience. He is, however, aware of many of his structural vulnerabilities and can ask for help in the right moment when he needs it. The analyst perceived that this is possible also because he has remained in John's mind as a positive father figure. Both the follow-up and the analysis of the sequence of the changes confirm the role played by the analysis in John's progress.

In my opinion, the 3-LM should make more extensive use of the assessment of the sequence of changes provided by these scales. Tracking the levels of change contributes to a better knowledge of the weight of the evidence that clinical material can provide (see Chapter 14). At the same time, this perspective bring new questions. John's clinical material allows a clear categorization according these scales. It is necessary to know if this kind of analysis is also possible in other cases. It would be interesting to compare the differences in the starting and final level and in the sequence in different cases. This kind of analysis can add useful information for understanding the adequacy of the foci of the analysis and of the mechanisms of change at stake, which are core questions at the third level of the 3-LM.

References

Basto, I., Stiles, W. B., Bento, T., Pinheiro, P., Mendes, I,. Rijo, D., & Salgado, J. (2018). Fluctuation in the assimilation of problematic experiences: A case study of dynamic systems analysis. *Frontiers in Psychology, 9*, 1119–1125.

Bernardi, R. (2014). The Three-Level Model (3-LM) for observing patient transformations. In M. Altmann (Ed.), *Time for change: Tracking transformations in psychoanalysis—The Three-Level Model* (pp. 3–34). London: Karnac.

Bernardi, R. (2015). What kind of discipline is psychoanalysis? *International Journal of Psychoanalysis, 96*(3), 731–754.

Bernardi, R. (2016). La formulación clínica del caso: su valor para la práctica clínica [The clinical formulation of the case: Its value for clinical practice]. In *La formulación psicodinámica de caso. Su valor para la práctica clínica* [*The psychodynamic formulation of the case: Its value for clinical practice*] (pp. 25–44). Montevideo: Grupo Magro Editores, Universidad Católica del Uruguay.

Fonagy, P., & Allison, E. (2014). The role of mentalizing and epistemic trust in the therapeutic relationship. *Psychotherapy, 51*, 372–380.

Leuzinger-Bohleber, M., Kaufhold, J., Kallenbach, L., Negele, A., Ernst, M., Keller, W., Fiedler, G., Hautzinger, M., Bahrke, U., & Beutel, M. (2019). How to measure sustained psychic transformations in long-term treatments of chronically depressed patients: Symptomatic and structural changes in the LAC Depression Study of the outcome of cognitive-behavioural and psychoanalytic long-term treatments. *International Journal of Psychoanalysis, 100*(1), 99–127.

OPD Task Force (Ed.). (2008). *Operationalized Psychodynamic Diagnosis (OPD-2): Manual of diagnosis and treatment planning*. Cambridge, MA: Hogrefe & Huber Publishers.

PDM Task Force. (2006). *Psychodynamic diagnostic manual*. Silver Spring: Alliance of Psychoanalytic Organizations.

Stiles, W. B. (2001). Assimilation of problematic experiences. *Psychotherapy, 38*, 462–465.

Stiles, W. B., & Angus, L. (2001). Qualitative research on clients' assimilation of problematic experiences in psychotherapy. In J. Frommer & D. L. Rennie (Eds), *Qualitative psychotherapy research: Methods and methodology* (pp. 112–127). Lengerich: Pabst Science Publishers.

World Health Organization (WHO). (2019) ICD-11 for mortality and morbidity statistics (Version: 04/2019). https://icd.who.int/browse11/l-m/en.

Discussion—Juan Pablo Jiménez

Some time ago, Marina Altmann de Litvan and, shortly afterwards, Ricardo Bernardi, asked me to review the discussion I had presented more than five years ago on Bruno Salesio's presentation of John's case to be included in this book. This case was offered at the FEPAL Congress in September 2014 in a panel on clinical observation. Discussion revolved around the epistemological and practical problem of whether it is possible to establish conditions for valid and reliable clinical observation, and the value in this sense of the working parties' methodology. On that occasion I did not write a text, but presented a PowerPoint document focused much more on the theoretical aspect than on the clinical one. It is clear that I will not be able to reproduce in this text what I said on that occasion, so the commentary I am writing now is an attempt to reproduce some central ideas, but from the perspective of my current ideas and concerns about the theory and practice of psychoanalysis.

The first topic I raised in the discussion back then was the question of what we psychoanalysts talk about in our clinical meetings. Allegedly, when we meet and present clinical material, we are talking about the patient in analysis. But experience shows that this is not always the case. Frequently we become entangled in discussions about the interpretation of what the analyst brings as clinical material, and it is not uncommon for the dialogue to shift from the patient to the preferred psychoanalytic theories or authors, without ruling out that some of the discussants may say that the case being presented is in fact "not psychoanalysis," meaning that the presenter did not adhere to the rules of a "standard technique." This still seems to be the case, even though in the past 30 years the most important change in psychoanalysis has been the increasing collective awareness that psychoanalysis does not constitute a unified field, in theory or in practice (Jiménez, 2009; Jiménez & Altimir, 2019). Certainly, there are authors who continue to defend "true psychoanalysis" (Blass & Carmeli, 2007, 2015). even though they themselves recognize that after more than 100 years we have not yet reached a consensus on what characterizes "true psychoanalysis" (Blass, 2010).

In these "postmodern times" psychoanalytic theory and practice seems to have become a tower of Babel, where the same words are used to refer to different concepts, where identical concepts have different names, and where many concepts can be validated only in the context of a given theoretical framework.

However, I think we are clear enough about the epistemological diagnosis, although many still think that the problem is not one of psychoanalysis, but of the model of science/discipline that we apply. Some have shouted "Vive la différence," as if to say, "I love living in Babel!" Others, however, are not happy with this situation. We are concerned about the lack of a methodology of observation that makes constructive clinical dialogues possible, and we are interested in the development of a psychoanalytic discipline that can be recognized as such by academia.

In response to this concern, and at the initiative of former IPA President Charles Hanly, in 2009 the IPA Board approved the terms of reference for two ad hoc project committees, the Project Committee on Conceptual Integration, and the Project Committee on Clinical Observation.

The purpose of the Conceptual Integration Committee, of which I was a member, was to find ways and means to enable members of the IPA to contribute to such integration of psychoanalytic theory as current, *reliable* knowledge of psychic reality makes possible to substitute conceptual and clinical enquiry for chronic controversy without diminishing critical questioning and without encouraging ideological orthodoxy or authoritarianism. In turn, the Project Group on Clinical Observation had a twofold purpose: (1) to *explore* how clinical observations are being used, how they can be used, and how they can best be used to test interpretations and theories; and (2) to *experiment* with testing hypotheses and theories by means of the methods of observation available to clinical psychoanalysis. For these purposes the use of working groups was proposed to enquire into specific methodological issues on the model of the EPF working parties, but with methodologies and tasks as required by the overall objectives of the Project Group.

The methodology of the working parties has innovative features with regard to the discussion of clinical material:

1 It does not start from a theory or a framework (frequency of sessions, couch, etc.).
2 It does not start from a hypothesis but from an open investigation.
3 It starts from the observation of what happens in practice when a psychoanalyst "is doing psychoanalysis." By the way, the question remains about when an analyst is "doing psychoanalysis." Nevertheless, if during the presentation of the clinical material the judgment of whether or not it is psychoanalysis is suspended, a window of opportunity is opened for the group to appraise "the practice of the psychoanalysts on its own merits" (Jiménez, 2009), following Joe Sandler's statement: "Psychoanalysis is what psychoanalysts practice" (Sandler, 1982, p. 44). Of course, this does not mean that "anything goes," but rather that the clinical theory that guides the analyst in the analyst's work is exposed.

The successful experience of small group work with long working sessions has shown that in-depth clinical work is possible (which contributes to the development of the clinical discipline), and that it is possible to learn from each other (collaborative work). In short, the working parties have made it possible to advance in the line of building a constructive clinical dialogue between analysts. (Many years ago, I was invited to present four analysis sessions at a working party's group in a EPF congress in Barcelona, where the material was discussed by a group of colleagues from many countries and different theoretical traditions for many hours in a row. The most impressive thing was how through the discussion of the material, and in a very tolerant and non-judgmental environment, the group was making manifest my own preconscious theories about the patient, even beyond what I myself knew about her. I remember that meeting as one of the most significant experiences of my life as a psychoanalyst.)

The clinical observation group has developed the Three-Level Model (3-LM), which borrows from the *Operationalized Psychodynamic Diagnostic* method (OPD, 2001) the dimensions in relation to which change can be observed and evaluated throughout a clinical process.

In my opinion, the work of the working parties of clinical observation, using the *OPD* dimensions, has made visible the importance of the psychoanalytic concept of psychic structure. *OPD* offers four dimensions to observe the changes in the patient throughout the process: (1) the subjective experience of illness; (2) interpersonal relational patterns; (3) conflicts and defence mechanisms; and (4) psychic structure, i.e., mental functioning.

I would like to stress the importance of considering changes in *mental functioning* throughout the process, because the clinical relevance of the psychic structure questions an idealized technique based exclusively on the exploration and interpretation of unconscious conflicts as they unfold in the transference. The concept of psychic structure enhances the point of view of psychic development and the relevance of mental deficit and structural vulnerabilities, and stresses the need to complement the viewpoint of the "clinical baby" with that of the "observed baby." However, and in the interest of fairness, as long as the psychoanalytic clinical researcher relies (as proposed by the 3-LM), on the analysts' reports as a starting point for observing and reconstructing the patients' transformations, the narrative character of these remains the critical point for scientific validity. But let's leave this thorny problem without delving into it.

Research in process and outcome in psychotherapy and psychoanalysis has shown the iatrogenic effect of a psychoanalytic technique that bases all its therapeutic action on the interpretation of supposed unconscious conflicts in patients with low mental structures unable to make therapeutic use of it. In practice, the analyst can often recognize that a basic conflict is unfolding in the transference, but understand that it is not possible to interpret it at that moment, because the patient is in such a state of emotional deregulation, that he or she will not be able to make use of that information; then, the analyst will remain silent or make an intervention so that the patient can recover the necessary emotional balance. The *OPD* calls for this type of intervention, structure-oriented interventions (ranging from supportive to mentalizing interventions). A theory of deficit, with emphasis on the relevance of non-interpretative interventions, deserves the official recognition that the institutional establishment has denied it since Ferenczi's time. The development of an adaptive technique, which takes into account the diversity of mental disorders, their pathogenesis, and their therapeutics, and which is able to coherently integrate interventions (whether these are oriented to the interpretation of unconscious conflicts or to enhance the psychic structure) that demonstrate their efficacy and are consistent with new scientific knowledge, remains as an unfulfilled task.

It could be argued that structure-oriented interventions have no psychoanalytic legitimacy. However, in this point I find it more productive to follow the suggestion of Gabbard and Westen (2003, p. 826, original italics) when they propose

> deferring the question of whether these principles or techniques are analytic and focusing instead on whether they are *therapeutic*. If the answer to that question is affirmative, the next question [they continue] is how to integrate them [officially] into psychoanalytic or psychotherapeutic practice in a way that is most helpful to the patient.

For these authors, a modern theory of therapeutic action needs to describe both changes and strategies that are probably useful for promoting these changes.

Let's now turn our attention to John's clinical material. In commenting on this case, I would like to emphasize three aspects: (1) John is a severely traumatized addict patient; (2) The material shows an analyst where the main concern regarding the interventions was guided by the diagnosis that John is a patient with important structural deficits and mental vulnerabilities; (3) The structure-oriented therapeutic strategy is without detriment to an analytical attitude aimed at understanding the unconscious functioning of the patient updated in the transference.

Early child adversity, drug addiction, and structural deficit

John was an abused and traumatized child and teenager. He suffered physically from an absent father who used to beat him up when he was present. He also witnessed sexual relations between his parents. Salesio's report shows an extremely negligent parental couple, who not only failed to protect their children, but directly harmed them. John started to use varied and excessive drugs in the beginning of his adolescence (marijuana, cocaine, and alcohol), and his addiction was a problem during the psychoanalytic treatment ("he came drunk to many sessions").

Recent research on the impact of early life trauma and adult psychopathology shows that, compared with individuals with no adverse childhood events, adults with five or more adverse childhood events are 7 to 10 times more likely to report illicit drug use problems, addiction to illicit drugs, and injection drug use. The population attributable risk fractions for these outcomes were 56%, 64%, and 67%, respectively. Results from the National Longitudinal Study of Adolescent Health and the National Youth Survey (USA) provide prospective evidence for a causal relationship between physical abuse and early adulthood substance abuse (Teicher & Samson, 2013).

Without going into detail, the relationship between John's traumatic childhood, his addiction to illicit drugs and alcohol, and the difficulties that Salesio faced in the psychoanalytic treatment with him is evident. From a psychopathological point of view, John is permanently excited and distressed, fighting against an internal experience of total abandonment, with which he cannot communicate. As Bohleber points out,

> Psychoanalytic trauma theories have evolved on the basis of two models, one psycho-economic, the other hermeneutic and based on object relations theory. To grasp the phenomenology and long-term consequences of trauma, we need both models. The psycho-economical model focuses on excessive arousal and on anxiety that cannot be contained by the psyche and that breaks through the shield against stimuli. The model is based on object relations and the breakdown of internal communication which produces an experience of total abandonment, precluding the integration of trauma by narrative means.
>
> (Cited by Leuzinger-Bohleber, 2015, p. 612)

John's addiction represents an unconscious attempt to psychically cope with unbearable psychic pain following severe traumatization: dissociative states, a chronic psychic state of shock, a disappearance of emotions, an emptying of the self and object relationships, as well as a disappearance of the psyche in the body are among the possible consequences.

From the OPD's point of view, John shows vulnerabilities in all structural dimensions

It was clear that John made changes in all four dimensions: in the perception of himself and of others, in the communication with himself and others, as well as in the regulation of his emotional states and behaviours and in the establishment of meaningful links both internally and externally. However, I am interested in highlighting the last dimension—the capacity to establish stable links—because it was this structural dimension, in my opinion, that guided the therapeutic attitude of the analyst during the treatment.

Salesio reports that John came to the sessions drunk several times at the beginning of treatment. However, he did not point out the situation. "Following my intuition, *as part of the more complex field that guided me*, I was comfortable with not mentioning my observation, as I realized that doing so could cause him to walk away from our sessions." For my argument it is interesting that the analyst says he followed his "intuition, *as part of the more complex field that guided me.*" I dare say the intuition that guided him throughout the treatment, "the most complex field" to which he refers, is his opinion that the first therapeutic task, to which any interpretation of unconscious conflicts should be subordinated, was that of establishing and developing a reliable, operative, and stable therapeutic bond. In the same sense, we must understand the very creative and timely intervention of offering John to keep the gun with which he was thinking of taking his life. By the way, such an intervention is not prescribed in any psychoanalytic text; however, I believe it was enormously therapeutic. John was moved by his analyst's offer and was able to communicate feelings that he had not been able to before.

The analytic attitude

As I said above, the structure-oriented therapeutic strategy is without detriment to an analytical attitude aimed at understanding the unconscious functioning of the patient updated in the transference. In the years of analysis that followed, Salesio shows how the therapeutic bond became increasingly operative and reliable so that he could, together with the patient, develop a new narrative based on the interpretative work of conflicts and unconscious representations as they unfolded in the transference. The analyst was always careful to take care of the link, but the strength of this link increasingly allowed for the interpretations that we normally consider the essence of psychoanalytic work.

Final comment

Thanks to John and to Bruno Salesio, his analyst, I hope I have shown the importance of considering non-interpretative interventions as an essential part of a psychoanalytic technique that does justice to the real psychoanalysts' practice.

References

Blass, R. B. (2010). Affirming "That's not psycho-analysis!" On the value of the politically incorrect act of attempting to define the limits of our field. *International Journal of Psychoanalysis, 91,* 81–89.

Blass, R. B., & Carmeli, Z. (2007). The case against neuropsychoanalysis: On fallacies underlying psychoanalysis' latest scientific trend and its negative impact on psychoanalytic discourse. *International Journal of Psychoanalysis, 88,* 19–40.

Blass, R. B., & Carmeli, Z. (2015). Further evidence for the case against neuropsychoanalysis: How Yovell, Solms, and Fotopoulou's response to our critique confirms the irrelevance and harmfulness to psychoanalysis of the contemporary neuroscientific trend. *International Journal of Psychoanalysis, 96*(6), 1555–1573.

Gabbard, G. O., & Westen, D. (2003). Rethinking therapeutic action. *International Journal of Psychoanalysis, 84,* 823–841.

Jiménez, J. P. (2009). Grasping psychoanalysts' practice in its own merits. *International Journal of Psychoanalysis, 90,* 231–248.

Jiménez, J. P., & Altimir, C. (2019). Beyond the hermeneutic/scientific controversy: A case for a clinically sensitive empirical research paradigm in psychoanalysis. *International Journal of Psychoanalysis, 100*(5), 940–961.

Leuzinger-Bohleber, M. (2015). Working with severely traumatized, chronically depressed analysands. *International Journal of Psychoanalysis, 96,* 611–636.

OPD Task Force. (2001). *Operationalized Psychodynamic Diagnostics: Foundations and manual.* Göttingen: Hogrefe & Huber Publishers.

Sandler, J. (1982). Psychoanalysis and psychotherapy: The training analyst's dilemma. In E. D. Joseph and R. S. Wallerstein (Eds), *Psychotherapy: Impact on psychoanalytic training—The influence of practice and theory of psychotherapy on education in psychoanalysis* (pp. 39–47). International Psychoanalytic Association, Monograph 1. New York: International Universities Press.

Teicher, M. H., & Samson, J. A. (2013). Childhood maltreatment and psychopathology: A case for ecophenotypic variants as clinically and neurobiologically distinct subtypes. *American Journal of Psychiatry, 170,* 1114–1133.

Part IV

Impasse

Chapter 8

Three hypotheses on impasse in the case of Janine

Robert White, Siri Erika Gullestad, and Bruno Salesio

Introduction—Robert White

"Impasse" as a technical term to denote analyses that stalemate or end prematurely has come relatively late in psychoanalytic history. In the *Oxford English Dictionary*, "impasse" is defined as a road or way having no outlet, a blind alley or cul-de-sac, a position from which there is no way of escape, a deadlock or stalemate. In an impasse, setting and frame do not change: the patient associates and the analyst interprets, but the process neither advances nor retreats (Etchegoyen, 1991). Impasse is the opposite of working through, which, when arrested, leads to impasse. It is a far more difficult technical problem in a clinical psychoanalysis than other negative reactions and negative therapeutic reactions, which can often be addressed with the usual psychoanalytic techniques; they are obvious and belong to the patient. Impasse is often difficult to recognize, remains silent, belongs to the analytic couple, and, when recognized, admits of no easy solution. "It tends to perpetuate itself: the setting is preserved in its basic constants; its existence is not obvious as incoercible resistance or technical error; it is rooted in the patient's psychopathology; and it involves the analyst's countertransference" (p. 795).

There are various routes to enter into an impasse (Maguire, 1990). There may be a gradual and insidious withdrawal of affective investment or contact, a loss of vitality, from the process. It is often more complicated, as the withdrawal is disguised by a pseudo-involvement that may be very difficult to distinguish from genuine involvement. The discourse is characterized by a subtle movement away from free association, characterized by obsessive, circular, and endless monologues that feel empty and numbing. Often neither patient or analyst is consciously aware of this process, and it is recognized only in the counter-transference when the analyst can recognize the same process within, of boredom, of lacking fresh ideas about the transference and making mechanical and stale interpretations. Or overt hostility may be more present, attacks on the frame, often around attendance, stereotyped complaints, or challenges to the analyst's competency. Depression may be used as a vengeful weapon, to maintain distance. Attempts by the analyst to bring the patient's attention to an impasse are often met with indifference or denial. Eventually a chronic sense of failure and hopelessness settles over the analysis. Interestingly, patients are often quite comfortable with this arrangement, and it can go on for years, neither making real contact nor wanting to end it. Impasse should be differentiated from slow or stalled analysis, where struggle remains alive and potentially solvable. As psychoanalytic work has extended to borderline and traumatic cases, impasse has become more common. We think most analysts have in their caseloads patients who require extremely long analyses with periods of impasse or near-impasse, as well as analytic failures and premature terminations. The experience of impasse in our work forces us to examine technique and the limitation of our work.

The case of Janine

This case was presented to a 3-LM group in New York City in 2013. Janine was a 25-year-old single woman in her last year of university studies when she started a nine-year analysis. The analysis was conducted in Germany and in German by an American analyst who lived and worked in Germany. The analysis was four times weekly, lying down. None of the present authors participated in the original 3-LM group; this report is based on a review of the clinical transcript of the hours presented.

The analyst had told the patient on the phone that she didn't have a waiting room. Notwithstanding, Janine rang the bell early, disturbing the analyst and a patient who was particularly sensitive to the analyst having other patients. When the patient opened the door to leave, a woman who looked like a pre-pubescent girl bolted in, pushing him aside. The analyst was angry, feeling that she wasn't ready for her yet, and Janine was fuming. It was almost impossible for either of them to find a way into a mode conducive for an analytic consultation. That was the "violent beginning." From then on, for many years of analysis, "there seemed to be little movement and almost no emotional involvement whatsoever."

Just as Janine had barged into the consulting room, she had bolted into her parents' world far too soon. Her father was still a student and her mother was working to support him. As a baby, Janine was cared for by the maternal grandmother, who lived in the same apartment building. Every evening the grandmother brought the child to be with her mother for two hours, which, she said, "neither liked." The father spent many years building a house for the family. When Janine was 7, twin sisters were born, who lived with the parents from birth, but the family did not move into the new house until Janine was 9 years old. Moving away from the grandmother was very difficult for her. At about this same age she swore a secret oath with a couple of other little girls that they would never become women. She lay in bed all night, stiff as a board, trying to prevent her period from happening and felt devastated when it did.

Janine's sexuality seemed to be a mixture of pain and pleasure. She described her first experience of sexual intercourse, an event she had carefully planned, as a "rape," and phantasies of rape seemed to accompany all her sexual experiences. She was successful in her studies, but complained that she had not really chosen her career. In fact, she never made any decisions, but seemed to fall into situations and activities. She felt she was always in a temporary state of affairs—"in an anteroom of life." Decisions were a problem because she always seemed to have two areas that played themselves off, one against each other. This either/or situation constituted itself immediately in the analysis. As soon as she decided to do an analysis, her boyfriend, X, left her, and she was convinced it was because of her decision. X said that it was because she could not be passionate, and she agreed—it was true that she could not be passionate. She had never felt an orgasm, except as a simple mechanical happening. She thought X had constantly caused her pain, perhaps on purpose, by flirting with other women. It was the excruciating pain of the separation, however, that now made her all the more determined to proceed with the analysis. She also had a symptom that she felt embarrassed to tell the analyst about; she regularly pulled out the hairs on a small section of her head and—as she told the analyst much later—ate them.

Janine made two interesting points in a session soon after the start of the analysis. She differentiated conspiracies from relationships. A conspiracy appeared to be a shared secret that holds two people together but each remains quite detached and unstable. It could fall apart or deceive at any moment. She longed for a relationship—commitment—but it seemed impossible. Janine explained,

> *My feelings scare me, make me helpless, powerless, exposed—it's as if the ground is pulled from beneath me. It's embarrassing, really devastating to lose face like that. I'm sworn to a child-like nature, that's my mainstay in life. Absolutely uncompromising, smashing my head through walls—brutal, relentless, severe . . . adamant, ambitious. But also fear. Fear of failure pushes me forward.*

All of this was fascinating, but the sessions were deadly. Janine lay completely still, session after session. From the analyst's perspective she seemed to have a huge head with a very tiny body below it, something like an embryo. Janine's clothes did not fall naturally around her body, but seemed to hover slightly over it, her bluish opal ring perfectly matching her dress. It was as if her body underneath were not alive. It was next to impossible to find a way to talk to her, the transference interpretations seeming mechanical and devoid of meaning. The analyst noticed how Janine would compliantly move into the mechanical interpretations she gave her, and often she would hear her saying things that were reminiscent of old interpretations from her. The analyst realized that counter-transference reactions (during the first two years especially) were missing, which made her analytic work, from her point of view, almost impossible.

In a series of hours in the second year, the analyst noted a persistent transference where Janine was dutiful and the analyst felt dead. The analyst wondered if she had gotten too close, and Janine described how she blocked any need by a rigid fantasy of being completely in control, by her defiance, and her feeling of being imprisoned. The analyst had an image of fighting a horrific prison warden. She tried to convey this sense in her interpretation of gnawing and nagging need—some awareness of wanting but catching hold of the punishing, hateful side as well. Janine responded with feeling understood—a sense of relief. In the next hour, she reported that she was glad to be heard and the analyst interpreted relief. But Janine responded with feeling tortured and the wish to be passive and dead. The analyst wondered about torture when there was silence. Janine disagreed; she did not allow any torture, she used the silence to move farther away and feel in control again. In the next hour, the patient reported how she destroyed any needs before they arose and suggested a paranoid transference—the analyst who withholds on purpose. Janine responded with self-torture, pulling out her hair, which brought relief. She was entirely self-contained; the analyst did not exist for her.

In the next five years, the analyst felt encouraged. Desire showed up in small ways and Janine began to talk about her hunger. In year eight, her father died unexpectedly. Janine had felt her father was the one and only person who had always stood by her. At the end of that month, the analyst found herself in a terrible conflict involving the bill: she did not want to charge Janine for the missed session on the day of the funeral, although they had the arrangement that all missed sessions were the patient's responsibility, regardless of the reason for her cancellation. She finally decided to charge for the day and withstand the horrible feelings of guilt and shame—she felt like a horrific monster.

In the next session, Janine responded with rage and the analyst said,

A: *I seem to have broken an unspoken agreement between us. I no longer am someone you can trust, like your father, who was always there for you. Instead I have become like your mother who would seem to be very understanding but then suddenly turn on you and stick a knife in your back. You feel I have betrayed your trust.*

P: *Exactly. You ride your principles—put principles above needs. I can never forgive you, never! I'll never trust you again. And this analysis is over!*

To the analyst's surprise, she did show up the next day and expressed relief that she could fully express herself. After this session, the analyst understood that what had happened between them in these two sessions was what Janine called an illusory analysis; in her mind, the analyst had promised she would never leave her, and she had held her in a special role above all other patients. However, over the remaining months of the analysis—it was a total of nine years—they drifted back into the illusory analysis again. The patient decided to marry her current boyfriend and moved to another country.

Impasse: An object relations perspective—Robert White

Janine fits Rosenfeld's (1987) description of destructive narcissism. In destructive narcissism, it is the omnipotent destructive parts of the self that are idealized. The self feels free to hate any positive relationship and any parts of the self that desires or needs objects. Both external and internal objects are permanently devalued. Envy is more violent, and there is a wish to destroy the analyst and any of the analyst's goodness. Such patients feel superior to the analyst in being able to control or withhold parts of their self that want to depend on the analyst. This is accomplished by a need to triumph over the analyst, through persistent indifference, withholding behaviours, or open belittlement. Yet this is quite frightening to the patient, who will then be entirely alone, resulting in violent self-attacks. Death can be idealized as a solution to all problems; patients may prefer to die, become non-existent, or deaden any desire.

In this sense, Janine rigidly controls her internal objects through shared secrets that bind but do not involve any commitment, any ties. She expects to be raped, deceived, and abandoned. Any physical or psychic growth threatens separation and abandonment—she remains as an embryo, never quite born. She cannot attack her objects directly, but indirectly through withdrawal and layers of protection by fluids and membranes. This is undoubtedly what the analyst feels in her counter-transference—nothing. Janine is dead and frozen—blue is the colour of death—she cannot be reached. She describes the violence in the fantasy of smashing her head—brutal and relentless. But at the bottom is persistent fear—of being deceived and humiliated, of being abandoned and left helpless and alone.

The danger for the analysis is illustrated in the first encounter. Janine, by disregarding the analyst's instructions, arranges to violently and intrusively attack the analyst's work, and, at the same time, feels abandoned and hated when the door does not open when she rings. We can easily hypothesize how this becomes a chronic but unrecognized enactment for the first years of the analysis. The analyst, in feeling nothing, is well protected against the projected hate, while Janine has withdrawn into a death-like state where she cannot be reached. Janine has arranged for a conspiracy of shared secrets. The enactment is likely that the analyst has secretly, even to herself, joined this conspiracy. To form a real relationship would be to experience shared rage and pain. Janine will resist any movement toward relationship, and the analyst passively accepts this. Only if a relationship can be established can we think of the analysis as truly starting, with a feeling of shared goals and shared work. The analyst reports Janine's persistent attitude: "boycott the analysis, block it whenever she could." Any other alternative would be "a catastrophe."

Two years into this work, the analyst reports a change. The work begins in the counter-transference. The analyst is struggling with her usual feeling of withdrawal and sleepiness when she suddenly has the image of herself as "a horrific prison warden" and she feels more free to respond. We guess that the analyst has started to get in touch with her own sadism. But, in speaking to Janine, she does not take up imprisonment, but rather what it must be like to feel abandoned:

> *When I am not there with you, your feeling of needing me is gnawing and nagging. Yuck, she's not there again. . . . Oh, how I wish she were here right now—it's punishing: Ugh! She's not there again. . . .*

It is not just the words. The interpretation is playful, full of emotion, engaging. Note that movement in the dynamic engagement is possible only when the analyst can free herself from the persistent deadness. Janine responds:

> *It's all about how it should be because I feel entitled to it. . . . I don't think I actually know at all what my desires and longings really are. . . . [R]ight now I feel very understood by you. But that doesn't make me happy the way I imagine that I should feel. It simply makes me feel some relief.*

We see in Janine's reply a condensation of the promise and the perils of analysis. She first restates her narcissistic position of total control, then admits to not knowing, a new feeling but more vulnerable, but then will use the analyst as a lavatory, without any concern for her, a move away from vulnerability (Rosenfeld, 1964). Janine in this period clearly outlines the impasse:

> *I really want to come to see you today. But I can feel myself destroying that before it really comes up. Right away I now have the feeling that you could give me what I want but that you don't and won't do it—on purpose.*

The absent analyst is quickly converted to an angry and attacking analyst, who must be immediately dismissed:

> *The only thing I know how to do is to damage and hurt myself and run away from it all.*

Here is the central challenge: how to interrupt this endless and vicious cycle of hate and withdrawal. The analyst then notes several years in which there were slight movements. Janine could, at times, voice an idealizing transference, the mother who will give total care and never leave.

Here is an hour from the fifth year. Janine arrives tortured and feeling full of shit. She sees the analyst as withholding goodness. The analyst, too, feels tortured and says, "That's just what I was thinking—you constantly feel plagued by a tormentor." Note that already there is a slight move away from transference, a tormentor rather than me as tormentor. Did Janine unconsciously pick up on this, as she gets angrier and angrier, but also aware of hunger?

Can we see this hour at two levels simultaneously? The first level is what is talked about between the pair. The themes are paranoid, an internal persecutor, who is projected into the analyst, which we see in the beginning of the hour. But later in the hour, we see the other side of the split, the idealized maternal object who loves unconditionally:

P: *I would like to . . . to force you to be helpful to me. Hmm—somehow it seems to me that you should have to prove how you're actually worth something . . . [the patient appears more comfortable]*

A: *Actually, it seems as if, when I do say something, it evaporates into nothingness. . . .*

P: *That's because I never get satisfied. Nothing is ever enough. I am endlessly hungry. Even if there were a whole buffet there, it wouldn't be enough. My hunger can't be satisfied—it will never stop tormenting me.*

Throughout the hour, there is an exploration of these fantasies and Janine genuinely appears to feel better and more in contact with the analyst. At the end of the hour, she reveals details about a good interaction with her current boyfriend, which seems to confirm a positive shift.

The analyst reports further progress in the next two years. Janice vacillated between two versions of herself, one loving and feeling loved, and the other bitter, rejected, and unhappy. The analyst, too, has a new countertransference, feeling deeply jealous. Janice states,

> *If I try to get both together I get really frightened, and that's when everything gets cut off and the anesthesia comes.*

The analyst comments,

> *She felt I betrayed her at the end of every session by sending her away. It was very painful, for it was as if I had promised her I would always be there for her, but then threw her out after all. She told me how her grandmother had promised her she would never leave her, but then did. She also reported for*

> *the first time that there had been a great-grandmother in her first two years of life who actually had remained constantly at her side and whose sudden death caused a traumatic separation for the 2-year-old. She said she couldn't help it, she felt I was constantly betraying her and lying to her and when she was at home, there was a devil version of me constantly with her. The only solution would be that I would remain with her 24 hours around the clock.*

We now see more elaboration of the transference, especially a greater awareness of the idealizing fantasies and their constant enactment at the end of sessions. Does the analyst get pulled into the enactment, of feeling she must be the ideal mother who never leaves?

Impasse often takes the form of what Bion (1963) calls "reversible perspective." Bion is referring to drawings that can be perceived either one way or its reverse. He applies this to analytic work of the psychotic parts of the personality—destructive attacks on any links and emotions.

The negative contained enters the container in order to strip and destroy it, and feels the container will do the same to the contained. The analyst has one point of view while the patient takes the opposite point of view, a manifest accord and a latent discord. The aim is to avoid pain at any cost. The reversal, however, is silent, as the patient consciously agrees with the analyst's interpretations, but unconsciously holds to the opposite view (Etchegoyen, 1991; Hart, 2012). The patient is constantly reinterpreting the analyst's interventions in accord with his own ideas. This leads to what Bion (1963) calls "static splitting," where the splitting quietly operates in the background, never changing, insulated from the analyst's awareness.

Janine's father died unexpectantly, the one constant person in her life. The analyst had a "terrible conflict" about charging her for the missed time on the day of the funeral, wanting to maintain how she usually bills, but feeling like a horrific monster in doing so. Janice arrives the next day enraged, wanting to quit the analysis. The analyst is under great countertransference pressure, wanting to maintain the frame (agreement on fees) but invaded by the patient's projection of the internal monster. The patient predictably is enraged; we now see the split in the patient in full force, the idealized mother who will never leave, and the abandoning mother who hates and deceives. To her credit, the analyst does not back away from the frame and absorbs the full force of the patient's attack, verbalizing Janine's fantasy that she (the analyst) could turn on the patient and stick a knife in her back. Janine's dilemma is that she is dependent on the analyst whom she desperately wants to leave and get rid of. The analyst interprets a transference fantasy: "You think I am exhausted by you and want to get rid of you." Janine responds with what may be the key to the impasse: "Silence is the only means I have to distance myself from you." That is, she must silence herself, deaden and kill off any links to the analyst and any need in herself. The analyst misreads this as punishment, but it is more likely a primitive defence against an analyst who she does not feel understands her needs. What may be missing is the analyst's examination of her own counter-transference; is she in fact exhausted by the patient's never-ending wish for total care, a kind of fusion with no separation? Is there a hate in the counter-transference (Winnicott, 1947) and relief at the end of sessions? The analyst must find a way to move out of her own deadness, defending against her own hate, in order to truly reach this patient.

Gullestad calls this "deficit transference," leading to a loss of the "as-if" quality of transference: the rejecting and horrible analyst is really horrible, not a fear that may or may not be true. I fully agree. The only solution that the patient can see is total fusion, and anything else is felt as a real abandonment and hate. Gullestad suggests affirming as a partial solution. In my experience, affirmation, in this kind of case, verbalizing as deeply as possible the patient's inner state of hatred and pain, often fails. The patient thinks the analyst is using the same reversible perspective, pretending to be empathic, while secretly continuing to hate the patient and be glad to get rid of her. The patient is an expert at reading the unconscious of the other and will glean any hate that may be present even if the analyst is unconscious of it. I suggest what we try to do is offer a mix of affirmation, containment (not retaliating to the patient's attacks), and work in the counter-transference (being aware of the extraordinary strain of caring for such patients and finding genuine compassion for their pain). I have found that at these times of crisis it is my work on my own distancing and hate that makes the difference and needs repeated working through.

Janice does continue the analysis, but she has now deadened herself, and she imagines the analyst to be equally untouchable. I think this is where her true self resides, walled off, untouchable, silent. The noisy paranoid interactions are the illusion. She came to the analysis in silence and leaves in silence. The patient decides to terminate in order to marry and move away.

The analyst, at this point, has grasped something: she now thinks of an "illusionary analysis," where "I had promised I would never leave her, and in which I held her in a special role above all other patients." Janice is still organized at a psychotic level: both split-off transference fantasies are felt as equally real, the wish for idealized merger and the fear of being attacked and abandoned.

What seems true is the deadly silence where she really lives. The patient left the analysis in the next year. The analyst does not state how the ending came about, but the analyst was left "with a horrible feeling that I had not really helped her enough in this analysis."

Impasse: A plea for affirmation—Siri Erika Gullestad

Conflict and deficit

Janine's analyst admits to a challenge that I think we all recognize: to find a way to talk that gives meaning. Janine experienced that the transference interpretations were devoid of meaning. The question of what is meaningful for the patient is in the centre of Killingmo's (1989a, 1989b, 1995, 2006) discussion of affirmation as a form of intervention supplementing interpretation. If Janine's personality structure is characterized by developmental deficits (e.g., defective self-structure, lack of object constancy, identity diffusion, splitting, and lack of capacity for emotional relating to objects), she may not be able to profit from ordinary transference interpretations. A patient organized on a conflict level, implying that the self-representation has been constituted as a responsible centre of the personality, may profit from interventions to confront impulses and affects towards internalized object representations that are projected onto the analyst. Such an undertaking presupposes an alliance between analyst and patient in finding out, searching for concealed meaning. In contrast, working with derivatives of deficit,[1] the analyst cannot take for granted that the patient will experience her invitation to explore as a benevolent helping act. It is more likely to be interpreted in terms of critique, provocation, or attack, with the risk of weakening the working alliance, and ultimately threatening continuation of the therapy. In such cases, where the perspective is to bring about structuralization of aspects of object relations which has not been accomplished in the previous development, the therapeutic endeavour is not primarily to unveil repressed meaning, but rather to assist the ego in experiencing meaning in itself (Killingmo, 1989a, 1989b). Here, the interventions have to be, not interpretive, but affirmative.

Affirmation

Affirmative feedback may be defined as a communication that removes doubt concerning the validity of the subject's experience (Killingmo, 1995). By using an affirmative mode of intervention, the therapist seeks to communicate to the patient that she understands what it feels like to be her, and that it is understandable that the patient feels the way she does.[2] Affirmation, communicating a sense of being seen, understood, listened to, and accepted, legitimates the patient's self-experience and strengthens the I-feeling (Killingmo, 2006; Gullestad & Killingmo, 2020).

Janine's analysis

As a baby, Janine was cared for by the maternal grandmother, but brought to be with mother for two hours every evening. At the age of 9 the family moved away from the grandmother, which was "very difficult" for Janine. These early separations seem to have left Janine with a feeling of not wanting to grow up, of remaining a child—a feeling embodied in the way she looks (pre-pubescent girl) as well as in the manner in which she lies on the couch. The child within Janine is "endlessly hungry" for a mother who will give total care and never leave, and at the same time enraged for having been abandoned. Maybe there is a fantasy that by remaining a child—staying in "an anteroom of life"—she may, magically, get what she deeply longs for? Janine says about her feeling of self,

> *My feelings scare me, make me helpless, powerless, exposed. It's as if the ground is pulled from beneath me. It's embarrassing, really devastating to lose face like that. I'm sworn to a child-like nature. That's my mainstay in life: absolutely uncompromising, smashing my head through walls—brutal, relentless, severe . . . adamant, ambitious.*

Commenting on this, the analyst says, "All of this is fascinating, but the sessions were deadly," Janine lying completely still session after session. Counter-transference reactions were missing, which made analytic work almost impossible: "It was next to impossible to find a way to talk to her, the transference interpretations seeming mechanical and devoid of meaning." It would seem that the analyst here understandably feels excluded and rejected by Janine's frozen attitude on the couch.

Of course, as an outside observer I cannot know how it felt being in the room with Janine. Nevertheless, in my reading, Janine's statement also contains an attempt at reaching towards the analyst. What she expresses is that to *feel* is extremely frightening: feelings imply shame and humiliation, and losing face. By saying this, she—slightly—opens a door to her inner world. To do so, however, makes her vulnerable. Implicitly, she also tells the analyst that in order to protect herself from this vulnerability, she has had to withdraw into a state where she cannot be reached emotionally. Although longing for a committed relationship she has settled for what she calls a "conspiracy"—a kind of relationship where the two people remain detached, thus guarding against the possibly catastrophic feeling of being abandoned. Could the analyst simply have affirmed that she understands Janine's fear, i.e., what it must feel like to be her—and that it is understandable that she feels this way? Given that expressing what she really feels is terrifying for Janine, no wonder that she has had to withdraw.

Arguably, Janine is not ready for "taking in" this kind of affirmative understanding. Later, the analyst in a most empathic way, comments on what it must be like to be abandoned: "When I am not there with you, your feeling of needing me is gnawing and nagging." Janine responds that she feels "very understood by you." However, that does not make her happy, it simply provides her "some relief." This statement seems to express a move away from the vulnerable position of closeness implied in feeling understood. At the same time the unconscious and aggressive message seems to be that the analyst shall feel that she is not able to really help her. Thereby, Janine punishes a hated mother-representation projected onto the analyst. Indeed, the analyst is faced with the challenge of handling pervasive feelings of distrust and destructiveness:

> *I really want to come to see you today. But I can feel myself destroying that before it really comes up. Right away I now have the feeling that you could give me what I want but that you don't and won't do it—on purpose.*

That the analyst is thus converted to an angry and attacking analyst, who must be immediately dismissed, White sees as "clearly outlining the impasse." But is this necessarily an impasse? As I see it, the analyst here should affirm the need to destroy along the line of "Wanting to come and see me today frightens you, because the feeling of needing me makes you vulnerable. So no wonder you protect yourself by destroying that feeling." Of course, I cannot know whether Janine would have felt such a comment as affirmative—the therapist never knows in advance. My point is that an affirmative strategy seems the best option is such a case.

The funeral crisis

A grave crisis in the analysis occurs when Janine's father dies and the analyst charges the patient for the missed session on the day of the funeral. Janine is enraged, claiming that the analysis is over: "I'm through with you." When the analyst asks what she has done, Janine answers,

P: *Yesterday in the session you said something to the effect that you thought that you found it impressive how I always experience you as having promised me you would never leave me, that you would always stay with me. I suddenly realized that if you can say that to me, all I am for you is a scientific object. Nothing other than that. You don't care about me at all! I'm nothing special for you—just another patient for you to examine and treat. . . . I can never trust you again!*

A: *You feel I have betrayed your trust.*

P: *Exactly. You ride your principles—put principles above needs. I can never forgive you, never! I'll never trust you again. And this analysis is over!*

How can we understand Janine's extreme rage and despair? The analyst tells us that Janine felt that she (the analyst) "betrayed her at the end of every session by sending her away, for it was as if I had promised her I would always be there for her, but threw her out after all." Janine's wish to have a mother always there, 24-hour hours a day, and available, leads to a dominant symbiotic transference, exerting a pull on the analyst. The analyst is dragged into feeling that she ought to provide such mothering and feels like a failure when she does not—expressed in the feeling of being a "horrific monster" if she charges Janine for the missed session.

To be sure, the analyst does not act on this feeling—she bills as usual. Nevertheless, it seems to me that the analyst is "trapped" by the pull to be the good mother in a way that hinders her from analyzing the symbiotic transference pattern as comprising needs that must be comprehended as understandable, given Janine's history, and affirmed as such, yet without being gratified. Distinguishing between different patterns of transference (Killingmo, 1989a) is important here. Obviously, in the case of Janine we are dealing with a transference pattern derived from structural deficit, the so-called deficit transference, which has to be distinguished from conflict transference (pp. 68–69). For a patient to function on a conflict level means that aspects of the object have been internalized and transmuted into personal enduring structures, implying that the patient has obtained a relative independence from the direct presence and gratification of the object. As affirmative functions of the objects are structuralized, the compulsive dependency on the object's approval will diminish. Most significantly, the patient is, in principle, able to recognize the object representations projected onto the analyst as *her* representations; that is, she is able to recognize them as transference.

In contrast, if internalization of object representations and object functions has not been completed, the patient will remain more or less in a functional relation to the object—the essential aspect of the transference originating from deficit. Importantly, the patient in this kind of transference pattern will *not* be able to recognize that object representations projected onto the analyst are *her own* representations and projections. There is a lack of mentalization (Fonagy et al., 2002), implying what Fonagy calls an equivalent mode of psychic functioning. This means that the patient will have problems recognizing her relational pattern as transference. The rejecting, horrible analyst *is* horrible. No transference interpretation seems possible.

To my mind, this is exactly what we see in the funeral episode. Janine tells her analyst, "[Y]ou said something to the effect that you thought that you found it impressive how I always experience you as having promised me you would never leave me, that you would always stay with me." It seems that the analyst, probably with the purpose of pointing to a transference need, must have said something (in the previous session) like "You always feel that I promised never to leave you, and that I will stay with you forever." However, Janine is not able to use a comment of this kind to explore her inner world. Rather she feels criticized for having such childish, unrealistic needs. Feeling as if she is being treated like a "scientific object" whose needs are just "analyzed," she feels humiliated and enraged.

Could a more affirmative mode of intervention have been an alternative, conveying to Janine that it is understandable ("no wonder that. . .") that she has an insatiable hunger for someone to hold her without leaving, as she has never experienced this? Affirmation, by establishing a causal relationship between current experiential states and life history legitimates the subjective feeling. The analyst simply communicates that this is how it is and that she can contain the intolerable feelings, be it greed or rage, without demanding that the patient should have felt otherwise.

What about the rage? We can imagine that even if the analyst had tried to communicate affirmatively that she understood Janine's longing for the 24-hour mother that she never had, she might still have been furious for being billed for the missed hour. The challenge, then, would be to contain the anger and hate. When Janine—in fury—exclaims, "I can never trust you again," the analyst responds, "You feel that I have betrayed your trust." This is "exactly" how Janine feels—betrayed. To have her feeling put into words does not, however, provide relief. At this point, functioning on a deficit level, in an equivalence mode, there is no "as if" to the distrust—the analyst *is* a traitor. Again, my feeling about the dialogue is that Janine would have needed to have her feeling of betrayal validated as understandable and legitimate, e.g., by the analyst conveying that when she charges the missed session, she becomes just like the mother—not being there when Janine most needed it. No wonder that Janine feels betrayed—she never felt that mother really was there for her.

Conclusion

Destroying what is good, or making the analyst a persecuting tormentor, expresses actualizations in the transference of inner relational scenarios that must be worked with as part of the analytic process. Moreover, there seems to be no difference between White and me in understanding the patient's destructiveness as expressing primitive self-protective relational strategies. Janine's statement that "silence is the only means I have to distance myself from you," White states, is likely a primitive defence against an analyst whom she does not feel understands her needs. I agree. I would like to add that his is the only kind of relationship that Janine is able to maintain, given her level of functioning—and this needs to be understood by the analyst.

As the analysis is presented in this chapter, it seems—sadly—to have ended in chronic but subtle enactments. It is the privilege of an outside observer to be able to reflect, post hoc, on possible alternative therapeutic strategies. White points to the need to work with one's counter-transference, to be aware of the extraordinary strain of caring for such patients and of finding genuine compassion for their pain, and to work on one's own distancing and hate. I agree, this is a precondition for affirmative interventions to have a chance to be taken in by the patient. Affirmation is not about "saying the right words"—it has to be felt by the analyst as a genuine stance (Gullestad & Killingmo, 2020).

Impasse: Anal narcissism in the analysis—Bruno Salesio

I will attempt to introduce examples from a psychoanalytic point of view that corroborate or are related to the impasse, *sensu lato* and *sensu stricto*.

In the comments below I use my experience as a Three-Level Model moderator. I will emphasize the theories that most resonated with me. Clinical material can be seen by various theories, each addressing a partial point of view. Like Green (1995), I think the role of theory is not to resemble the clinic, but to think it. "Theory" is a word that represents the thing (*Das Ding*), but the word itself does not look like the thing.

Some metapsychological considerations

The logic of Janine's narcissism was that she lived in fear, the threat of losing her organization, the intense fear of depending on someone, the loss of trust in relationships, the vulnerability, the anger, the boycott, the conspiracy—all this was deserving of the analyst's attention and care. Janine's analyst wrote ". . . and she was fuming" and "*[She smells strongly of nicotine].*" In the first session Janine associated to a secret language, secret words for "secret smoke" and for "masturbation." I think (1) the analyst was not comfortable with Janine's narcissistic expressions; (2) Janine expected to be accepted and understood; and (3) there was a lack of mental space/reverie in the analyst, which could have contributed to the impasse.

To consider sphincter control as having a role in psychic structuring means taking into account both the sources of erogeneity and one's own narcissistic constitution (Janin, 2017, p. 150). The delicacy is important for developing the ability to exchange anal bodily functions for dirty substitutes (in the child/mind) and for neutralizing aggression through language acquisition. A relationship of containment, an eroticism in experiencing the passage of content, an opposition to passage or a retention of passage—all are feelings based on anal mucosa and feces (Green, 1993). The transaction between "child"/Janine and "mother"/analyst, implies the analyst could understand Janine's nicotine language as a gesture of confidence, a gift to be understood and appreciated.

In the stage of anal narcissism, the child gives the body's internal contents as a valuable gift to the mother (Freud, 1905). In the transference Janine was actualizing her primitive trauma—through a secret language expressed in the sessions. Janine's language can be understood as an action, when "she smells strongly of nicotine" and, at the same time, as a primitive experience of exchanging "feces and urine" for language. When the anal narcissism progresses smoothly, the child symbolically recovers the lost objects that were lost by naming them—exchanging one pleasure for another. When Janine's analyst interprets that the analytic relationships could be exciting, but also threatening, she adds that the analyst's role would be to help her remember the forgotten pieces. To remember means to put her primitive traumas into words. Words and speech allow detachment and symbolic possession (Janin, 2017). But in Janine's speech one can see wishes for closeness mixed with feelings of being threatened: vulnerability and dependency. Janine suffered traumas that resulted in failures in the formations of her psychic stability and, consequently, in the structuring of her ego functions. What was not symbolized appears as a deficit in mental capacity. The analytic function will need first to comprehend and second to explain (Winnicott, 1956; Kohut, 1984; Killingmo, 1989a; Storolow & Atwood, 1992). To comprehend is a kind of understanding, the process of structuring. Frequently the analyst interpreted in a way that Janine could experience as a demand for a symbolic functioning that she did not yet have. Current theorizations go beyond thinking about narcissism as a phenomenon from libido to ego; neither are they centred on grandiosity; nor do they equate narcissism with an aggressive ignorance of the other (Bernardi & Eidlin, 2018). Narcissism has its own evolutionary line (Kohut, 1984). The antinomy between narcissistic and object libido is only a part of our clinical thinking. It is necessary to include in the narcissistic pathology painful experiences of vulnerability, inferiority, emptiness, annoyance, fear, and lack of confidence in oneself. Before interpreting, it is necessary to create meanings.

As intersubjectivity in childhood is initially pre-verbal (Stern, 1985), Janine didn't understand her analyst and felt that she was inappropriate. Children show an intuitive awareness of the other's feelings and purposes; this is innate and may or may not have cognitive or symbolic elaborations. I think Janine's speech presents two kinds of events: Janine's *reliquat* (a residue) of the primitive trauma that was enacted in the transference, and her repetition of the same trauma (Storolow & Atwood, 1992); I suggest that her analyst didn't understand these two levels of functioning.

Anal narcissism is a crossroads where narcissism and object relations are constructed. Janine felt she was "not worth it" for her analyst. In her words, "Quit your silence! . . . Ach! It's so hopeless! . . . How can I convince you that you should do something? . . . I can't force you. I would like to—to force you to be helpful to me." Janine felt lonely and received no response to the messages she delivered to her analyst (five years into analysis). Janine did not receive "affirmation" (and validation) from the analyst of her needs, as pointed out by Gullestad. The process for establishing a relationship (affirmation of the self and validation by the other) was interrupted, causing pain and intra-systemic failures. In such cases, opposition is a key defence for Janine: it further delineates her identity and makes her feel alive.

On a rare occasion when the analyst recognized her impositions, Janine calmed down:

A: *I think that I'm asking a lot of you by sending you away every day according to what the clock says and not according to your needs.*

P: *[She is very moved, and she calms down and is silent awhile] You don't know how good it makes me feel to hear you say that. It's as though I have waited an eternity to hear you say it.*

What was conveyed by the imposition of a schedule can build a need that can lead to a reaction/protest or to a masochistic submission.

Janine lived a fusional relationship that coexisted with a secret and internal communication. To name or reflect on her primitive bodily experiences and to symbolize them was linked with the feeling that this would bring to an end her symbiotic omnipotence.

A: *And when you do have a good moment with me and feel I understand you, then I suddenly throw you out and—*

P: *[interrupts] —and all of it is then erased. None of it was good, it was all a lie. That's just it, that's exactly what happens. And so nothing can grow and nothing can become solid and stable. [Associates with her mother.] It was terrible. I would trust her and confide in her, and then she'd turn around and stab me in the back.*

Often the analyst can experience this anal opposition as negativity: an unconscious negativism, unperceived by the subject. But this can mean the repetition of a wounded narcissism that seeks a "solid and stable" relationship in the transference.

The deep resistance to carrying out what has been proposed sounds as if the analyst were the prisoner subject/poop of a constricting mother/mucosa.

To give up the primitive bodily experiences and to exchange them for language, Janine needed to work through the mourning of the "thing" before the symbolization (Roussillon, 1995). In the analytical relationship, Janine lived out the impossibility of this mourning process because there was a heightened helplessness of not being recognized. As a consequence there was a permanent splitting between her and her analyst/world. The ambivalence was not in question but a decision to defend her narcissism:

P: *I don't want to choose; I want both the thing and its opposite.*
A: *[In fact, she never made any decisions, but seemed to fall into situations and activities].*

For example, the "violent" beginning of the analysis may have been a silent/speechless enactment (Benjamin, 2009) of a dramatic situation between analyst and patient in which both participated. When the analyst couldn't understand, decipher, or interpret, the communication occurred more through what was being acted out than in actual words; Janine brings her real problem of much anguish to her non-place, which is also repeated throughout the transference. We can imagine that the analyst was probably experiencing a complementary and indirect countertransference (Racker, 1953; Borensztejn, 2009), feeling undervalued and incompetent (Bernardi & Eidlin, 2018).

In the first session, when the analyst said that Janine might also be frightened of growing up, Janine says "Very!" "She's frightened that she will lose her structure, that she will be vulnerable at someone else's mercy, that she will lose confidence, that she will be totally vulnerable"—a description of the outcome of her anal primitive and narcissistic exchanges with her primary objects. She seeks conspirators rather than real friends.

Janine says that she uses detachment to protect herself against panic, "But at the price of feelings." I think these paranoid feelings express Janine's conviction that she is not being taken into account, but is only seen as an object of study by her analyst. Would this explain the dilemma between the secret and the conspiracy as a pathology of hidden meanings and how to experience feelings?

After two years of analysis, the analyst noticed Janine's static psychoanalytic process and lack of desire. Janine would say, "Boycott the analysis" . . . ". . . refuse to allow analysis." Janine found herself in a desperate impasse and unable to find what she was looking for. In terms of anal narcissism, everything Janine gave to her analyst, seeking to establish a relationship, did not find a receptivity capable of establishing the place of a meaningful and stable experience (Rosenfeld, 1988; Baranger & Mom, 1983). The primitive impossibility of creating a narcissistic relationship was repeated. She considered herself very "bad" as a result, and the analyst couldn't help.

Around the eighth year of analysis, Janine misses a session when she attends her father's funeral and the analyst decides to bill her, as was their agreement:

P: *All I am for you is a scientific object. Nothing other than that. You don't care about me at all! I'm nothing special for you—just another patient for you to examine and treat.*

To put principles above needs! Principles are impersonal, an object, dead, not emotion or love, just hate. Needs are expressions of an extreme and humiliating dependence. But the analyst is in an impossible situation: if she charges her patient, she is greedy and unloving, but if she doesn't, she is weak and powerless. The patient feels at a similar impasse. Again, the situation presents a frustration and an offence to Janine's narcissistic needs: principles above needs! Janine expected more an affirmation of her uniqueness, more than of originality. In this experience, the analytical relationship began its end.

Janine complains about the analyst:

> *I have the feeling that I am imprisoned here by you and by the analysis. You make me have bad feelings—and it's always when you're not there—although if you were there, then I wouldn't be able to complain.*

Janine perceives her analyst as withdrawn, like her father, and in reaction, she demands a good mother. Janine's transference may seem paradoxical, with opaque, empty, stagnant, talkative bitter sessions of complaining. The analyst experiences very strong feelings of aggression caused by the boredom and seeming uselessness of their work. The transference *is* the past; the present goes back to the past. Counter-transference usually reflects the subject's problem as in a mirror. The failure of the analyst must be understood as a failure of the past.

Final comments

I commented on the possibility of understanding the impasse as rooted in a pathology that has to do with anal narcissism. This term refers to the characteristics of a previously wounded and destroyed narcissism that is shaped in the moment when the patient has to live the experience of delivering or not delivering (retaining, keeping) her internal contents, to someone outside herself or to a space outside of her narcissistic body. I call it an "other/space" because the other might be a person, but will always be another space, outside the subject's narcissism. Janine struggled to build an identity of stable meanings. Janine felt the analyst's interpretations as a failure of understanding, as criticism and as distancing. This analyst couldn't be internalized with her implicit theory and her way of listening. I think this was reason for the analyst's failure.

Notes

1 In clinical practice we are faced with combinations of derivatives of deficit and conflict, in complex patterns of character. It is almost impossible to distinguish the one sharply from the other. We are always in the world of "both/and,"

constantly dealing, and in turn, both with the Oedipal, where there is a coherent self, and the pre-Oedipal, where there may not be (Killingmo, 1989a, 1989b).

2 Affirmation should not be confused with praising or complimenting a person's achievement or self-image, which is better characterized as gratification.

References

Baranger, M., Baranger, W., & Mom, J. (1983). Process and non-process in analytic work. *International Journal of Psychoanalysis, 64*, 1–15.

Benjamin, J. (2009). Sobre a ideia de que os analistas deveriam admitir aos pacientes as falhas cometidas: um debate clínico [Translation]. *Livro anual de psicanálise*, tome 25. São Paulo: Editora Escuta,

Bernardi, R., & Eidlin, M. (2018). Thin-skinned or vulnerable narcissism and thick-skinned or grandiose narcissism: Similarities and differences. *International Journal of Psychoanalysis, 99*(2), 291–313.

Bion, W. R. (1963). *Elements of psycho-analysis*. London: Heinemann.

Borensztejn, C. L. (2009). El enactment como concepto clínico convergente de teorías divergentes. *Revista de Psicoanálisis, 66*(1), 162–177.

Etchegoyen, R. (1991). *The fundamentals of psychoanalytic technique* (Trans. P. Pitchon). New York: Karnac.

Fonagy, P., Gergely, G., Jurist, E. L., & Target, M. (2002). *Affect regulation, mentalization and the development of the self*. New York: Other.

Freud, S. (1905 [1901]). Fragment of an analysis of a case of hysteria. *S.E. 7*, 3–122.

Green, A. (1993). La anualidad primaria. In *El trabajo de lo negativo* [*The work of the negative*] (pp. 393–402). Buenos Aires: Amorrortu Editores.

Green, A. (1995). Pensar la epistemología de la práctica [Think about the epistemology of practice]. In *La metapsicología revisitada* [*Metapsychology revisited*] (pp. 369–380). Buenos Aires: Eudeba; translation 1996.

Gullestad, S. E., & Killingmo, B. (2020). *The theory and practice of psychoanalytic therapy: Listening for the subtext*. Abingdon: Routledge.

Hart, H. S. (2012). Reversible perspective and splitting in time. *Psychoanalytic Quarterly, 81*(1), 111–126.

Janin, B. (2017). *El sufrimiento psíquico en los niños*. Buenos Aires: Noveduc libros.

Killingmo, B. (1989a). Conflict and deficit: Implications for technique. *International Journal of Psychoanalysis, 70*, 65–79.

Killingmo, B. (1989b). Conflicto y déficit: implicancias para la técnica [Conflict and deficit: Implications for technique]. *Libro Anual de Psicoanálisis* (pp. 111–126). Lima: Ediciones Imago Londres.

Killingmo, B. (1995). Affirmation in psychoanalysis. *International Journal of Psychoanalysis, 76*, 503–518.

Killingmo, B. (2006). A plea for affirmation: Relating to unmentalised affects. *Scandinavian Psychoanalytic Review, 29*, 13–21.

Kohut, H. (1984). *How does analysis cure?* Chicago: The University of Chicago Press.

Maguire, J. (1990). Notes on stalemate: A particular negative reaction affecting therapeutic outcome. *Annual of Psychoanalysis, 18*, 63–83.

Racker, H. (1953). Los significados y usos de la contratransferencia [Meanings and uses of counter-transference]. In *Estudios sobre técnica psicoanalítica* (pp. 153–201). Buenos Aires: Paidós.

Rosenfeld, H. (1964). On the psychopathology of narcissism: A clinical approach. *International Journal of Psychoanalysis, 45*, 332–337.

Rosenfeld, H. (1987). *Impasse and interpretation: Therapeutic and anti-therapeutic factors in the psychoanalytic treatment of psychotic, borderline, and neurotic patients.* New Library of Psychoanalysis. Abingdon: Routledge.

Rosenfeld, H. (1988). *Impasse e Interpretação* 1 (pp. 63–76). Rio de Janeiro: Imago Editora.

Roussillon, R. (1995). La métapsychologie des processus et la transitionnalité [Process metapsychology and transitionality]. *Revue française de psychanalyse, 59*, numéro spécial Congrès, 1375–1519.

Stern, D. (1985). *The interpersonal world in the infant: A view from psychoanalysis and developmental psychology*. New York: Basic Books.

Storolow, R., & Atwood, D. (1992). Varieties of therapeutic impasse. In *Contexts of being: The intersubjective foundations of psychological life*. Hillsdale: Analytic Press.

Winnicott, D. W. (1947). Hate in the countertransference. In *Through pediatrics to psycho-analysis* (pp. 194–203). New York: Basic Books.

Winnicott, D. W. (1956). *Variedades clínicas da transferencia* [*Clinical varieties of transference*] (pp. 483–489). São Paulo: Libraría Francisco Alves Editora; translation 1988.

Chapter 9

Change and impasse in a systematic case study

Foci of the analyst's interpretations

Margaret Ann Fitzpatrick Hanly and Andrea Rodríguez Quiroga de Pereira, based on 3-LM reports by Margaret Ann Fitzpatrick Hanly, Carolyn S. Ellman, Michael Singer, Andrea Rodríguez Quiroga de Pereira, Adela Leibovich de Duarte, and Monica Eidlin

The psychoanalysis of R conducted in the late 1990s took place in the context of a research project on psychoanalysis and creativity conducted by a research foundation, which offered psychoanalysis free of charge to a selected group of creative writers, who agreed to have the analysis tape-recorded and to participate in testing and interviews.

This chapter will present a brief history, a clinical narrative guided by the Three-Level Model, a review of the systematic research on the case of R, and a comparison of these findings with the 3-LM observational research. From this joint perspective, the goal of this chapter is to evaluate the evolution of R case from clinical and empirical perspectives.

R's psychoanalysis continued for four and a half years, four times a week. This is a naturalistic case study; the materials used were the tape-recorded sessions. Eight sessions at six-month intervals were transcribed, and eight of these from different points in the analysis were studied independently by two 3-LM groups of psychoanalysts, one in Buenos Aires and Montevideo and one in New York. The verbatim sessions referred to in this chapter are sessions 1 and 2, beginning of analysis; session 308, at two years; session 504, at three years; session 586, at three years, five months; sessions 76 and 77, at four years; session 708, at four years, five months. Reports were written based on the Three-Level Model, in Buenos Aires and Montevideo, and in New York and Toronto, and this case study is based on those reports.

The research methods evaluated the evolution of the patient through shared methods and different measures at different periods of the patient's analytic process. The Rorschach (Rorschach, 1921), the Adult Attachment Interview (AAI) (George, Kaplan, & Main, 1985), the Therapeutic Cycle Model (TCM) (Mergenthaler, 1997), and a structured work interview were carried out (Kaslow et al., 2015).

The patient's life and some facets of his psychic functioning showed signs of positive change as well as absence of change and impasse in the analytic process in the last phase of the interrupted analysis. The clinical narrative highlights three presenting problems or anchor points, which both groups saw as central in the developing process. The narrative explores excerpts from later sessions, which indicate some change in the patient, describe a central enactment, and assess lack of change in specific dimensions of R's psychic functioning.

The 3-LM groups worked progressively and retrogressively to confirm the centrality of the selected presenting problems in the analysis, as they became landmarks from which change, no change, and the elements leading to impasse could be observed.

Anchor point 1: difficulty in distinguishing inside from outside and thus in judging what leads to destruction and what to survival, leading to paralysis

Anchor point 2: passive idea that nothing is in his control, aggression expressed indirectly or turned back on the self and suicidal depression

Anchor point 3: R's "inner voices" and harsh superego, guilt, suicidal depression, more questions about initial degree of difficulty with paranoia

The analyst's narrative on the case of R (from interviews with the analyst)

R entered psychoanalysis in his late 40s, saying he felt "depressed" and "alienated." His parents and grandparents had immigrated to the United States from Eastern Europe before World War II. R had grown up in a poor neighbourhood. He described his father as "yelling, and bullying" at home, while feeling he had "to submit to the bastards" in the outside world. R's father died three years before the analysis began. R said his mother was always depressed, "never getting over things," and doing laundry for the rich. His mother was diagnosed with cancer just as the analysis began and died six months into the analysis. R had an elder brother, and a younger brother of whom he was jealous; during the analysis, he told the analyst he'd imagined "throwing [his] little brother off the porch."

R went into the Marines shortly before graduating from university, with a plan to leave as a conscientious objector, so as not to go to the Vietnam war. The cruel treatment of some enlisted men in the Marines affected him deeply.

He lived with his elder brother for a while after leaving university and the Marines, and he helped care for his sister-in-law when she was dying of cancer. The analyst believed that it was as a result of watching over this painful treatment that R counselled his mother not to get treatment when she was diagnosed with cancer. R always felt guilty about the advice he had given her.

After his sister-in-law's death, R "drifted" around the country, writing short pieces on sports and travel, taking casual jobs, worrying that having a job and making money would be to participate in an "engine" charging toward "planetary destruction." One of his story/scripts was made into a successful movie. He tried, without success, to write other stories that would sell as film scripts.

His most important relationship was with his partner, Mary. They met (10 years before the analysis) in a bar; they left intoxicated, went out driving too fast, and the car flipped over. R talked of this event as a "turning point" and as a "suicidal experience" although they were not much hurt. Mary came from a poor rural family, but she had been to university. Mary agreed to act as "editor" of his stories for a time but stopped because of the depression R suffered when his stories were rejected. R never talked about sex.

The case of R: presenting problems, change, and absence of change

Overview: Nature of the clinical material

In the first two sessions of the analysis the analyst makes very few interventions. A 3-LM clinical narrative presents observations from the "bottom up," starting with verbatim data from the first sessions of the analysis. However, in the early sessions and to some extent throughout this analysis, the patient's speech is very difficult to follow, almost painful to read. The Rorschach results refer to the patient's "avoidant style of complexity," which is "a cornerstone of his defensive operations" (Lunazzi, 2015, p. 1). Kaslow et al. state (2015, p. 18), "Anger, derogation, and hostility appeared very high across both his personality profile and attachment style at the outset of treatment." The Interpretive Report on the Rorschach testing indicates precisely what both 3-LM groups discussed and reported on, that R demonstrates "a serious impairment of his reality testing abilities," which could designate "a psychotic degree of disturbance." The counter-transference of the two 3-LM groups of analysts who read and discussed the verbatim transcripts was the same in New York as in Buenos Aires and Montevideo: a sense of disturbance and at times dismay. The patient's life and some facets of his psychic functioning showed signs of positive change as well as absence of change and impasse in the analytic process in the last phase of the interrupted analysis. The following clinical narrative highlights three presenting problems, looks at excerpts from later sessions that indicate some change in the patient, describes a central enactment, and assesses lack of change in specific dimensions of R's psychic functions. R's speech is so full of false starts, hesitations, repetitions, and contradictions that, while this chapter presents some "raw verbatim," there are many elisions (. . .) to make the speech readable.

Anchor point/presenting problem 1: Difficulty differentiating inside from outside

R's expressions early in the first session of the analysis show his trouble in perceiving what comes from outside him and what comes from inside his mind.

P: *While I go to this job and I do this work . . . and I don't want to lose this work . . . there's a little part of me that says it's . . . it's . . . it's just . . . it's just adding more [chuckling slightly] to this to that great engine! . . . that . . . that . . . that I . . . I cannot trust, that seems to me to be working to be . . . to be charging toward a kind of d-o-o- . . . of a destruction not only of . . . not only a planetary! destruction but also that runs absolutely contrary to . . . to um . . . to what makes good sense for existence.*

R is struggling to exist and he cannot trust. He is unable to differentiate internal destructive impulses from external destructive forces. He is afraid the voice that's inside is an "obsession,"[1] leading him to waste his life.

These ideas led the group to discuss the severity of the patient's paranoia, with differences of opinion about his psychic structure and capacity for reality testing.

Six months into the analysis, R's mother died, and the analyst asked us to look at the session when R returned to the analysis.

P: *I try to come up with some . . . reasons for . . . these kinds of mood swings and this irritability . . . this real inability to feel as if I'm in my own skin . . . regardless of my decisions about her [advising his mother not to have treatment] my attitudes toward her, . . . that long-term connection being broken, is probably enough to . . . disturb and uh disorient . . . that means that I'm not the same me anymore.*

R's feeling that he is not "in his own skin," his sense that he is "not the same me anymore" after his mother's death suggest a lack of stability in his sense of identity, for he is disturbed and disoriented, and perhaps identifies with his dead mother.

After three years in analysis, R begins (with hesitation) to realize he could be ruthless. The patient agrees he has a conscious hatred for those who have power. The analyst speaks about a power that gives agency:

P: *I had the capacity! to be um at . . . you know at certain times pretty ruthless. . . . I was willing to take that kind of leadership roles occasionally. What . . . if I had!, say, exploited that—*

A: *[The analyst completes his sentence] —that power! is good, . . . that gives you a kind of an energy or strength, agency! . . . It's also kind of a uh either conscious, maybe unconscious, uh, hatred! of those people that have it.*

P: *Oh, absolutely! Try conscious.*

Change can be observed in that R is no longer projecting his hatred entirely onto the outside. But he still denies his own power and agency and reveals a belief that the powerful will always be arrogant and belligerent.

After four years of analysis, R brings an important dream about getting a ticket to an event and being able to go outside and get back inside.

P. *We finally got the tickets . . . I had to go outside again for some reason and, and I was worried that I couldn't get back in, but there was . . . no, I went outside and did something and came back in and there was . . . there was no problem.*

This dream and the associations indicate a change in this presenting problem related to his lack of reality testing. R associates to the dream, saying he had talked with Mary.

P: *I don't have to conceal the hurt . . . it's just right out there, and Mary understands what's going on, and I don't have to, um, you know, that I don't feel that I'm faking anything while I'm, I'm, you know, just talking to her.*

There is evidence here of change in R's ability to experience painful feelings. He is pleased to able to talk frankly to his partner, as an "other," not having to "conceal the hurt," no longer "faking."

Anchor point/presenting problem 2: Passivity, aggression, and depression

In the second session, R's idea that nothing is in his control is a dominant and almost determined position. He gave up two good jobs after university, when he succeeded in getting out of going to war: "When the goal became graspable, when it became within reach, I was turned away from it." The passive tense in R's expression is striking: "I was turned away from it [his goal]," as if he is controlled from the outside. Related to a cynical attitude, he sees himself as a passive victim and mistrusts those who could harm him, e.g., publishers, partner. In this second session of the analysis, R speaks of his own severe depression in terms of a financial "depression" when everything will be taken away:

P: *When I was growing up in the house there was a tremendous sense that another depression was going to come, and take everything away or another war! . . . tremendous amount of fear there, and there was no sense of the future.*

R's passivity, signified in these presenting complaints, closely linked in his associations to his self-defeating acts, are connected to the father he was so angry with:

P: *My father was . . . well my father died [sic] when he was in high school so, . . . he quit high school to go to work um, you know these were things that were forced upon them, . . . they didn't have choices!*

The group took note that R's active but unconscious murderous aggression to the father comes out in this parapraxis in saying his father died in high school rather than his father's father, evidence that R's aggression was turned back against himself resulting in his guilt-ridden, self-defeating, and self-inhibiting acts. He disparages the idea that women need a "magic dick" to restore a sense of self. This metaphor expresses R's unconscious fixation to a passive desire for power to be given to him by a male and the unconscious belief that he is unable to assert his own agency.

In the third year, there is some change evident in R's ability to express his feelings and wishes to the analyst.

P: *When I was yelling at you a few weeks ago about the healing component, even about wanting me to, or um, to find a way out of this, out of this, um . . .*
A: *Suicidal depression?*
P: *Yeah, yeah. I mean, uh, uh, my feeling! is that that you we . . . you're here to sort of watch and monitor, um, but in terms of you know, um interceding!, I don't . . . feel! much of that.*

R makes a strong complaint, sometimes "yelling" at the analyst, angry with him because he was not "interceding" actively to save him from his "suicidal depression." After three and a half years, more aggressive and insistent in his demands, R does persuade the analyst to be his actual partner in editing his stories:

P: *You're the only one who's reading it. . . . You're the only one . . . from whom I can get a response . . . the whole idea of this is that there's no response, I mean, . . . you know, something is better than nothing in this situation.*

R pressures the analyst, who said he was very "insistent." He's the "only one" from whom R can get a "response"; he's "better than nothing." R insists on concrete help rather than analytic help, even while damning the analyst with faint praise. The analyst does read the stories and offer his suggestions.

R vividly enacts an unresolved conflict between his powerful longing for help, his negative expectations and anger towards the analyst, none of which is addressed in the interpretations. R creates an extended metaphor for his experience of the creative process, which ostensibly attacks the whole writing project.

P: *That whole idea of, of creative people . . . it's something that could be analyzed away with everybody. You know, that it's a . . . it's* an irritant. . . . *It's like th, . . . sand in the oyster. You know, it makes the pearl, but it's still a fucking irritant [laughs], and it probably hurts the oyster . . . one purpose of analysis would be to . . . wash the. . . the speck out so that the oyster could just be a bloody oyster. Um, you know,. . . that might be a purpose of analysis, or . . . hope in analysis . . . you get rid of that . . . that irritant, . . . or you recognize it as an irritant.*

In tracking change and absence of change, the psychoanalysts studying this oyster allegory observed a greater coherence in R's speech and some increased capacity for symbolization. His metaphors are vivid and speak to his involvement in the transference. However, R's negativism is strong as he rejects what was, explicitly, a mutual purpose of the analysis. Although R has "insisted" that the analyst "respond" to his movie scripts, R now attacks him for not getting rid of the "fucking irritant," the urge to write those scripts, revealing an unconscious contradictory perspective. As the session ends, R gives away, in confused and grandiose phrases, that he wanted his work to "transcend meaning" and that a person may want to hide so that there's "not evidence *[laughs]* of . . . of your *[his]* obsession with meaninglessness."

In the last session of the analysis, R is still trying to come to grips with his dependency wishes, voicing conflicted wishes for independence with his ongoing negativity.

P: *I need somebody to help me do . . . do things, you know. I want somebody to . . . to be my partner in these endeavours. . . . I mean it's* not that it's *no . . . it's not that it's, uh, not worthwhile, or hasn't, you know, or, or, tha- that it's* been useless *or anything like that, but it's, um, just might be time to stop talking about it . . . someone who will be really, you know, a, an active partner, in, in, in the thing.*

R demands a concrete partner in the analysis, whom he can diminish under his negations: "Not that it's . . . been useless," he says, "just might be time to stop talking about it." R's identifications with his depressive indulgent mother "who never got over things" and didn't know right from wrong, and with the father who was bullying to his sons, telling his sons to "suck it up" while expressing rage at the "bastards" who had it all, led to transferences filled with Catch-22s. R's aggressive impulses to the analyst intensified in the last six months. There is a change from passive to active and an expression of aggression to the other, with the aggression not turned back so often on himself, indicating a reversal of direction but not a change in the dynamic. But the aggression was not addressed in the analyst's interpretations.

Anchor point/presenting problem 3

In the first session, R tells the analyst that his "inner voice" is his "real fundamental problem."

P: *This voice that's inside of me . . . that that that I, I cannot trust . . . "put it aside . . . put it away."*

R's way of talking about his irritating "inner voice" evoked a strong response in the psychoanalysts studying the sessions (in two different cultures) as they questioned his capacity for reality testing (later corroborated by the finding in interpretive report on the Rorschach tests "a serious impairment of his reality-testing abilities") (Lunazzi, 2015). These "inner voices" were brought up repeatedly over the four and a half years of the analysis.

Both groups of analysts questioned whether R experienced "this voice that's inside" as an auditory hallucination. The analyst/participants questioned how serious R's loss of contact with reality could be, and how severe R's paranoia was. R struggles with the relentless moral prohibitions in the voice, against holding a job: was the prohibition a moral "triumph" or did it lead to a "waste"?

Tracking change in the patient, the analysts in both 3-LM groups focused on a verbatim passage in session 308, in the 21st month of the analysis, which showed that at this point R thought of his "inner voice" as his "moral stance" and one that paralyzed any action he might take on his own behalf. R's passivity seemed to be rooted in his belief that any action could be destructive.

P: *You know when I was looking for a reason not to do something I could always find it in this ostensible moral stance. . . . I can't untangle those . . . they're . . . absolutely simultaneous.*

R elaborates his moral paranoia, passivity, depression, and lack of agency, while chuckling, when he describes Kurt Vonnegut's story *The Sirens of Titan*. His negativity, his cynicism, his "bleak," "hopeless" inner states (denied by his chuckling) emerge in a type of dark poetry.

P: *I mean his stuff is so black. . . . You'd better laugh because . . . otherwise you'll go out and kill yourself . . . it's so black, it's so bleak, um it's so hopeless [chuckles] . . . [Y]ou know as I said the . . . the . . . the . . . the successful people in his stories are all . . . buffoons . . . and they're the ones . . . who are delusional . . . it's the . . . it's the ones who are who are broken and beaten and . . . either cynical or . . . or oblivious . . . just blown out, literally wrecked, um who are . . . those are the real people.*

The analyst asks, "The damaged people are real people?" and interprets that R's thinking that he has no control is his "rationalization." But R ignores the analyst's interpretation and continues with his cynicism: "And the bad guys win *[chuckling]* a lot." The analyst focuses on what might block R's creativity, while R finds some satisfaction in "the bad guys" winning. (See the finding of the systematic research on R's "intellectualization" and "avoidant style of complexity" as "a cornerstone of his defensive operations" below, pp. 204–205).

After three years of analysis, in session 504, R seems to show some insight into his harsh, self-punishing superego inner voice. He seems to have an insight when he hears the "same tone" in voicing his contempt for others and for himself:

P: *When I read something that I think is, really is stupid . . . and . . . and I want to . . . condemn the perpetrators, it's in the same tone, the same sound as the one I use on myself.*

The impasse in the process results when R's contemptuous voice is turned on the analyst, along with R's fear that the analyst will desert him, a half-hidden contempt left unaddressed by the analyst in the negative transference.

In the last session of the analysis R shows the derogation, dismissiveness, and lack of gratitude towards his analyst. R reports that he has "upped" his "intake of the drug," changing the dosage of the antidepressant by himself, not consulting the analyst who is prescribing.

P: *I was taking enough to just kind of quiet, the voice . . . and I realized that, um I could take enough to shut it up, you know? just shut it up!*

Here, R is telling his analyst that the irritating "inner voice," which he presented with in the first session, has finally been "shut up," not by the analysis, but by R's increasing the antidepressant medication himself. R then brings what he calls "another lost dream."[2] The analyst makes an interpretation:

A: *I'm wondering if this dream of losses suggests . . . the disappointment in the past four years . . . that you've done some writing, and . . . not, really gotten too far . . . with the writing, to be recognized.*

The participants/psychoanalysts were struck with this moment when the analyst's intervention focused once more on R's lack of success in his creative writing and not on his feelings about the loss of the analysis ("this little spot . . . that I was, you know, comfortable in, for a minute").

R associates to the dream, telling the analyst that he's talked to Mary about the dream:

P: *I talked to Mary about this . . . the whole thing seemed to be, loss, loss, loss, loss, loss. . . . I had finally made some, active . . . movement against . . . the depression, then . . . someone else came along and said, "Well you're not only going to lose what you've had but you're going to lose whatever else you have, in the future." ["Now we're going to sue you."]*

Is there a reversal in the dream situation, with R imaging unconsciously that he will sue the analyst? At this point in the session, R suddenly tells his analyst that he'll "just finish it [the analysis] off here," end "here," because "the drug" has "calmed" his "inner voices":

P: *As far as our meeting, um I think that um . . . um I think that we should just, finish it off here . . . because I felt fairly comfortable, you know, um . . . uh the drug is . . . has calmed that . . . voice.*

The analyst does not address R's passive experience of "loss, loss, loss, loss, loss," even though R will lose the analyst, who has helped to bring about some positive changes in R's inner states and life. R attributes his gains to himself: "I had finally, made some, active . . . movement against . . . the depression."

Level 2 conceptualization of presenting problems, changes, and partial impasse

Difficulty distinguishing between inside and outside

The opening session presents a verbal plunge into his disturbed symptomatic speech, with simultaneous opposite outcomes difficult to hear and to interpret. Having a job could mean "charging toward a kind of d-o-o- of a destruction not only of . . . not only a planetary! destruction," "but also, that, runs absolutely contrary to . . . to um . . . to what makes good sense for existence." R cannot judge what would lead to destruction and what to survival. In conceptualizing these interconnected difficulties, we reflect on specific mental capacities and primitive defences, asking "Is R able to adequately perceive his own internal states and those of others?"

P: *Our language and our philosophies drive us toward confrontation and conflict and aggression and . . . and . . . and our language and our philosophies and our economic system demand ah, antagonism and fighting and a struggle . . . from . . . subatomic particles to galaxies . . . there is a-a-a-a clashing, . . . competition . . . a fight.*

R uses metaphors such as "fighting," "struggle," "chaos," "clashing," "planetary," "destruction," "narratives in two directions" to describe the outside world in the first two sessions. R does not know that the metaphors also describe his inner world and unconscious fantasies. The intensity of his projections distorts his perception of inner and outer reality. The images of war are mirrored in his fragmented speech, full of attacks on his own thoughts, making his speech difficult to follow and to interpret. Thoughts are spoken and then rejected or qualified or denied. R's speech is striking in his high number of fillers and hesitations. He ruminates with long, detailed, intellectualizing, obscuring narrations. He theorizes and philosophizes about himself with minimal insight, and with obsessive isolation of content and paralysis. Bodily symptoms or character traits border on stammering, with perseveration of words and syllables, interrupted sentences, repetitions, hesitations, and various sighs, coughs, ums, and chuckles, all presumably arising from anxiety and serving as hypertrophied defences.

In session 676, R composes the extended metaphor of the oyster:

P: *it's like the . . . sand in the oyster. You know, it makes the pearl, but it's still a fucking irritant [laughs], and it probably hurts the oyster . . . one purpose of analysis would be to . . . wash the . . . the speck out so that the oyster could just be a bloody oyster.*

Although R's associations imply the denial of his own conscious goals in the analysis as a writer, as if the goals were only the analyst's, there is a change in the improved coherence of his speech. (We will see that changes in this dimension are the first finding of the report on the "Adult attachment, personality and patient-analyst communication" by Kaslow et al., 2015, p. 15.)

In session 676, four years into the analysis, five months before ending the analysis, R's dream also reveals R's increased mental capacity to symbolize inside and outside.

P: *I was out of the building, and, and, um, back in again, . . . and then we finally got the tickets, . . . and then I had to go outside again for some reason and . . . and I was worried that I couldn't get back in, but . . . there was no problem, . . . I was inside, holding this ticket, and I could . . . I could go outside again, and I could also come back in.*

R's dream images and associations represented a more defined "inside" self, differentiated from an "outside" other, or situation, an ability to symbolize more sense of a differentiated ego and object and more sense of belonging.

R's passivity and suicidal depression

In conceptualizing this presenting problem and changes in it, we can track his major conflicts over dependency and the effect on his interpersonal relations: "How does the patient experience others and how does he experience himself in relation to others?"

In the second session, and in the second year in the Vonnegut passage, R's sense that nothing was in his control was a dominant and almost determined position. We noted that he gave up two good jobs after university, when he succeeded in getting out of going to war, as if he had been controlled by an outside force: "When the goal became graspable, when it became within reach, I was turned away from it."

The use of the passive tense was striking: "I was turned away from it [the good job]," as if he is controlled from the outside. He sees himself as a passive victim and mistrusts those who could harm him, e.g., publishers, partner, taking on a cynical attitude. Probably as a response, he does not share intimate thoughts and feelings with those close to him.

R came to analysis trapped in a struggle between desperately wanting a "partner" and hatred of any partner he depended on, as "useless," a struggle played out in the central enactment described above: "There is a piece of me that you just preferred to ignore . . . and . . . it's real important for me . . . to get rid of this dependency." As the analysis proceeds, R complains urgently that his partner and his analyst "ignore" his needs, and that this only makes him more dependent, while he desperately wants to get rid of "this dependency." R's demands for magical omnipotent care are countered simultaneously by his hostile wish for omnipotent control over, and exposure of, his "useless" helpers, in the transference, the analyst.

In asking how he experiences himself in relation to others, and how others (including the analyst) relate to him, we observe his insistence that he be given concrete help and that the help from the other is never enough and is rejected as stupid. R insists that the analyst act as an editor: "So, tell me about the story." The analyst complies, unconsciously colluding as R sets him up to fail and to be exposed. R seems identified with his bullying father at this point, projecting his own sense of failure, keeping his envy of the advantaged analyst repressed. Shengold (1994) has explored a patient's need to have the analyst fail as an expression of "malignant envy." R insists that the analyst's advice about how to revise his story will be better "than nothing," but later in the analysis, he implies that not only has the analyst been "useless" but has added to his "pain" by focusing on his writing.

Perhaps the analyst has come into a complementary counter-transference, the role of the mother who is "all for her boys" and "doesn't know right from wrong," and if he "murdered someone, wouldn't care." After four years of analysis before the summer break, before offering antidepressant medication, and before discussing the ending of the analysis, the analyst tries to bring into the open and discuss the issue of his "wanting" R to be "successful" in selling his stories.

A: *You said, once, jokingly . . . about that* New Yorker *cartoon, "What I need is an agent, not an analyst". . . . I kind of want you to be successful. . . . It would make me feel good to . . . to have you come in and . . . so that says I'm not very neutral.*

In reflecting with the patient on his being "not very neutral," the analyst tries to leave the constricted place in which the patient has tried to control him.

P: *You thought that with some success in my writing that . . . the trigger mechanisms for my depressions wouldn't occur so quickly? or, uh, disappear?*
A: *Yeah, I thought . . . [if] the world was [to] give you some . . . opportunity to be successful again, that would definitely help.*

From the analyst's point of view, for R "to be successful again . . . would definitely help." But we can hear the patient's skepticism: "You thought that with some success . . . the trigger mechanisms for my depression" would "disappear"?

The guilt that generates R's impulse to fail, in conflict with his wish to succeed, seemed rooted in a powerful guilt and an aggression turned back against the self (Fitzpatrick Hanly, 1995). Success meant not only to surpass his immigrant father, but to abuse his power as a guilt-ridden son. The failure of R's story/scripts (written with grandiose "moral" objectives and hidden contempt for the reader) led to bouts of suicidal depression and rage at those whom he had insistently drawn in to help him, but whom R, unconsciously, set up to fail, indicating the underlying negative maternal transference, in which R feels unloved, full of rage, and attacks.

R's wish to expose the analyst/father/mother as failing to help him continues to the end of the analysis. Nonetheless, the analysis has helped R in lessening his paranoia, alleviating his severe inhibitions, and reducing his self-sabotage. The analysis had helped him to own his feelings in his relationships, and with the analyst, and to find suitable work using his talents.

R's "inner voices" and harsh superego, guilt, suicidal depression

Both groups observed that the irritating inner voice continues to the end of the analysis and R believes that only the antidepressant has "shut it up." But in conceptualizing the inner voices related to the harsh restricting and humiliating superego, and in noting changes in these dimensions of psychic functioning, we can ask, "Which are the dominant unconscious fantasies that can be inferred from conflicts and relational patterns?" R's grandiose, furious, child's fantasy of destruction can be seen in the idea that he might cause a planetary destruction by getting a job. His childhood fantasy/desire to be provided with a "magical penis" that will give him a missing sense of self, agency, and power can be inferred from this repeated theme in his language.

In the third year, R shows more ability to reflect, and addresses the "pain" he has been "inflicting" on himself.

P: *I'm just trying to stop inflicting pain! on myself and it seems that um, that you know writing stories is, in some way . . . a source of pain, if not a cause of pain. And . . . you know that's my goal right now . . . to try to stop anything that . . . that causes me pain that* I! *can control.*

R sets up minor enactments in the analysis, to play out the impulse to make someone else (the analyst) feel the pain of failing, or he inflicts pain on himself and expresses contempt for the other or contempt for himself. However, by the end of the analysis, he was no longer so trapped in the self-defeating way of using his creative talents, nor paralyzed from all activity. His coherent aggressive complaints against the analyst can be seen as an advance from his passive, self-defeating, paranoid, near-psychotic difficulties observed in the opening sessions. However, his dismissing the analyst expresses, overtly, his tendencies to be rejecting and negative that were there all along.

Discussions at Level 2 addressed the question "Were R's prevailing defences adequate and flexible or dysfunctional, distorting, or limiting internal and external experiences?"

Both groups concluded that R suffered many overlapping primitive and higher-level defences: excessive projection, splitting, denial, intellectualization, rumination (with defensive throat clearing, self-interruptions, sighs, chuckles), paranoid elements with moralization, compartmentalization, isolation of affect, and turning active to passive. He suffered from strong unconscious guilt, with unconscious fantasies generating a need for punishment (he can't use what he is given), and suffered survivor guilt in surpassing his parents and leaving the other soldiers to go to war.

Level 3: The foci of the analyst's interventions

Did the analyst's interpretation effect changes in R's difficulties distinguishing what was inside from what was outside his psyche, his conflicts over dependency, his struggles with control and submission, his passivity, his suicidal depression, the obsessional symptoms in his speech?

What do the analyst's interpretations address?

In the first session of the analysis, the analyst interpreted "Some guilt?" about R's getting out of going to war when others had to go. Three years into the analysis (session 504), the analyst interprets R's "envy" and "hatred" of those who had "power," not just those who "abused their power," and the patient seems to acknowledge his hatred. But let us look closely at the precise associations to the interpretation.

A: *Hating them for something they had that was good, not because that was bad.*
P: *Well, hating them for, um, I guess for the . . . the . . . the . . . the way that it was often manifest! I mean the way power is used! and abused . . . the way power is used! and abused.*
A: *That may be a rationalization. Maybe the first layer was just pure hate that they [the rich] had it.*
P: *Sure.*
A: *The immigrant situation.*
P: *Absolutely.*

R seems to accept that he feels "pure hate" for the rich just because they have the "power," but the word "sure" shows a hesitant and acquiescent attitude. It is only when the analyst adds that the hate and envy belong to his situation as an immigrant, not specific to him, R can say, "Absolutely."

The analyst interprets the separation anxiety in R's wish not to succeed as a "mountain of resistance," because he fears being cut off, "separated," from his internal immigrant family. The analyst understands R's sibling rivalry (he reported R's fantasy of throwing his little brother off the porch). He acknowledges that R experiences bouts of "suicidal depression." The analyst makes supportive interventions, noticing when R tries to stand up for himself with a friend whose work he is editing and who takes advantage of him, or when he pursues a publisher after she has rejected him.

What aspects of the clinical material do the analyst's interpretations not address?

One key moment in the analysis about which to ask but was not addressed was when the enactment occurred and the analyst was persuaded to read R's movie scripts. R's experience as a humiliated, frightened, little boy in a poor immigrant household with a yelling right-wing father lay far underneath the multiple overlapping defensive systems. The analyst did not address R's wish to expose the analyst and the desperate need for help with his writing that would never be enough. The problem with interventions directed mainly to therapeutic action of corrective emotional experience is that they don't address the patient's ambivalence and the Oedipal envy of the analyst and the patient's wish to steal what the analyst has. This makes the need for "support" and corrective "support" never enough. R's envy of the analyst as the "seat of power" came into the associations displaced in this fantasy that was not interpreted.

The analyst's interpretations did not address R's dismissive attitude to the analyst, and the absence of this interpretation may have increased the angry derogation of what the analyst had to offer, and the turn to medication, self-administered in the ending.

The analyst may have acted as a container for the patient's need for catharsis; he listened to R's depressive affects and his criticisms, expressed in a difficult speech, without retaliation. However, he did not analyze R's deeper dependency conflicts, demand for concrete magical help, and derogation of helpers and rage that something in him was ignored. This core conflict was enacted in the transference and enactment.

Hypotheses on alternate interventions that could address the clinical material

R dismisses a transference interpretation related to a dream in the fourth year, insisting that Dave (the analyst) is "disappointed" because R is leaving, not R disappointed that the analysis is ending. R makes a denial: "It wasn't as if I wanted to ditch him and, you know, take his car." The denial seems to ask for an interpretation: "Maybe you did, in some way, want to 'ditch' me, and 'take [my] car.'" The fantasy, an aggressive wish, unanalyzed, could have increased R's guilt. The symbolic theft of the father/analyst's "magic penis" is an aspect of aggression in the positive Oedipus complex. We might consider whether this alternative explanatory and interpretive hypothesis is counter-factual, but the clinical material gives evidence for quite specific interpretations.

Counter-transference blind spots to R's unconscious aggression in the transference contributed to the impasse. The analyst told the moderator about an incident that occurred one day when R ran over the analyst's cat in the driveway of his home office. The analyst knew his old cat often "got out" and "might be run down." So when the patient entered the session saying, "Your cat is probably dead in the driveway," the analyst went on with the session. Afterwards, he felt that this may have deepened R's sense that the analyst "did not care." Going to see if the cat was dead or alive, and asking the patient how he felt about running over the cat, would have led to alternative interpretations.

The analyst's attitude of listening without retaliation, his owning that he was not "very neutral" about R's success, indicates that he wished to present himself as a new object, a kinder and more resilient father, and there are positive gains through the analysis. However, in the verbatim material, R turns the analyst into the weak father, perhaps the weak mother, and seems to act out the role of the bully-father in the last months of the analysis. This provides evidence both for the therapeutic effect of corrective emotional experience and its insufficiency.

Discussion of the impasse

R's negativism and multiple primitive defences all played a part in absence of change in R over the long term. The analyst's over-engagement with the "success" of R's creative writing seems to have inadvertently played into the struggles with dependency, aggression, and guilt that were predominant in the derivatives of R's unconscious fantasies and impulses. Given R's primitive guilt (clearly presented in the initial sessions), the inadvertent effect of being offered a "free" analysis, may have been to exacerbate R's masochism.

Added light can be shed on the impasse in the analysis of R when we consider it as a "pathology of the process" (Etchegoyen, 1991). The verbatim reveals an ongoing negativity in the patient, and extended periods in which the analyst has one point of view on the purposes of the analysis to help R write script that would sell, while the patient has a different, unconscious, and concealed point of view, a "reversible perspective" in the analytic situation (Etchegoyen, 1991). The groups observed multiple overlapping defensive "processes of thought": a "special form of thought which tries to avoid mental pain at any cost" and "locates oneself along a particular perspective and not to move from it," so that every experience is "understood from a position already taken, and which we can define as tendentious" (Etchegoyen, 1991, p. 767). The analysand "holds fixedly to his premises, without expounding them, and without even knowing them, because they are unconscious" (Etchegoyen, 1991, p. 768). We observe these defensive modes and unconscious positioning in R's responses to the analyst's interpretations, which sidestep, ignore, or reject them.

The analyst is focused on addressing what he perceives as a mutual point of view: to help R work through the psychological difficulties that block him from writing successful stories. But R's perspective remains unconsciously to attack a "connection" with the analyst as someone powerful but useless. R's punitive superego (father's "suck it up") initially seemed directed against expressing any emotional vulnerability to the one he depended on, and against an authentic search for insight. R conveys a profound feeling of meaninglessness, which he feels his "partners" ignore, but also a barely hidden wish to dwell in the meaningless. However, there is evidence that there was a more trusting dependence on Mary at the end of the analysis.

The central enactment generated by R's insistence that the analyst act as his editor may have had some positive function in R's demanding what he wanted and articulating how disappointed he was, for the analyst did not retaliate and accepted some responsibility. In this "third look" we are aware that we do not have sufficient evidence to come to conclusions about the analyst's functions as a container, positive and negative (Etchegoyen, 1991). The analyst does not appear to analyze R's projections and his paranoid thoughts, and seems to miss the struggle over control between them. R speaks about himself in displacement as a Vonnegut protagonist, "completely wrecked," controlled by others, hopeless, suicidal, the bad guys winning, and those who "succeed" as "delusional."

Discussion

Systematic clinical research on the psychoanalysis of R

The changes observed in R's life, and absence of change in several dimensions of his psychic functioning, described with detailed verbatim evidence in the 3-LM reports, were corroborated in the systematic clinical research. Assessing a patient's evolution is a difficult task, not only clinically but also empirically, as it involves processing the patient's material and identifying any biases that may remain as unresolved issues. Bernardi et al. (2016) suggest that the factors contributing to therapeutic efficacy may sometimes be the same ones that contribute to the failure of treatment, such as the positive therapeutic relationship. We highlight that certain errors are specific to each therapeutic process and have a variety of effects and manifestations, including dropping out of treatment. In this case, the core pathology of the patient needed a deeper exploration for establishing precisely the ways in which the analysis helped the patient (Bernardi, in press). (For a more detailed analysis of limitations, omissions, and biases see Chapter 14 on clinical evidence.)

The semi-structured work interview was set up to study the patient's creative process. The relationship to work coding system was used to evaluate, such as to what degree the patient is motivated by his desire to work through his psychological problems (Baucom et al., 2000).

The course of the analysis has been described in two publications. The paper written by Stern et al. (2000) reviews R's perception of his treatment, his main relationship with Mary, and the state of his professional work over the first 18 months of the analysis. These instruments were completed by the patient, by the therapist, by his significant other, or by some combination of the three. The patient evaluation of the therapy (Stern & Baucom, 2000) describes the patient's rating of the "depth" of the therapy using the Intimate Bond Measure (Wilhelm & Parker, 1988), which was also completed by R's partner, Mary. The work interview (Daniels, Stern, & Baucom, 2000) and Relationship to Work Coding System (Baucom et al., 2000) were completed. The paper was focused on the analyst's rating of the patient's self-analytic capacity and the analyst's rating of the quality of the therapeutic alliance using the analyst's session evaluation (Stern et al., 2000).

The second study by Kaslow et al. (2015) evaluates the patient's attachment style, personality characteristics, and communication between the patient and analyst throughout the analytic process. In addition to the Mergenthaler quantitative data scoring system for patient–therapist communication, this study used the Adult Attachment Interview (AAI) (George, Kaplan, & Main, 1985) and the Minnesota Multiphasic Personality Inventory—version II (MMPI-II) (Butcher et al., 1989). The following will highlight some of the findings in these studies.

Comparison of the systematic research findings with 3-LM observations

In the long-term study, the finding was that after three years, "the patient's AAI scores revealed that he had greater coherence of his narrative, which was evidenced in terms of more coherence within transcript and in state of mind" (Kaslow et al., 2015, p. 15). The 3-LM reports were corroborated by this result, as they presented verbatim session material designating the change from R's long, detailed, intellectualizing, obscuring narrations to a more coherent speech in the associations and his ability to use metaphor expressively, such as in the "oyster" metaphor.

The most remarkable and telling correspondence with 3-LM reports came in the Rorschach tests, which were administered in 1995 at the beginning of the analysis and in 2006, about 15 years after the end of the analysis. The interpretive report from the 1995 Rorschach test (Lunazzi, 2015) (done at the beginning of the analysis) states,

> He demonstrates a serious impairment of his reality-testing abilities, tending to misperceive events and to form mistaken impressions of people and what their actions signify. . . . This confusion in separating reality from fantasy and the inappropriate behaviors to which it can lead appear to constitute a chronic and pervasive source of adjustment difficulties in his life. The extent to which he distorts reality is likely to prevent him from maintaining adequate adjustment for any length of time in most situations. Many people with this degree of impaired reality testing . . . meet criteria for a psychotic degree of disturbance. . . . This person tends to think about his experience in an inflexible manner that results in his clinging rigidly to previously held convictions and resisting any reconsideration of his beliefs in light of new information. . . . Such inflexibility frequently impedes progress in psychotherapy. . . . [R] appears to be a person who uses intellectualization as a cornerstone of his defensive operations.
>
> (Lunazzi, 2015)

The 3-LM reports (made prior to reading the research) noted these difficulties with reality testing signified in the "inner voices" and the grandiose projections of destructive impulses, with the idea that for the patient to work was to be "charging towards . . . a planetary destruction." R's dream images in a session in the fourth year and his associations represented a more defined "inside" self, differentiated from an "outside" other.

The outcomes reported in the Rorschach tests 15 years after the end of the analysis, "The integration of the client's own identity has achieved only partial synthesis"; his "avoidant style of complexity" still "very active." The interpretive report on the Rorschach tests in 2006 indicated "limitations" in results because "the protocol does not report responses to Card X." "The findings that can be observed in 2006 show a better adjustment to reality testing." However, "the integration of the client's own identity has achieved only partial synthesis," and his "avoidant style of complexity is corroborated, and again observed to be very active." The 3-LM reports noted a lessening of the speech pathology and of the grandiose ideation. Both 3-LM groups focused on R's ability to voice aggression, but also on R's continued negativity, his rejection of the analyst, and the uninterpreted negative transference in the ending phase.

Kaslow et al. (2015, p. 17) report simply that there was a "decrease in the perceived quality of his relationship with the analyst in the last six months." The paper had no observations about why this occurred but speculated that the "decrease in quality" was linked to the perception of the approaching termination. The 3-LM reports provided detailed verbatim data to reveal the uninterpreted affects and impulses in the ending phase, as well as R's passive aggression and desperation:

> I need somebody to help me do . . . do things, you know, I want somebody to . . . to be my partner in these endeavours. . . I mean it's not that it's no . . . it's not that it's, uh, not worthwhile, or hasn't, you know, or . . . or . . . that it's been useless.

The 3-LM observations corresponded with the systematic research concerning R's improved subject–object differentiation. After R expressed anger to the analyst that he wasn't "interceding" to help, he was able to share vulnerable feelings with Mary. The 3-LM had insufficient data to see more about the nature of his relationship with Mary but did track the ways he related to the analyst: R came to the analysis trapped in a struggle between desperately wanting a "partner," and hatred of any partner he depended on, as "useless," a struggle played out in the central enactment described above: "There is a piece of me that you just preferred to ignore . . . and the other part of it is that, um, it's real important for me . . . to get rid of this dependency."

The patient's relationships outside the analysis were evaluated through his attachment patterns and discourse about his childhood and adult relationships as well as with the Intimate Bond Measure completed by the patient and his significant other, Mary. The patient started analysis with an insecure-preoccupied attachment, and this remained the same throughout the analytic process. The 3-LM reports did note that that R was able to confide feelings that he felt "hurt" to his partner in the sessions at four and four and a half years of analysis, and he was able to voice strong complaints against the analyst.

The study by Stern et al. reports that the patient felt as if he were cared for by his partner when the levels of "connection" increased in the analysis. However, Mary's perception was the opposite: she felt better about their relationship when R displayed negative emotions in the analytic process. The 3-LM data did not provide observations from this point of view.

> The systematic research indicated that anger, derogation, and hostility appeared very high across both his personality profile and attachment style at the outset of treatment . . . his use of anger or aggression as a reflexive strategy may have been reduced, since he did express less anger and derogation in his attachment narratives by the end of psychoanalysis.
>
> (Kaslow et al., 2015, p. 18)

However, "unfortunately, the remainder of his scores remained consistent with an insecure-preoccupied attachment throughout the treatment. For example, he showed very low loving scores and very high rejecting and neglecting scores for the duration" (Kaslow et al., 2015, p. 15).

> Despite this positive attachment style shift, a number of his scores on the AAI reflecting his relationship with his father were not ideal and reflected very low loving and very high rejecting and neglecting feelings toward his father even at termination.
>
> (Kaslow et al., 2015, p. 17)

The 3-LM observations corresponded to the systematic research findings that R presented with "anger, derogation, and hostility." The 3-LM reports reviewed the verbatim passages conveying R's anger at, and derogation of, the analyst, implicit and explicit in the transference, and very clear in the ending of the analysis. The coherent expression of anger at the analyst was accompanied by a denied insight and a resistive derogation of the analyst even with the kernel of truth.

The 3-LM observations lack data on R's relationship with his father; however, the AAI showed that that patient "decreased role reversing" in caregiving and what had started out as a "less preoccupied attachment" concluded as a "secure autonomous attachment" with his father.

There were "some positive shifts in his state of mind toward his mother, including reported lower levels of anger and derogation by termination" (MMP-II). The 3-LM did not have session data on this point.

The systematic research states,

> The patient showed elevations on Scales 4 MMPI-II Individuals who score highly on Scale 4 tend to have difficulty with authority figures,

> stormy and superficial relationships with loved ones, and trouble maintaining a job. High scorers on this scale . . . often demonstrate impulsivity, hostility, and narcissism. These individuals may report feeling sad at times, but do not usually experience deep emotional responses or strong emotional turmoil. They tend to blame others for their difficulties and intellectualize problems in treatment, making it difficult to see change or successful treatment.
>
> (Kaslow et al., 2015, p. 17)

These descriptions of the patient's difficulties correspond to 3-LM observations of his associations to his "faking" it in relationships, afraid of disclosures (R never spoke about sex to the analyst). The 3-LM observations are corroborated: "Difficulty with authority figures," "superficial relationships with loved ones," and "trouble maintaining a job."

Change and impasse in the analysis of R

The childhood object relational experiences seemed to be repeated in the transference, as R experienced "no response" and bullied the analyst to respond more concretely. He evidenced ongoing unconscious motivations to control the primary object (father, mother) along with inhibitions in his ability to love and to work. R remained "preoccupied" with a persecuting superego, his "inner voices," which comprised an important factor in the impasse in the analysis (Etchegoyen, 1991). Bleger (2012) wrote that we need to assess the degree of difficulty at the start of the analysis because some analyses start where others end. R's lack of reality testing in the early sessions was a presenting problem that could be related to his severe obsessional character, or to a serious deficit in the structure of the self, or as the two are linked (Rosenfeld, 1987). The data for making a decision on this were not available in the verbatim material. However, we have good reason to say that the observational research done guided by the Three-Level Model in two groups to build a clinical narrative has found important confirmation of its main points in the systematic clinical research.

Notes

1 P: *This voice that's inside of me, either to . . . either to . . . let it talk and trust it, um or to put it aside and put it away because I'm afraid sometimes it's um . . . it's an obsession . . . waste of time and a waste of my life or else a kind of . . . triumph? . . . is there a truth in there or not, or is it . . . or is it simply where you put your camera, ah is it simply a matter of . . . of perspective?*

2 P: *I'm on the very edge of the road and this truck comes over, a pickup truck, parks against me and there's a load of gloves in the back seat. . . . I became really angry because . . . you know, I've had this little spot [laughs] that I was, you know, comfortable in, for a minute, and then . . . and so I started throwing the . . . the . . . the . . . the gloves out, . . . just in anger and yelling at the driver. And then a lawyer came up to me and said, "Well, well, you know, now we're going to sue you."*

References

Baucom, D. H. Stern, A. J., Allen, E., & Sullivan, L. (2000). Relationship to work coding system. Unpublished.

Bernardi, R., Varela, B., Miller, D., Zytner, R., de Souza, L., & Oyenard, R. (Eds). (2016). *La formulación psicodinámica de caso. Su valor para la práctica clínica* [*The psychodynamic formulation of a case: Its value for clinical practice*]. Montevideo: Grupo Magro Editores, Universidad Católica del Uruguay.

Bernardi, R. (in press). Moving from clinical inquiry to clinical research. *In Clinical research in psychoanalysis: Using working parties and metaphors in research and practice.* Abingdon: Routledge.

Bleger, J. (2012). Theory and practice in psychoanalysis: Psychoanalytic praxis. *International Journal of Psychoanalysis, 93,* 993–1003.

Butcher, J. N., Dahlstrom, W. G., Graham, J. R., Tellegen, A., & Kaemmer, B. (1989). *Manual for the restandardized Minnesota Multiphasic Personality Inventory: MMPI-2—An administrative and interpretive guide.* Minneapolis: University of Minnesota Press.

Daniels, L., Stern, A. J., & Baucom, D. H. (2000). A semi-structured work interview for creative writers. Unpublished.

Etchegoyen, H. (1991). *The fundamentals of psychoanalytic technique.* London: Karnac.

Fitzpatrick Hanly, M. (1995). Introduction. In M. A. Fitzpatrick Hanly (Ed.), *Essential papers on masochism* (pp. 15–17). New York: New York University Press.

George, C., Kaplan, N., & Main, M. (1985). Adult attachment interview protocol (rev. edn). Unpublished.

Kaslow, N., Fischer, N., Pollard, S., Powers, A., & Reviere, S. (2015). Adult attachment, personality and patient-analyst communication: A case study. *Journal of Projective Psychology & Mental Health,* 22(1), 9–23.

Lunazzi, H. (2015). Interpretive report on the Rorschach tests provided by the Lucy Daniels Foundation. Unpublished.

Mergenthaler, E. (1997). The therapeutic cycles model in psychotherapy research: Theory, measurement and clinical application. *European Psychiatry, 12,* 143s–143s.

Rorschach, H. (1921). *Psychodiagnostik: Methodik und Ergebnisse eines warhrnehmungsdiagnostischen Experiments (deuten lassen von zufallsformen)* (Vol. 2). Bern: E. Bircher.

Rosenfeld, H. (1987) *Impasse and interpretation.* London: Karnac.

Shengold, L. (1994). Envy and malignant envy. *Psychoanalytic Quarterly, 63,* 615–640.

Stern, A.J., & Baucom, D. H. (2000). A measure for assessing a patient's reaction to psychoanalysis. Unpublished.

Wilhelm, K., & Parker, G. (1988). The development of a measure of intimate bonds. *Psychological Medicine, 18,* 225–234.

Part V

New uses of the 3-LM in the transmission of psychoanalysis and in professional development

Chapter 10

The 3-LM's contribution to developments in analytical treatment

Beatriz de León de Bernardi, Luisa Pérez Suquilvide, Marina Altmann de Litvan, Nancy Delpréstito, Marianne Leuzinger-Bohleber, Lisa Kallenbach-Kaminski, Rosemarie Kennel, Anju Labuhn, Luise Laezer, Susanne Landsiedel-Anders, Sebastian Ohlmes, Gertrud Reerink, Sarah Römisch, Jörg Scharff, Karin Schwind, Erwin Sturm, Heike Westenberger-Breuer, Liliana Fudin de Winograd, and Mayela Falvy

Introduction—Beatriz de León de Bernardi

This chapter will show the uses of 3-LM in the transmission of psychoanalysis and in professional development. Experiences in Montevideo, Frankfurt, Buenos Aires, and Peru have integrated candidates into 3-LM group workshops. In this chapter, a variety of these experiences with candidates will be described. The different institutional contexts have adapted the 3-LM to the realities and demands of psychoanalytic communities. Various modalities are used in setting up the 3-LM groups: some only for candidates, others in which the candidates participate together with members of their psychoanalytic society and institute, and in some cases qualified members are brought in as consultants. There have also been formal modifications in the time allotted for group discussion, which needs to be adapted to the institutional schedules. On several occasions the 3-LM group process has been carried out in two or three meetings with intervals of several months. Sometimes, parts of the model have been used. In some cases, the transformations of the patient have been studied and described on the phenomenological level. In other cases, the transformations of the patient have been discussed considering the Level-2 dimensions of the changes that have occurred, and the theoretical-clinical conceptualization of how the changes came about, at Level 3. New questions on the analyst's interpretative foci and mechanisms of change have recently been incorporated into the work of the 3-LM third level.

These experiences have been productively evaluated by participants and have raised new questions to be explored. The most valuable aspect of these experiences lies in contributing to the creation of a space for analysts-in-training that allows them as participants and careful observers of the clinical material presented to reflect and intervene without the pressures of institutional evaluation, thinking about the transformations or absence of transformation that have occurred in the patient, promoting internal evaluation in relation to the ways they work with their patients. The priority given by the model to the richness of the clinical phenomena favours an attitude of research that becomes the basis for candidates' future personal development, offering a complementary starting point to the demands of psychoanalytic training.

The Montevideo experiences

Part I: Analyst's focus and mechanisms of change in analysis: New questions in work with the third level of 3-LM— Luisa Pérez Suquilvide and Beatriz de León de Bernardi

We present clinical material that shows one experience in Montevideo, Uruguay, with modifications to the questions in the third level of conceptualization of the 3-LM. The Education Committee and the Scientific Committee of the Uruguayan Psychoanalytic Association supported this activity.

Two groups, comprising 12 analysts-in-training and analysts with different levels of training, worked with one moderator each and on the same clinical material in two stages, with a three-month interval between them. In the first stage, the groups addressed Levels 1 and 2. In the second, participants in both groups merged into one of 14 participants and worked with the two moderators.

The patient

Joseph is a 30-year-old professional, married, with three children. The first child was the product of an unwanted pregnancy during his late adolescence. In the first meeting, the analyst describes him as a very rational person, correctly and formally dressed in an overcoat, suit, and laced leather shoes. This clothing surprised the analyst as unusual and unexpected in a person of his age. He found Joseph's discourse lacking in emotion, meticulous, monotonous, and dull, in contrast with the content: Joseph felt overwhelmed and had difficulty in organizing his life. He linked his feelings of guilt and anger to the birth of his first child. When the pregnancy occurred, he felt that he had no choice and submitted to the situation as well as to the family's demands: "You have to graduate." He victimized himself in the face of this situation and blamed himself for his absence during the first months of this child's life, when he devoted himself to his career. He still maintains a conflicted relationship with this son.

In the transference, the analyst experienced the patient's hostility while the patient did not make any contact with it. He made his analyst feel stupid and worthless. He responded to the analyst's interventions repeatedly, with "It's not that." At times, he placed the analyst in the role of the idealized figure of his grandfather, with whom he could think.

Levels 1 and 2 of 3-LM

Phenomenological observation and discussion of the patient's transformations

Both groups observed positive changes linked to Joseph's subjective well-being. His experience of being overwhelmed disappeared; he began to feel that he could manage his life. His contact with his emotions, his ability to express them, and his capacity to relate to his children and friends improved. He moved from a position in which he did not allow himself to choose, often subject to the desires of those around him, to a position in which he began to make professional and emotional choices. He moved on to "playing at the big table," a metaphor that became an anchor point throughout the process. The two groups highlighted different aspects of the material. For one group, the narcissistic aspects of Joseph showed less change. The other group emphasized the weight of his moral ideals, which led him to assume altruistic behaviours that were detrimental to him. This aspect changed in the course of the analysis.

Dimensions of change that occurred in the analysis (Level 2)

The group worked on the changes in Joseph's "experience of illness," his interpersonal relationships, the predominant conflicts, and the structural aspects of his mental functioning.

Joseph appeared initially overwhelmed: "The wave passed me by." This expression represents a first anchor point. He could not cope with his work, his home, or his children. At the same time, he had an experience of confinement and of a house in disarray, of being on hold. He made his wife, parents, partner, and children responsible for his problems and felt misunderstood and subjected to the desires and decisions of others: "I didn't choose it"—an expression that he repeated throughout treatment.

After he had spent a year and two months in analysis, having increased the number of sessions, an anchor point containing a metaphor for Joseph's subjective situation showed modifications. He was anguished, afraid of the very changes he wanted, like "throwing oneself into the water" without knowing how to swim. Pleasant childhood memories, such as bathing in the sea with his father and his son also appeared as "murky waters," showing conflicts in his experience, e.g., the son being "lost in the sea" in a dream. The analyst referred to aspects of the child inside that Joseph feared to modify: "You got stuck in that child who could not say 'I don't want.'" The fear of loss concurred with the possibility of losing what he called "this space," referring to his analysis (for financial reasons), but also with a fear of deepening the relationship with his wife, which, although the analyst persisted, Joseph did not want to address.

Both the death of his paternal grandfather, an idealized figure, and his wife's affair had substantial impacts on him. While Joseph was open to address his grief over his grandfather's death in the analysis, he could not make contact with his pain and anger regarding his wife's affair, nor recognize his defensive denial and avoidance.

The group discussed how far the patient and analyst agreed on the transformations expected through the analysis. For the analyst, the expectation was that Joseph would be able to get in touch with his emotions, while for Joseph, the purpose of analysis seemed to be to put his life in order and to be able to choose.

Interpersonal relationships

At the beginning of the analysis, Joseph was more inclined to submit to others as figures of authority and did not show bonds of intimacy—problems that changed throughout the process. He maintained distant relationships characterized by submission to his wife and father. He felt cared for by his mother, but criticized: "What she gives you she charges you for." The rivalry with his sister seemed to cover up incestuous aspects: "We were unbearably on top of each other, but never in a positive way."

The second anchor point was "the *Truco* table"[1] in which he visualized the "big guys," family, and professionals. In the beginning, he felt he could not take part in the game as he felt less than they were, with no ability to compete in the way he wanted. At the beginning of the analysis, the transferential relationship was ambivalent. He was asking for help while he devalued the analyst for his interventions and the handling of fees. This relationship changed throughout the process: the analyst felt less controlled and became less bored. Joseph could recognize that he needed help and that the analytical space was important to him. He could voice his pain and anger and could hold onto the relationship with the analyst as a man who did not "slap him down." There were changes in the relationship with his son, whom he could previously approach only from the "cramped" position. He was able to play and have fun with him. He could relate this with the relationship he had with his father. The group questioned the extent of changes in his emotional distance and to his capacity to experience intimacy, especially with a woman.

Predominant conflicts

Submission vs. control and conflict with the demands of excessive superego moral ideals led Joseph to assume masochistic positions. An intense Oedipal rivalry emerged with the father, but, throughout the process, he could ask him for help and dared to grow and compete in his work. The

Truco game (card game) metaphor, in addition to this Oedipal rivalry, showed his conflicts about greed: he wanted to take it all. There was a predominance of defences of repression, denial, intellectualization, and isolation. They became more flexible throughout the analysis, as did the projection. The patient was able to perceive his internal states such as pain, rage, and pleasure better and began to recognize them in others (e.g., his son's and his wife's discomfort). His capacity for empathy increased.

Mental functioning

Joseph showed a strong identity but with secondary conflicting identities linked to hostile aspects with his father and negative oedipal aspects with the mother. At first he had difficulty regulating his impulses and emotions. Joseph could not control his anger and grumbling about his son for every small thing and could cry at a client's observation about his work. However, he appeared very controlled in his speech and presentation in the analysis, without emotions, moving in an all-or-nothing pattern of emotional regulation. At the end of the analysis, he regulated his self-esteem better, being able to face challenges with "the big guys" of his profession and being happy about it. He began to do things that he liked, that felt he deserved and could enjoy, in contrast to the image of his late adolescence, crushed by obligations. He brought dreams, associations, and childhood memories to the analysis, which opened up the possibility of thinking about himself. However, the group wondered if Joseph achieved a genuine capacity for symbolization. The relationship with his internal objects ceased to be so persecutory. With respect to his external objects, he improved his relationship with his son, he managed to get a new partner, and the analyst gave him an affectionate pat on the back at the end of the analysis.

Finally, both groups agreed that Joseph had a neurotic organization of his personality at the beginning of the analysis.

The Third Level of 3-LM seeks to understand the mechanisms implicit in the patient's changes. How and why have they occurred? The group analyzes the foci of interventions and interpretations of the analyst, their variation throughout the analysis, what kind of interventions worked best, and aspects that the analyst left out.

The foci of the analyst and their modification

The first focus of the analyst was on Joseph's masochistic functioning. The group understood some of the analyst's interventions as provocative and aimed at easing the patient's rigid defences. In some interpretations, the analyst's discomfort was evident, understood as a counter-transferential aspect linked to the patient's aggressiveness.

The interpretative foci (what in the patient's mind and problems the interpretations addressed) varied. The analyst sought to ensure that Joseph did not deny reality (his wife's affair) and could get in touch with his emotions: "What seems to be falling far short in our work here is your bond with your wife." "Is it comfortable for you not to work on this issue with me?" "Where did she come from?" "Didn't she go back to sleep?" "It's all very reasonable, but you got angry." "You're very angry and very hurt." "You get pretty disconnected, huh?"

The analyst supported Joseph in discriminating and separating his childhood objects and his current bonds throughout the analysis. His work helped Joseph to think more freely about himself, able to choose according to his interests, while still taking care of those around him. At the end of the analysis, the analyst enabled Joseph's decision to end the analysis, despite thinking that some conflicts needed further analytic work.

Types of interventions by the analyst and mechanisms of change in the patient

The group analyzed the possible mechanisms of change, discussing whether the analyst offered himself as a "new object," representing for Joseph a new emotional experience in containment and support. The transferential relationship changed from one in which Joseph repeated a way of being with someone in which he viewed himself as passive and the analyst as active through his interventions and interpretations. In the first stage of the analysis, he felt that the analyst "slapped" him with his interventions, repeating an aspect of his relationship with his father. Joseph stopped slapping his son, showing that the experience in the transference had affected his bonds with others. His ideals changed with transformations in trans-generational ideals represented by endurance, resistance, and work. Joseph showed ideals that were more flexible. Thus, he developed personal interests, which brought him significant changes and satisfaction in his professional life and relationships, and a more appropriate location in his chronological age.

Another mechanism of change was the introjection of the analytical function. This permitted Joseph to move from the obsessive rumination of the beginning phase to the reflexive function in the ending phase. The analyst acted as an auxiliary self, mirroring the split affects, adjusting to the transferential movements that Joseph proposed, including his proposal to end the analysis. The patient managed to incorporate the desire to know about himself and to have a less naive view of himself.

Aspects of the material left out of the analyst's interventions

The group highlighted the patient's slip of the tongue—"Thinking that this is what I want as a woman"—which the analyst noticed but did not explore. Following the slip would have opened a path to enable contact with a passive, unconscious desire, "me as a woman," and to approach homosexual ambivalence. In the clinical material offered, it seems that the analyst could not work on the bond between Joseph's mother and father in depth. The internal image of the mother was of someone who crushed him and did not allow him to make his own decisions, resulting in a persecutory mother to the extent that there was no discrimination: "the mother hen who later charges you." In the transference, the analyst also gives and charges. The father appeared devaluated, despite Joseph's recognizing his help. He changed from submission to the authority figures to competition in his professional growth:

> They told us that they consider us competition and on the one hand, it generated a little fear in me, and on the other hand it gave me a lot of pride in what we are achieving. . . . It is like they tell me to play but at the same time I feel, "Be careful not to bother the big guys."

The group discussed the fact that his aggressiveness did not appear more directly in transference with a male analyst. The analyst pointed out that there were changes in the patient's physical presence and in his way of expressing his emotions, such as the "soft hand" Joseph gave him at the beginning of the treatment turned into a "firm hand" at the end.

As an alternative hypothesis, the group raised the question of how the patient would have reacted if the analyst had proposed an adjustment of the fee, adapting the fee to the increase in his income. Some participants suggested that the analyst might not have proposed this change because the patient was under supervision in the training program, and he feared the patient would leave treatment.

Alternative theoretical hypotheses

Finally, we discussed ideas from different theoretical frameworks as alternative explanatory hypotheses for the patient's changes.

Joseph arrived with a rigid presentation, obsessive defences, and a masochistic enjoyment. The group discussed which theory it would be more appropriate to select in working on these difficulties. The analyst preferred the Freudian theory about Oedipal conflict, castration anxiety, and desire. At the beginning of the analysis, Joseph's ego appeared suffocated, crushed by superego ideals and the external reality in which he lived. The analytic work sought to make defensive functions and the permeability between psychic instances more flexible.

Members of the group proposed a Kleinian perspective to understand the patient's conflicts. They suggested a transformation in a schizo-paranoid functioning with the integration of split-off aspects of idealization-devaluation, giving place to depressive affects. An alternating dynamic between schizo-paranoid and depressive positions, or, as Marucco (1999) describes it, the coexistence of different psychic levels of functioning. From this perspective, the incorporation of the good object allowed him to finish the analysis.

From a Winnicottian perspective, Joseph acquired the capacity to be alone in the absence of the analyst. From a Bionian perspective, he was able to incorporate the reverie function of the analyst, which would allow him to consult in the future if needed.

Conclusion

In both groups, participants worked intensively. In the second meeting, they took up the new questions proposed to discuss in Level 3. The integration of the two groups showed different emphases on the problems of the patient, although there was agreement on the changes observed. The three-month interval between the groups' meetings allowed participants a retrospective reflection and a resignification of the material. This schedule had a positive influence on the psychoanalytic conceptualization of the patient's transformations.

The new questions proposed in the third level contributed to rethinking the theoretical-clinical problems raised in the first levels and complemented the discussion of alternative theoretical hypotheses. They allowed critical reflection on central aspects in the analysis, which the analyst had not addressed, on the ending of the analysis, and on the explanatory theoretical hypotheses on the mechanisms of change.

Part 2: Working in changes of the different foci of analyst interventions with the third level—Marina Altmann de Litvan and Nancy Delpréstito

In this space we seek to show a work experience aimed at candidates, using the Three-Level Model. The clinical material belongs to a candidate-in-training who, out of generosity and curiosity, suggested to start penetrating this work model. This is an ongoing analysis material that poses certain questions to the analyst, which are connected to the patient's change process. This was discussed by a group in which both candidates and analysts participated.[2]

It is interesting, then, to observe what this new experience of using the model for a group to understand, think, and rethink the material offered, considering what the analyst added as well. We believe this last point to be extremely important because, at the beginning, we all held a personal view on the material, and, in the course of the exchange about the first two levels, our view on the patient was modified.

For this purpose, we will use the clinical observation of Level 3 as an example, the aim of which is to understand how and why changes occurred (or did not occur). Therefore, it discusses the explicit and implicit theories (Sandler, 1983; Canestri, 2006; Bleger, 2012) by which transformations can be explained, starting with those that are revealed in the analyst's interpretations. Participants were asked to propose alternative hypotheses or points of view coming from their own theoretical and technical frames (Bernardi, 2015). We will focus on groups of questions:

1 What were the foci of the analyst's interventions and interpretations? Did the interpretative foci change throughout the analysis? Which interventions worked best?
2 What parts of the clinical material were not pointed out by the analyst? Would you consider another type of intervention or alternative hypothesis that might have been useful to the patient?

Characteristics of the work proposal

The clinical material (four sessions: first interview, a session that took place two years later, and two more interviews) was given to the participants prior to the beginning of the discussion, and previous readings and videos were recommended to learn how the 3-LM works.

At the beginning of the first module they had to complete the form to first respond individually and, at the end of the work, they had to complete a new form to respond after the group experience.

In the discussion group, in view of the fact that the changes that had taken place were slight, it was suggested they meet again a few months later to see if what the group had contributed had resulted in modifications to the analysis. This was a novel experience that yielded very good results. This situation is quite rare in this type of approach.

The analyst accepted this new challenge, and, after a few months, we met again to continue working, particularly on Level 3 of the model.

As previously mentioned, we chose Level 3 to reflect on different alternative hypotheses, upon having observed slight changes in interpersonal and proximity relationships, as well as in the transferential bond, and taking into account the two years of analysis that the patient had undergone.

Presentation of the patient

J consulted because his partner, with whom he had a little child, told him she wanted a separation. Faced with this situation, he consulted at his partner's behest, yet unaware of his partner's problems, which he did not perceive as threatening. Although they were constantly fighting and making up, their relationship stayed the same.

His discourse was of marked disconnection from his affections. J said, "It is hard for me to express affection." When he expressed negative affection, he did not seem to consider its impacts. This could be seen very clearly in his relationship with the analyst. J displayed a series of obsessive symptoms: "I do not tolerate yawning." He pushed away or rejected smells, or anything related to the other's body. He presented "rituals," such as going to the bathroom right before starting every session. At the beginning of the sessions a method was developed, by which he remained silent unless the analyst started talking. He markedly controlled the analyst, by comparing her clothes with those of his partner. When his analyst got pregnant, it could be clearly observed that he rejected her, as he made hostile comments that she kept receiving by not answering accordingly. He made a bodily use of the analyst.

A distinctive feature of this patient was that, in each stage of his life, he had a different name. His first name was linked to his childhood, the second one to his adolescence, and the third one was his current name. Consequently, depending on the peer group he was with, he called himself differently, thus interrupting his existential continuity.

He came from a vulnerable economic background, but he currently was a professional who has overcome these hardships. However, when he contacted his old friends, he changed his clothes, thus hiding what he has achieved and displaying marked feelings of guilt.

Another key point was the death of his father, which clearly showed a "frozen" mourning. For example, his father's car had not been used since his death, and it had been hidden in the garage, out of sight. At this point of the treatment, he could open up and work on his loss. We think that it was through the work on the mourning for his father that his positive affections of love and sadness began to appear.

Over the course of almost three years of treatment, very slight changes in the closeness and proximity to his partner occurred.

In the discussion of Levels 1 and 2, the group agreed that the patient had a neurotic organization, with very rigid obsessive-type defences, yet still did not form a clear obsessive structure. Since his identity was fragile, there was a dependence conflict, a marked mistrust, and submission. Additionally, he had a poor capacity for empathy.

1 What were the foci of the analyst's interventions and interpretations? Did the interpretative foci change throughout the analysis? Which interventions worked best?

During the first years, the analyst's focus was to generate a high-trust environment between the two of them. J was a patient with a rigid defensive world, who attended his sessions thinking about everything he was going to say, all prepared, and distant from his affections.

Later, mourning for the dead father emerged. The analyst changed the focus of her interventions by trying to soften the hardness of his father perception, for all his references to his father were negative, which prevented him from the mourning that had been frozen until that moment.

The father had left a car, which had remained covered in his garage, so no one used it in over 10 years. The analyst used this object as a metaphor for what was frozen, and the patient could work differently on the relationship with his dead father, who was also dead inside him. Therefore, this prevented J from being a father to his own son. The analyst focused on the repression of representations linked to positive affects. She interpreted, for example, "It seems to me that today you talked about the love you feel for your father and the good he left in you."

The group, in complete agreement, proposed that during a whole period the analyst should place herself as a "new object," containing his cold, distant, and hostile stories. This was meant to promote a space of trust and a relationship of proximity, mainly as part of the transferential relationship, when the discourse became hostile towards the analyst.

2 What parts of the clinical material were not pointed out by the analyst? Would you consider another type of intervention or alternative hypothesis that might have been useful to the patient?

Sessions began once the analyst began to speak. In turn, the patient always asked to go to the bathroom before entering the office. This style had become a ritual, making it hard for the analyst to study these actions and look for a meaning in the affects that appeared in his actions.

Another thing observed by the group was the omission of sexuality and his relationship with the female figure and with the analyst in transference. This focus appeared clearly in a dream the patient had. It was a long dream, so only some parts are discussed: "I sort of had a lover . . . and at some point I gave her a kiss and we went down . . . and she asked me if I still was with that woman, my partner. . . . We went up and down a narrow path." The analyst's interventions were aimed at breaking down the dream into questions, omitting interventions that targeted the forbidden, incestuous childish sexuality that he kept repressed.

In another moment the patient said, "The contact with the semen: I ejaculated but not inside her; I went to the bathroom to wash my hands for fear that I could have sperm and thus get her pregnant." This way of telling the story in a stark way made it difficult for the analyst to find the right words to express the content of fantasies or fears that were typical of the mapping of his childish sexuality, which were deeply rooted rituals.

Members of the group only read the analyst's interventions, and finding that the analyst had intervened mostly in an interrogative way was revealing. This method made the group think that she was implicitly using a classic Freudian model, which promoted associations such as those that arise from dream analysis.

The group proposed an alternative mode to try to make the patient talk about his feelings. Therefore, instead of using an interrogative mode in relation to his thoughts, like "What do you think?," "What are you thinking about?," the analyst was asked to encourage his talking about his emotions: "How do you feel about this?" Considering that J was highly disconnected from his affects, the analyst's interventions further strengthened his rationalization mechanisms. The analyst was surprised by these observations, while at the same time perceived her difficulty in formulating interpretations that evoked and touched on unconscious content.

Final reflections

As opposed to the initial question—"What does the use of a methodology such as the 3-LM to discuss clinical material offer to analysts-in-training and to analysts who have completed their curricular training?"—we can say the following.

Addressing the analytical training, different authors (Altmann & Franch, 2006; Altmann et al., 2015) have pointed out that "the analytic function" is consolidated over the years through a construction of the analyst that is supported by the tripod: seminars, supervision, and personal analysis. In this construction of the analyst as such, which occurs during training, the analytical thinking achieved is emphasized.

In training, the "analytic function" is amplified and enriched when the group produces new outlooks that amplify the internal dialogue of the analyst with themselves and with their own clinical thinking and the one generated by the workgroup. This links personal theories with different theoretical frameworks, thus enabling dialogue from the most concrete clinical thinking to the most abstract.

However, this emphasis on the subject-in-training sometimes leaves the patient aside, yet the emphasis is key to methodologies such as the 3-LM. The model of the three levels allows for observation of external and internal relationships and psychic changes of different degrees and qualities.

The weight of the unconscious transmission, in groups or individually, should not leave aside inclusion of the working models that have been developed by the different working parties of the International Psychoanalytical Association and the Federation of Psychoanalytic Societies of Latin America. These group experiences provide a new perspective in training by establishing a third group view of an analytical process over long treatments.

We continue ratifying what the 3-LM offers. It provides the opportunity to analyze clinical material that spans several years with a protocol that invites reflecting analytically, with questions that look at separate dimensions of a psychoanalytic process, thus helping to locate aspects in which psychic changes were or were not produced (in the descriptive level and in the second level of the dimensions of change). Additionally, it enables the formation of alternative hypotheses that can promote delving into conflicting aspects of the patient and of the analytic relationship. Working with different levels of conceptualization allows the candidate to reconsider concepts with greater accuracy. The model strongly focuses on the patient, and how the patient has benefitted over the analytic process or how the process could be modified, by delving into the material and establishing a more rigorous structure.

Thus, we find that "mini partial theories" arise from analysis of the analyst's interpretations, which are directly linked to the problems presented by the patient. This is what we mean by "clinical thinking."

Therefore it is enriching for the analytic training to have these methodologies introduced, following what Bohleber (2012) and de León and Bernardi (2005) claim about the importance of the free circulation of alternative ideas and their discussion in a respectful, critical, and creative environment.

The Frankfurt experience

Part 3: The Three-Level Model for Observing Patient Transformations: The Frankfurt Psychoanalytical Institute—Marianne Leuzinger-Bohleber, Lisa Kallenbach-Kaminski, Rosemarie Kennel, Anju Labuhn, Luise Laezer, Susanne Landsiedel-Anders, Sebastian Ohlmes, Gertrud Reerink, Sarah Römisch, Jörg Scharff, Karin Schwind, Erwin Sturm, and Heike Westenberger-Breuer

Institutional context

The question of how psychoanalysis educates its next generation is as old as psychoanalysis itself. After the IPA decision that in the future, three to five weekly sessions in psychoanalytic training will be accepted, many controversies have been rekindled (see, inter alia Bohleber, 2019).

In 2000, under the presidency of David Tuckett, the European Psychoanalytical Federation (EPF) initiated groups to discuss and optimize training and exchange among psychoanalysts of different traditions and cultures. After 10 years, a mid-term review was carried out at the EPF Congress in Copenhagen (2011) to decide which groups should be continued. The Clinical Comparison Methods (CCM) groups, for example, used detailed reports of psychoanalytic sessions to examine how psychoanalysts work with their patients, what specific treatment techniques they use, what models they have in mind, and how they are influenced by their conscious and unconscious identifications with specific psychoanalytic groups, concepts, etc. One of the most important results of the CCM groups, in my opinion (MLB), was that a new culture of mutual listening to each other was created. Instead of the unfruitful "wars of faith" about which psychoanalytic theory was "the best," "the true and only," it was now necessary to critically reflect together on the opportunities, but also the risks of theoretical pluralism in contemporary psychoanalysis.

In view of these achievements, I (MLB) proposed in a panel at the EPF conference in Copenhagen that this culture of mutual listening and understanding in times of theoretical, clinical, and scientific pluralism should now be made fruitful for our central concern in psychoanalytic treatment: to focus on the changes of patients in psychoanalysis. As important as the analysts, their theories, and treatment techniques are, psychoanalysis is not an end in itself. Ultimately they always serve the desire to initiate lasting psychological transformations desired by our patients (Leuzinger-Bohleber & Arnold, 2020). Only because patients are suffering and wish that they would feel better after psychoanalysis or psychoanalytic treatment do they seek us out. This also applies in a particularly challenging way to training cases.

The Project Committee on Clinical Observation of the IPA (formed in 2009) faced up to this complex task and developed the Three-Level Model for Observing Patient Transformations (3-LM) in the last nine years, which is presented in great detail in this volume (see also Altmann, 2014). The application of the 3-LM to observing patient transformations in international groups has become very popular among psychoanalysts in the IPA. On the one hand it is based on tried and tested forms of case discussion (supervision/interview) and, on the other hand, an invitation to systematize discussions and assessments within a formal framework. It offers the possibility for psychoanalysts with different theoretical orientations to refer to common criteria.

Our group in Frankfurt used these promising opportunities of the 3-LM in two different institutional contexts.

Supplement to the quantitative research in the LAC Depression Study

We used it as a supplement to the sophisticated quantitative research of the large outcome study, the LAC Depression Study, in which 252 cognitive-behavioural and psychoanalytic long-term treatment with chronically depressed patients have been investigated (see Leuzinger-Bohleber et al., 2019a, 2019b). With the help of the 3-LM we investigated the transformations in several psychoanalyses in detail and systematically in the weekly clinical conference. The 3-LM enabled us to conduct a series of single case studies to improve the quality of the narrative summaries of these treatments focusing on different aspects of the transformations of the patients. Some of these narrative case studies now will be published in *Was nur erzählt und nicht gemessen werden kann. . . .* [What can only be told and not measured. . .], edited by M. Leuzinger-Bohleber, U. Bahrke, and A. Negele (2020).

Tool for understanding transformation processes in training cases at the Frankfurt Psychoanalytic Institute

Based on these inspiring clinical and research experiences in the frame of the LAC study, the idea was born to offer the 3-LM to a group of training candidates. The aim was to discover together if and how the 3-LM is suitable to discuss training cases systematically and creatively in a mixed group of candidates and training analysts. The aim was to examine in clinical psychoanalytical terms whether and how transformation takes place in the hope that the insights gained will prove helpful for the candidates involved.

Application of the 3-LM in psychoanalytic training

In the last three semesters, weekly evening sessions were held, in which about six candidates and four training analysts took part. After an introductory session in the 3-LM, one candidate presented one of her ongoing psychoanalyses in four sessions each. We discussed seven psychoanalyses. In the first session, the initial interviews, the health insurance report, and a psychoanalytic session from the initial phase were presented in detail, leading to the definition of "anchor points" (Bernardi, 2014, p. 8; i.e., central issues and conflicts) that are important for the patient, whose transformation, i.e., change or modification over the course of treatment, is to be studied. In the second session—each time after a short summary of the analytical process since the discussed session—a psychoanalytic session from a later phase—in the third session a recent psychoanalytic session—was discussed in detail. The fourth session served to discuss the transformations that had taken place with reference to the third level of the 3-LM.

Impressions of group members involved in working with the 3-LM

All members of the 3-LM group at FPI found the 3-LM experience an intense, enriching experience. The intensive study of detailed clinical material from the same psychoanalysis over four evenings proved to be worthwhile and expanded insight into conscious and unconscious dimensions of the analytical process. Although the detailed documentation of the often intensive and sometimes controversial group discussions was time-consuming, it resulted in a valuable report of the successive understanding of the clinical material. It proved to be helpful for the candidates as well as for the participating group members not to lose sight of the forest for the trees.

It took some time for the group to find a productive way to discuss Level 3 and the attempt to illuminate the transformations that had taken place from different theoretical perspectives. These discussions became increasingly fruitful. To mention just one example, discussing Level 3 of the third psychoanalysis, which we had discussed, the training analysts tried to apply a developmental-psychological, gender-specific approach, trauma-specific considerations, Kleinian object relationship theory, and a drive theory explanation to the same clinical material. It remains an open question whether this can offer the candidate a helpful orientation in times of theoretical pluralism, or whether it represents an excessive demand. One candidate described how she struggled in her treatment to avoid theoretical "top-down" views ("putting theories on top of each other"). The differentiation of the three levels of 3-LM is intended as an aid in dealing with this danger. First, an attempt is made to discuss transformations on a phenomenological level (Level 1). Level 2 is about individual dimensions of observation, which are to be described with clinical material, very concretely (e.g., looking at the changes in the patient's relationship with his external libidinal objects, his inner objects, his transference relationship with the psychoanalyst, etc.). Only in Level 3 is an attempt made to "play with the theories," in the sense of dealing with the richness of theories in contemporary psychoanalysis. Depending on the setting of the (theoretical) kaleidoscope, other structures become visible in the complexity of the clinical material.

One specific problem area should be mentioned briefly. One teaching analyst had feared that our seminar could lead to conflicts with the supervisors of the training cases. This concern was not justified. The 3-LM offer is intended as a supplement, not as an alternative to regular supervision and technical seminars within the psychoanalytic training. It is well known that the continuity and the holding function of a (responsible) supervisor for a training case is needed to provide a safe, holding, reflective "home base" in the sense of case-based learning. However, the downsides of such a personalized learning model have been the subject of repeated critical discussion within the IPA (e.g., by Otto Kernberg). The master–student relationship carries certain dangers, such as submission to authority, hindering one's own innovative and creative development, etc. It sometimes reminds one of religious as opposed to scientific institutions. The experiences in the small 3-LM group are especially interesting against this background, as they enabled the recurring experience that perceptions, perspectives, understanding of sense structures, etc., could be quite different among the four training analysts (as well as the candidates), sometimes complementing or contradicting each other, etc. However, it is always important to stress that the 3-LM discussions are about expanding psychoanalytic understanding in an open space of creative clinical thinking. Its aims are not evaluations and assessments! This is particularly important in difficult treatments: the responsibility for the treatment lies, of course, with the treating analyst and his or her supervisor!

We also discussed whether the great amount of time and intergenerational commitment is really worth it. In this context a modification of our approach in 2019/2020 proved to be useful: the four training analysts each committed to only four evenings (the discussion of one case). This limited the commitment and time of these colleagues. An additional advantage was that candidates lying on the couch of one of the training analysts could participate in those evenings where other training psychoanalysts were present.

It is also very important that the 3-LM is accepted as a regular component of psychoanalytic training, because today's candidates are very busy. Therefore it is also helpful for some candidates if they can use the 3-LM seminar as a direct and indirect preparation of their case presentation to conclude their analytical training.

The following is just one exemplary feedback from one of the candidates.

Making lived psychoanalysis tangible for the next generation—Luise Laezer

While even the best-case seminar, in which one presents one's own case once during the semester, remains an important experience, and the considerations coming from the group and from the lecturers refer mainly to the respective presented session, the 3-LM model seminar with four sessions per case offers the opportunity for an in-depth exchange, in which the entire treatment, from the beginning to the current phase of treatment, and even beyond that comes into view. This is something very special and valuable.

Not only was I able to experience what the training analysts were thinking clinically and conceptually about one specific session, I also had the opportunity to observe the different trains of thought of the experienced training analysts throughout the complete analysis of the treatment. I was able to feel how training analysts, drawing on their experience and including past and current cases, deal with the wealth of transference/counter-transference observations, how they would react professionally in difficult clinical situations, how they would "digest" them and embed them conceptually. I could observe that some working hypotheses have to be discarded, that it is always a challenge to acknowledge ignorance and that we analysts can nevertheless trust the analytical method, the "talking cure," again and again.

What was unusual about the exchange was the composition of the group. While the team teaching in normal clinical seminars of our psychoanalytical training with two, sometimes even three lecturers for 15 candidates is a great gain, the distribution of four training analysts and six candidates was almost a 1:1 supervision and felt like an authentic meeting of the generations at eye level. Throughout the two semesters of the 3-LM seminar in which I have participated, the hard work of the candidates in their treatments was recognized at every moment, which was a balm for the analytical psyche in training. My analytical superego also found relief in the two semesters, because it no longer pressed so hard for "the one correct" interpretation and "the one correct" theory, but increasingly enjoyed the variety of psychoanalytical concepts.

From the perspective of a candidate I can say that through the 3-LM seminar the lived and even suffered psychoanalysis, as a profession in its most diverse facets and its great moments, became tangible, and tangible for me. Just as good surgeons can only pass on their experience to the next generation in their joint practical work at the operating table, the 3-LM seminar enabled me to participate in such a practical transfer of psychoanalytic experience and experience. Many thanks to you, my dear teachers!

Notes

1 *Truco* (trick) is a card game from Río de la Plata, the most popular one in Uruguay, in which two individuals or teams compete against each other to gain points by beating the other's cards based on a given hierarchy and lying to fool their opponents.

2 Psychoanalytic Association of Uruguay. Three groups of 10–14 analysts and candidates. Clinical observation group organized by the Committee of Clinical Observation, the Education Committee, and the Scientific Committee. Levels 1 and 2 were developed over two sessions, and Level 3 was developed three months later during one session.

References

Altmann, M. (2014). *Time for change: Tracking transformations in psychoanalysis—The Three-Level Model*. London: Karnac.

Altmann, M., & Franch, N. (2006). La formación analítica y la actividad analítica profesional en América Latina [Analytic training and professional practice in Latin America]. Sub Comité de Investigación-Educación de FEPAL [FEPAL Training Research Sub Committee]. Unpublished.

Altmann, M., Marucco, N. Devoto, T., Andrade, A., Franco, G., Minuchin, L., Mion, C., Petrucci, J., Rojas Urrego, A., Yamhure, E., & Baptista Franca, J. (2015) ¿Cómo ven los analistas el futuro del psicoanálisis en América Latina? [How do analysts see the future of psychoanalysis in Latin America]. Comité de Educación de FEPAL [FEPAL Training Committee] Research. Presented at FEPAL Congress.

Bernardi, R. (2014). The Three-Level Model (3-LM) for observing patient transformations. In M. Altmann (Ed.), *Time for change: Tracking transformations in psychoanalysis—The Three-Level Model* (pp. 3–34). London: Karnac.

Bernardi, R. (2015). What kind of discipline is psychoanalysis? *International Journal of Psychoanalysis*, *96*, 731–754.

Bleger, J. (2012). Theory and practice in psychoanalysis: Psychoanalytic Praxis 1. *International Journal of Psychoanalysis*, *93*(4), 993–1003.

Bohleber, W. (2012). The use of public and of private implicit theories in the clinical situation. In J. Canestri (Ed.), *Putting theory to work: How are theories used in practice?* (pp. 79–81). London: Karnac.

Bohleber, W. (2019). Die Geschichte des Eiitington Modells und seine Bedeutung für die psychoanalytische Ausbildung. *Psyche – Zeitschrift für Psychoanalyse, 7*, 477–496.

Canestri, J. (2006). Implicit understanding of clinical material beyond theory. In J. Canestri (Ed.), *Psychoanalysis from practice to theory* (pp. 13–28). Chichester: John Wiley.

de León, B., & Bernardi, R. (2005). Contratransferencia y vulnerabilidad del analista [Analyst's counter-transference and vulnerability]. In S. Lewkowicz & C. Laks Eizirik (Eds), *Verdad, realidad y contribuciones Latinoamericanas al psicoanálisis* [*Truth, reality and Latin American contributions to psychoanalysis*] (pp. 23–41). Montevideo: International Psychoanalytic Library.

Leuzinger-Bohleber, M., & Arnold, S.E. (2020): Introduction: outcome research and the future of psychoanalysis. In M. Leuzinger-Bohleber, M. Solms, & S.E. Arnold (Eds), *Outcome research and the future of psychoanalysis: Clinicans and researchers in dialogue* (pp. 1–26). Abingdon: Routledge.

Leuzinger-Bohleber, M., Hautzinger, M., Fiedler, G., Keller, W., Bahrke, U., Kallenbach, L., & Küchenhoff, H. (2019a). Outcome of psychoanalytic and cognitive-behavioural long-term therapy with chronically depressed patients: A controlled trial with preferential and randomized allocation. *Canadian Journal of Psychiatry, 64*(1), 47–58.

Leuzinger-Bohleber, M., Kaufhold, J., Kallenbach, L., Negele, A., Ernst, M., Keller, W., & Beutel, M. (2019b). How to measure sustained psychic transformations in long-term treatments of chronically depressed patients: Symptomatic and structural changes in the LAC Depression Study of the outcome of cognitive-behavioural and psychoanalytic long-term treatments. *International Journal of Psychoanalysis, 100*(1), 99–127.

Leuzinger-Bohleber, M., & Bahrke, U. l., & Negele, A. (Eds). (2020). Was nur erzählt und nicht gemessen werden kann. . . . Veränderungsprozesse in Psychoanalysen der LAC Depressionsstudie [What can only be told and not measured. . . . Change processes in psychoanalysis of the LAC Depression study]. Giessen: Psychosozial Verlag.

Marucco, N. C. (1999). Las neurosis hoy: en las vías de acceso a las "zonas psíquicas." In N. C. Marucco (Ed.), *Cura analítica y transferencia. De la represión a la desmentida*. Buenos Aires: Amorrortu.

Sandler, J. (1983). Reflections on some relations between psychoanalytic concepts and psychoanalytic practice. *International Journal of Psychoanalysis, 64*, 35–45.

Experiences in progress

Part 4: A Buenos Aires experience with candidates of the Argentine Society of Psychoanalysis—Liliana Fudin de Winograd

Introduction

For a few years we've been implementing the 3-LM in the Argentine Society of Psychoanalysis' (SAP) Training Institute, as we consider it a significant tool to help our candidates (psychoanalysts-in-training) deepen and expand their capacities for observation in their practice.

In 2019 we realized that it would be impossible to have all participants use our original format of two consecutive meetings of four to eight hours. We couldn't burden our students with 12 additional hours of training, given that they worked long hours, spent significant time in training, and had family commitments.

For this reason, we arranged a format of two five-hour sessions, one in May and one in October. For both we used the same clinical material: a first interview consisting of the candidate's notes, and two sessions, one before the patient completed her first year of therapy and one when the patient began her third year. We used transcripts for the latter two sessions.

We focused on Level 1 in the first five-hour session, and on Levels 2 and 3 in the second session. Most of the psychoanalysts-in-training already knew the 3-LM because they'd worked with it in prior years. We also invited two experienced SAP psychoanalysts to participate, one in discussions at Level 1 and one in discussions at Levels 2 and 3. We shared the clinical material with them, and they joined the group after the candidates had discussed the material by themselves for two hours. For Level 1, we asked the expert to focus on phenomenological aspects. For Levels 2–3, we asked the expert to adapt the 3-LM as appropriate.

We invited these two experienced psychoanalysts because the 3-LM coordinators thought it important that our candidates learn from psychoanalysts who emphasized observation of what was happening during a session. Both had worked with David Liberman, who had included a focus on the linguistic aspects of the clinical material, based on the hypothesis that changes in the patient's linguistics corresponded to changes in the patient's psychical structure. Besides, both experts had made unique contributions to the understanding of the interactions between patient and therapist.

Conclusion

The experience led to significant insights for all participants. We realized how important the coordinator (or coordinating function) was to help students categorize their observations, as categorizing observations improves the analyst's ability to follow and understand the patient's transformations.

LEVEL 1

The observations made by the candidates as a group agreed with those of the experienced guest analyst. The latter remarked that students' observations that might have seemed unrelated were delicately intertwined, and such intertwining created what could be considered, epistemologically, a "coherent" empirical understanding. He also emphasized how important the therapist's phenomenological descriptions were when integrated into the interpretations, for the patient to begin to understand his own problems.

LEVEL 2

The expert asked for more clinical material to better understand the candidate's work. We gave him transcripts of two sessions that took place in between the two sessions, the transcripts of which we had already provided. We shared the additional two transcripts with the candidates in the Level-2 meeting.

At this level, we coordinators didn't refer to the questions in the 3-LM protocol but observed that the group discussion answered most of them spontaneously. The experienced guest analyst, also an experienced educator, explained how to diagnose and evaluate a therapeutic process, demonstrating with examples from his own observations regarding the clinical material discussed.

We conclude that both meetings using the variation on the model enriched and consolidated our candidates' competences in observing patients' transformations.

The Peruvian experience

Contribution of the 3-LM Model to the psychoanalytic training in the SPP—Mayela Falvy

The opportunity to conduct a Three-Level Model group with the analysts-in-training of the Institute of the Peruvian Psychoanalytic Society was promoted by Oscar Rey de Castro, the scientific secretary of the institute, and there was a very good attendance.

The 3-LM group experience had a variety of aims: importantly, to make the model more widely available, especially with respect to its objective to refine observational skills in the clinical work of the candidates, and more broadly, to develop their imaginations and creativity in the psychoanalytic field.

From the beginning, the group was both interested and perplexed. The clinical material was handed out in advance and raised concerns and also curiosity about the numbered lines, in accordance with the model. The importance of considering the different phases of the analysis (beginning, middle, end or recent) in order to visualize the changes or absence of changes that occurred during the treatment was discussed.

The clinical material was read without interruption, with the goal that the candidates would be engaged by what they perceived, and the effect was to arouse a certain unsettledness, since analytic material is usually read in paragraphs, with pauses for discussion and understanding of certain lines in the text. It was possible to continue without interruption, and that modified the group's way of attending and analytical listening.

The candidates' contributions took place spontaneously and highlighted the content of the material that aroused interest. Little by little the connections between the lines in the sessions were made and observations and comments arose freely among the group. There was no difficulty in getting into the task; although it was important to present the model as a very valuable kind of work to expand analytic openness and deepen clinical thinking, it was also to contribute to the enrichment of the candidate's individual process in becoming an analyst. It was pointed out that the experiences and the concerns arising while working with the 3-LM would contribute to the candidate's incorporation work as psychoanalysts of the Peruvian Psychoanalytic Society.

As the group work went on, the commitment to the task became stronger. Comments and open contributions flowed among the participants; they entered dialogue, making references to the lines in the material, showing consistencies and inconsistencies with ideas on difficulties and change being discussed. Although some comments referred to analytic authors and theories, these were translated in order to return to the observations and creative reflections that were arising. There was a natural affective tone, and differences were respected. The analyst-in-training who presented the case maintained her role, intervening or not intervening, according to what was presented in the clinical material. It was interesting to witness the active participation and natural exchanges among the group members, which continued during the breaks.

I believe that the 12 hours of work over two days motivated all the analysts-in-training. Throughout the work, the group maintained interest in the way change happened in the patient, her expressions and verbalizations, and also kept highlighting the dispositions and abilities of the candidate to stay with the difficult moments that the case offered. With respect to the transference and counter-transference, there were variations and developments in the discussions, which modified the group's perception of the patient. The observations evolved from a generic view based on the symptoms, towards recognition of the presence of a person in deep anguish, with unresolved conflicts, and the urgent demand to be tolerated in the real world.

The articulations of the analysts-in-training also underwent transformations. The language evolved and became more open and colloquial, expressing affects and emotions, and even doubts and uncertainties were shared with curiosity and commitment.

It was a wonderful experience that generated positive feedback. It is also important to notice that the intensity of the training seems to make it difficult to increase the frequency of this kind of encounter. I would take this into account for future projects.

Chapter 11

A dialogue between 3-LM presenters and moderators

Margaret Ann Fitzpatrick Hanly and Marina Altmann de Litvan, with Ricardo Bernardi, Natalia Goungian, Mette Hvalstad, Bernadette Kovach, Luisa Pérez Suquilvide, Pilar Raffo de Lavalle, and Beth Steinberg

Introduction—Margaret Ann Fitzpatrick Hanly and Marina Altmann de Litvan

The moderators of 3-LM groups have been impressed with how important it has been to work with psychoanalysts while they were in the process of writing a brief history and thinking about selecting sessions to present to a 3-LM group. The analyst was asked to send us detailed verbatim material from the first (or very early) sessions, two sessions from a middle phase of the analysis, and two from a late (or recent) phase of the analysis. The moderator and reporter read the first draft and had a discussion with the analyst via Skype, asking for clarifications and beginning to observe major difficulties and points of change. The analyst could then decide to bring a different session or a counter-transference reflection showing an additional important aspect of the analysis.

This first stage in setting up a 3-LM weekend group gave us the opportunity to get to know analysts and patients from different countries, languages, histories, and contexts. Our discussions before and during the group experience increased curiosity about different ways of practising psychoanalysis, both in the moderators and in the presenting analysts.

The dialogues with presenters have been fruitful, as we learn more about analytic traditions, differences, and similarities, and get a sense of which papers and theories are important to each analyst. Also, in working with the detailed clinical materials, we have been able to identity weaknesses in our training. For example, we could see that analysts (moderators as well) seldom used crucial information from the first sessions of the analysis or the assessment interviews that were effective in formulating the case. The moderators found that in some cases the analyst did not keep in mind questions that arose from the history or accepted just what was in the analytic session without reflecting on certain life situations that appeared quite traumatic to the listener/participants but had not been in the foreground in the analyst's mind.

Presenters evaluated their experience in a questionnaire, and almost all presenters have been very satisfied. The editors decided to ask presenters to send later reflections on their experience in order to include them in this book:

> We need to assess the strengths of the evidence or checks that arise from clinical observations, but also must therefore decide on which aspects of the material can be relied on to provide them. This involves examining the omissions or biases that limit the value of the evidence.

The presenters articulated their reflections and we place them in a dialogue with moderators' comments.

Presenters' comments—Natalia Goungian, Mette Hvalstad, Bernadette Kovach, Luisa Pérez Suquilvide, Pilar Raffo de Lavalle, and Beth Steinberg

Preparing the 3-LM clinical text in the months before the meeting

One presenter writes,

> During the weeks before the 3-LM group met, I and my clinical material were prepared through discussion and clarification on Skype calls with the moderator and the reporter. This working through was essential for me to feel safe presenting verbatim sessions to a group of analysts.

Another presenter observes,

> In my view, to prepare a clinical material to present in a 3LM group is to begin the very exercise proposed by this model: to recognize, in taking a "third look" at one's work, that the model explores the longitudinal changes, observes the analysis at intervals in the process, at transversal cuts, at certain moments, certain sessions. In preparing the material, I chose to observe the process through the lens of the transferential moments that I had lived as intense emotional experiences. I tracked the metaphors expressing the patient's affective states and those involving the analytic field, and the way they changed. Contrasting my ways of thinking with different perspectives in the group expanded my understanding of the patient´s mental functioning and changes in it, in the course of the analytical process.

A moderator comments,

> The analyst's process in preparing and selecting sessions is important. The model recognizes a "bias" in having the presenter choose the sessions that he or she thinks best demonstrate initial difficulties and points of change. A dialogue ensues over the next months with the moderator, reporter, and then the group, through which the analyst gains some clarity about specific changes not clearly seen before. A presenter may say during the preparation stage, "But I left out something really important," which is then reflected on. We encourage the presenter to bring very detailed typed verbatim sessions: the patient's words and the analyst's interpretations. We ask that presenters remove any theoretical comments that may have been included. The clinical material is sent (via encrypted message) to all members of the group about two weeks before the meeting.

The participants receive a line-numbered transcript with all sessions, prior to the group discussion, along with a series of questions that guide the description and identification of the transformations and the main diagnostic dimensions of change. Although the transformations are observed through a transversal look at sessions selected at intervals in the analysis, because they come from the first phases and throughout an analytic process, the experience is of a longitudinal look.

The analyst needs to feel safe but also to be authentic and open-minded in presenting this kind of analytic material. We ask the analyst to find sessions that convey periods of the analysis in which there were typical problems for the patient or the analyst.

In accordance with the objectives and methodology of this model, the preparation of the clinical material and the group's receiving it in advance are crucial steps.

Presenters' thinking on anchor points

One presenter who is also a researcher writes,

> Using the Three-Level Model as a form of research and as a method of understanding clinical material using anchor points as a guide lends itself easily to creating a greater volume of research that evidences transformations that occur in psychoanalysis. . . . The effect on my work of being a presenter for the 3-LM Clinical Observation Group was that I began to use the 3-LM model outside of the clinical setting. Using concepts of the 3-LM model in a research class with candidates increased their curiosity about our work as observational

research. They also found the method to be helpful when considering their written 6-month summaries and how to choose material that demonstrated their own as well as their analysand's growth. The concept of using anchor points to determine areas of transformation is being incorporated into a course that focuses on case writing for graduation.

Presenting more than once

Two analysts presented the same analysis more than once, in different 3-LM groups in local, regional, or IPA meetings:

One writes,

> I presented the analysis of my patient twice, the first time in a national group and some months later in an international group. The second time was more comfortable, possibly because I knew more about the method. Both groups were guided by the same moderator, leading the group discussions using the Three-Level Model thoroughly, to bring out the phenomenological description of transformations, the dimensions of change and hypotheses on links between interventions and observed changes.

Another writes,

> I have had a unique and wonderful experience presenting using the 3-LM model. I presented three times—first with a group of local analysts, then in Boston at the IPA meetings, and then in Austin during the APsaA meetings. With each presentation I expanded the number of years that I presented, not only in terms of time going forward, but also earlier in the treatment (even before we were meeting 4x/ week). My experience was that each time I presented, listened to, and participated in this guided conversation with colleagues, the appreciation of my patient's dynamics, as well as my analytic work with my patient deepened. It was an amazing experience to present the same case multiple times with different groups and experience the analysis deepen each time.

The moderator comments,

> For the moderators, it was important to have follow-up conversations with the analyst about the patient and the analysis. Usually as analysts we do not have the chance to experience a follow up on our

> patients This is an area in assessing change that needs further development. The 3-LM is the most complete and updated tool (outside of systematic research) for studying patients' transformations during long periods of analysis.

In discussing the third level, participants are asked to consider alternative hypotheses on the nature of the difficulties and changes, such as to look of evidence of the patient's subjective experience of her illness or the transgenerational transmission of trauma from which the patient is suffering, unrecognized by the analyst and the patient. Participants explore how the changes in the patient's mental functioning have been brought about, what interpretations have helped with regulation of their impulses, affects, or narcissism, or have led to an increased capacity for symbolization and mentalization of their problems.

Presenting clinical material: Usefulness of the model's methodologies

The 3-LM's use of evidence from the clinical verbatim text

One presenter writes,

> In part it is the method that promotes deepening. I have presented cases many times in groups, but the 3-LM ensures that the group will function as a workgroup. The method in Level 1 of requiring participants to provide evidence (referring to a line number in the text and reading from the verbatim material) for any statement that they make about the case provides a structure that ensures rigour. It creates a tight working experience with people thinking together about a case without anyone being able to privilege and impose their own theory on the material. This also ensures a level playing field among the group members; no matter how brilliant anyone's formulation, it has to be grounded in the text. The group builds upon Level 1, so that more abstract formulations come out of the grounded work of Level 1, and again this ensures a kind of rigour that is unusual in psychoanalytic groups.

Another presenter observes,

> The responses from the participants were accompanied by references to lines in the written verbatim text. This documentation done in a focused and systematic way made it easy for me to follow the evaluation process in detail and it did not feel too overwhelming.

Oral transmission of the patient

One of our presenters says,

> The group works as a sounding board in which the oral transmission and the reading of the material by the analyst is central to giving life to the analytical scene. This plays a particular role, complementary to the written text, because it gives participants the chance to integrate affects transmitted by the analyst's reading, and to compare this with reading the text on their own before the group meets. As with music, the voice of the analyst with its tones and rhythms introduces us to non-verbal aspects in the analytic verbatim material, reflecting (or not) aspects of the patient at different intervals in the process, vividly conveying to us the affective climate of transferences and counter-transferences.

Working with a moderator using the 3-LM's approach to observations on change and to clinical thinking

One presenter writes, "It was clear that a tight leadership by the moderator who was able to keep in mind the tasks of the group and to keep the members on track was more generative than free discussion."

Another presenter agrees:

> For me it was important to have an experienced instructor who focused on the procedures and principles of the model and kept the group participants following the method. This made it easier for me to observe and to absorb the comments and group discussion.

A presenter reports on the stress of being presenter: "Some discussions were stressful and ended quickly. During the group discussion, it would be very valuable to have time to write down important comments or to record them for further processing."

Use of 3-LM by presenters with ongoing cases to further understand their patient

One presenter writes about the traumatic experience that came to light in the group:

> One area that the group helped me take in more deeply was the intergenerational transmission of trauma in her family. At the beginning of the treatment, the extent of her dissociation, the degree of risk, as well as the amount of concern that this generated in me strongly suggested

> to me that there was some kind of repetition of trauma that was occurring, but it wasn't until more recently (and with the group's help) that I really explored her history several generations back. I learned more about her mother's history as the daughter of Holocaust survivor parents who lived in hiding in the woods during the war, her mother's subsequent affairs and two subsequent children with other men, her biological grandmother and grandfather's separation and her grandfather's remarriage, and the fact that her mother never saw her own biological mother again. I also learned more about her father's large, wealthy, Indian family, and the tremendous trauma that marrying someone from a different cultural and religious background caused in the family. However, none of this history nor the feelings about any of these painful events on either side of the family have ever been discussed in her family.

Another presenter writes,

> I found the process of looking at my work using the Three-Level Model to be at once challenging and satisfying. Observing both my patient and my interventions while writing the case material for group consideration was useful in making self-observations that I had not been aware of prior to writing the material.

One presenter reports new perspectives and new helpful formulations:

> New recognition from the group discussion of the patient's more primitive functioning leads me not to rush with the processes, not to demand, although sometimes, this is very difficult. Another important understanding, which the 3-LM group helped me with, concerns the relationship with the other. I recognized that I did not feel the patient had empathy for "the other," yet I saw that she can use others to feel accompanied or to have models to imitate.

Using the 3-LM with the group to understand the patient from new perspectives

One presenter writes,

> The model brings in an argumentation from observations to hypotheses and as long I agreed with the observations, it was very easy to follow the hypotheses of change. It is a valuable situation to experience colleagues doing research on my work and discussing the process of change. The method in the model gave me as a presenter a distance

to the material which made it easier to take in the different comments and perspectives.

A presenter to a pre-Congress of a Regional Congress, with participants from different analytic cultures, writes,

> The 3-LM helped me think about the different views of the participants, with several minds approaching the material. I could identify with some approaches more than with others. Some perspectives and clinical approaches were very different from mine but actually gave me new ways to approach the patient. It became clear to me that my patient has a structural deficit and I could strongly agree with this diagnosis. I recognized that with him we were at a very primary stage with a lack of ego-object differentiation, where the invasion of the other's mind is normalized and is represented in the analytic setting.

Another presenter writes,

> The horizontal perspective of the 3-LM, which looks across the years of an analysis, opens up a wide angle on the whole analytic process and its most striking characteristics, including blind spots, which remain in place over time. The observations of the 3-LM group concerning my patient highlighted both the metaphor of the analyst (the patient "on the edge of an abyss") and the lack of interpretations addressing the patient's sexuality. Several months after the group met, it was possible to hypothesize a link between the sense of an abyss and the absence of references to sexuality; insight into the link was triggered by a dream the analyst had.

The 3-LM as a unique kind of clinical research

A presenter from a scientific research background writes,

> Coming from a background in clinical chemistry, I have often found the idea of psychoanalysis as a research method consistent with my understanding of all clinical work as both aiding a patient, and as a method of observation and learning. . . . The 3-LM model looks at the intricate interactions of a dyad with changing hypotheses based on an increasingly detailed understanding of the individual and the associative links that are changed and created throughout the process. . . . The use of anchor points allows the observers to gain knowledge of the processes that result in change, in those that do not lend to change, and for the clinician, a language to speak with analysands.

Moderator's comment:

> It is possible to study a patient's transformations during the course of one session or through a long-term analysis. The latter is the path taken by the 3-LM. In discussion groups guided by the 3-LM, although participants may have different theoretical approaches, a common clinical ground develops through shared resonance with the clinical material. This is clearly observable in the first-level discussion. In the third-level discussion, it is also evident that the fruitful communication takes place at the level of implicit theories and operational models of the participants, in spite of their theoretical differences.

Clinical observation groups promote a participant-observer research attitude. Participants develop a sensitivity to meaningful unconscious material through participation in the shared resonance with other members of the group and with the analyst (Level 1); a critical conceptualization of clinical phenomena through Level 2 discussion; comparison of alternative hypotheses and interpretative strategies, and reflection about foci and mechanisms of change and testing clinical hypothesis through the analysis of the patient's evolution, combining prospective and retrospective (*après-coup, nachträglich*) perspectives. A new 3-LM discussion of a case after months or years checks the confirmation of hypotheses (predictive validity).

Ongoing gains from presenting

One presenter writes,

> The impact of this kind of working group on me was far-reaching. As psychoanalysts we mostly work alone in our offices. Sometimes we present our work to a consultant or a colleague for consultation; occasionally we present to a group of colleagues. It was profound to have a group of people spend over 10 hours immersed in the material from an analysis and over time have the experience of this group come to understand the patient and the work of the analysis. This experience made me feel deeply accompanied in a way that is extremely unusual, and it is a feeling that has stayed with me, not only vis-à-vis the patient I presented to the group, but in all my work with my patients.

As a result of added formulations, one presenter writes,

> The 3-LM group helped me to see (at Level 2) that there is also a psychopathic dimension in the patient's way of functioning, even though this is not an essential aspect of the patient. I also recognized the idea

> of a "narcissistic suffering" in my patient, with serious difficulties in his psychic development. Importantly in reflecting with the group, I realized that in the counter-transference I sometimes feel trapped in his speech and in a feeling of impotence both in him and in me.

Interpreting sexuality and triangulation

One presenter writes,

> She began to emotionally take in the significance of how she has used sex to get love and the sad awareness that she has never really had a real spontaneous sexual feeling with another person. With this, she has been able to perceive many more subtle feelings in the analysis around small disruptions, impingements, and the pressure that is always there to be precocious. The group noticed her beginning to show more triadic and sexual anxieties.

Becoming more rigorous in assessing change and no change yet

One presenter is able to use her observation of "no change yet":

> Nonetheless, although my patient has made many important internal changes, the smoothing pull is always there. It continues to assert itself again and again in the treatment; just as we open things up and encounter uncertainty, messiness, and pain, the next thing we know, she gets on top of it, tames it, smoothes it, dampens her feelings down, and makes her experiences meaningless, unreal, and vague. We are still dealing with this dynamic now.

Part VI

Clinical observation groups and the psychoanalysis of children

Chapter 12

Observing transformations and interventions in a child analysis through the 3-LM

The case of a 5-year-old girl

Marina Altmann de Litvan, Griselda Revella, and Patricia Singer

Introduction—Marina Altmann de Litvan

This section presents the clinical observation of children using the 3-LM by the IPA Clinical Observation Committee. The method was adapted for this stage of development by Altmann de Litvan, Miller, and Bernardi, and already presented in our first book, *Time for Change: Tracking Transformations in Psychoanalysis—The Three-Level Model* (2014).

Here clinical cases are presented that have been observed using the model, along with some reflection upon it.

Several childhood aspects were key in this process: the role of play, the influence of interpersonal factors, family, etc.

In this second book, we thought it interesting to present two examples of patients that—in the clinical material—reflect the evidence on the transformations they underwent during their analyses. One case shows in detail the work on different levels on a 5-year-old girl. The second is the case of a 5-year-old boy who lost his mother at a very young age.

Observing transformations and interventions in a child analysis[1] through the 3-Level Model: The case of a 5-year-old girl—Marina Altmann de Litvan, Griselda Revella, and Patricia Singer

Introduction

This chapter is about the use of a version of the Three-Level Model for Observing Patient Transformations (3-LM) designed for children. It was formulated by Marina Altmann de Litvan, Delfina Miller, and Ricardo Bernardi (2014) and published in *Time for Change: Tracking Transformations in Psychoanalysis—The Three-Level Model.*[2]

The model explores whether analytic intervention fosters intrapsychic, intersubjective, and structural transformations, taking into account the patient's stage of development.

In this section, we will describe the application of the model to clinical material of a girl in analysis from 5 to 9 years old. To apply the model, we selected clinical vignettes capturing different moments of her analysis.

We used the 3-LM as a guide, forming a working group to observe and evaluate the analytic process and possible transformations.

The girl was in analysis starting with two weekly sessions during the first three years, and one weekly session during her last year of analysis.

Introduction to the patient

Lorena, aged 5 years and 5 months, was referred to the analyst by her school because she was having a hard time getting along with her teacher and peers, displayed markedly oppositional behaviour, and was not open to learning.

When she was 3 years old, her parents were referred to a specialist because Lorena's teacher observed that she was flapping her arms, walking on her toes, couldn't step firmly on the floor, and avoided eye contact.

Concerned with Lorena's oppositional behaviour in school, the parents came to see the analyst. They choose to sit on the same couch, squeezing next to each other and leaving the other couch empty. They feel overwhelmed and lost and say, "None of the strategies ever worked," referring to Lorena's constant arguing with her parents.

The parents say that Lorena is unlike her older siblings, who did not cause any problems growing up, and the father says that it would be "impossible to uncover one in order to cover the other," when he refers to her constant attention-seeking behaviour.

The mother, anguished, asks herself what she can do to help her daughter. She describes aspects of her own life, a hostile relationship, and much rivalry with her mother and sisters—a chain of women in which she feels diminished.

The mother describes her past and how she was able to get through her childhood "doing whatever she could and without therapy." She seems to project it in her daughter, setting off a permanent tension between the intrusion and the absence of libido.

During the parents' narrative, the child is lost, without a name; an empty space is marked by the empty couch, to such an extent that, when the analyst needs to refer to the child, it is hard for her to remember her name. It feels as if the parents bring a dark shadow into the room with them. In response, the analyst did intense parallel work with the parents during the child's treatment.

When Lorena was 3, a series of traumatic family events occurred, and the girl was "thrown in school for various hours per day," according to the mother.

Since the initial sessions, Lorena shows not only how fragile but also how resourceless she is. When the analyst first meets Lorena, her rigid body, hypertonia, and dark look in her eyes stand out. She is short and slim, has a robot-like walk, a hoarse voice, and dark hair. Everything about her projects darkness.

In view of the above, the working group set out to explore Lorena's clinical material, applying the 3-LM, starting at a descriptive level, continuing with a second level to identify the main dimensions of the transformations, following with a third level testing the explanatory hypotheses of transformation. At each level, the group explored what transformations occurred in each of the points considered.

Level I: Phenomenological description of the transformations

The 3-LM poses a series of questions for this level, and the working group selected several for discussion: Which parts of the clinical material have special resonance within the participants of the clinical observation group regarding the transformation? How does the patient use her own mind and body during the session? Are there changes in the answer to these questions in view of the intensity of transference?

There are different anchor points (lines of force, as named by Marta Nieto, 1965) that capture complex problems in the psychic functioning, such as play, fears, fantasies of madness and death, body, and family interactions.

By applying the 3-LM, analysts can go back to the original hypotheses explaining central issues explicit or implicit in the points, moving back and forth between earlier and later sessions. By exploring these lines of force, we can better understand their dynamic meanings and vicissitudes in later phases of analysis.

Analysis of play

In the version for child patients, the 3-LM emphasizes the role of play, since it is a natural form of expression for the patient, as well as a valuable means of exchange with the analyst, where the patient displays desires, anxieties, fantasies, defences, and object relations. Not only can it be used to evaluate the patient's development level, abilities, and personality organization, it is fundamentally through play that we will foster the growth and emotional development of the child. Sexual drives, knowledge drives, infant sexual theories, and expression through play are clearly linked and displayed in a pleasant act, compromising the body during the enactment (Freud, 1905). Their nature allows us to understand the dynamic level of conflicts and structural aspects of the organization of the psychic apparatus. Their creative display separates them from the fixedness of the symptom (Freud, 1908).

Since it is an activity driven by desire, it allows the child to play out a script in which it displays unconscious dynamics without losing the commitment of the id with a reality that nurtures it and that they transform. Playing is therefore an expression of the psychic work that reveals and leads to structuring. It is a link between the hallucinatory realization of desires and the realization of desire by an examination and modification of reality, in that passage, never completely achieved, that goes from the reality principle to the pleasure principle (Volinski de Hoffnung et al., 1986). It was by precisely focusing on the study of play that Melanie Klein (1962) based a large part of her theories about the development of mental functioning, the nature of infant psyche, focusing on the close contact between conscious and unconscious anxieties, fantasies, and defences.

A child's play displays projection, elaboration, and unloading, so we emphasize the need to interpret the child's play. In order to do so, we play with the child and for the child, in transference, enabling the symbolic repair of internal objects and of the representation of the child's self. The interpretation, in turn, favours the display of the game, as it relieves the child's effort to withhold repression by helping to synthesize and integrate the different contents. The close relationship between fantasies and structuring allow us to influence mental organization through analysis.

By playing and interpreting play we are able to modify the fantasies about internal and external objects and the anxieties and defences attached to them. Thereby, we can generate a transformation in the child's functioning. We agree with Winnicott that, in order to carry out infant analysis, the analyst must know how to play, and the patient must be able to play (referred to by Volinski de Hoffnung et al., 1986). The play that takes place during analysis in that intermediate space between the analyst and the patient is a valuable creation for analyst and patient. Its structuring condition, especially of play that occurs during treatment, is the reason we focus on the analyst's observation, not only to understand the child but also, in this case, to evaluate the analytic process and the patient's development.

Communication during child sessions occurs mainly through action and play, sometimes accompanied with language. Even when action and play imply different levels of symbolization, we can identify a sequence tied to unconscious fantasies that goes from the more corporal expressions linked to release and exploration to other levels of increased symbolization.

This "making" is a precursor to thought, and this display of action and play allow the analyst to observe the child's functioning and evaluate changes.

One aspect of the analysis that stood out for the working group was the patient's type of play. On this subject, Paulina Kernberg (1996) asks some important questions. Is it age-appropriate? Are there changes in the type of play throughout the process? What themes does the child develop? What affects prevail? What kind of relationship is established with the analyst during play?

Play in this analytic process varied from symbolic to concrete body expressions.

The analyst explains:

> I realized that it was hard for her to start playing. For a long time, Lorena would begin saying, "I'm not sure what I want to play with." I felt that the freedom to choose a play and to use a space to play made Lorena uncomfortable. It was new to her. Later, she became obsessed with classifying things by size, ordering different spaces, and designating a particular space for each animal. The excessive attention paid to the smaller animals attracts my attention, and I wonder if it was her way of showing me her subjective experience of feeling very diminished, lost, and without a place.

Of all the animals, a small pig became her favourite object. In every session she worried about losing it. She says,

P: *Not again! Things got complicated with the cow and lion. . . . All the cows are mixed up. I'm going to line them up, so they look tidier and they don't fall down. The little yellow cow will go last. Things got a little complicated. The little elephants in front because they're so small.*

A: *You are trying to arrange the places in your family. This worries you a lot.*

P: *Yes, in my little head. My little head thinks a lot about what I need to do. This small one goes last, no, the mother last. And I'm not sure what to do with the shark. I'm going to think about it, in front of the crocodile, that takes the places. Since it's so small, small things, very small things, I mean very small things, very small, get lost. . . . Yes, I'm scared I'm going to lose my favourite toys because that's how small things get lost, or the tiles will open up and they'll fall through.*

Here Lorena shows clearly how she uses her mind and body during the session. The analyst's interpretative focus is on providing order for the child's confusion. Lorena says that her little head is full of complications as she tries to play. When she does, there is danger, mix-ups, and falls.

She seems to be able to put her confusion and fragility into words and she starts showing some of her important resources.

The narrative continues:

P: *Yes, the words have a shiny road. The words are here: book, table, food. I need to go to the bathroom to go poop. . . . The small ones are driving me crazy. . . . I need to go poop.*

A: *Perhaps poop is a way to show me the awful things you feel inside.*

The working group observes how her play expresses the strength of a pre-Oedipal sexuality, both oral and anal.

We believe that there are moments of much anguish, where the amount of symbolic play decreases and the child acts out her inner experiences.

Likewise, separating herself from the feces refers to distances that can be "illuminated" with language. Perhaps she feels that what she loses in letting go of her feces can be recovered with the "luminous" words she receives from her analyst.

Of the two levels that she uses to express her losses, verbal and action, we emphasize the following: "I would like to play what I never saw and what I always saw," as an auspicious sign of transference that brings to mind Christopher Bollas's phrase "the unthought known" (1987).

She says,

P: *I make a lot of noise because I don't like school. . . . Come on, help me build a house. No, instead, costumes for animals. One had to be the wolf, better yet dogs, better there's a girl, no, a monster. . . . I turned into a little pig, oink, oink. Do you want to jump in the mud with me? (Let's play that we're little pigs lying in the mud).*

Lorena stands up and says, "I'm full of bananas; the bananas are falling, the bananas are on my head."

A: *You're very worried. You don't know how your new teacher will greet you, but you're neither a little pig, nor a boy with bananas; you're a beautiful girl!*

P: *I'm going to draw before leaving . . . a girl.*

A: *A girl just like you! With a skirt, long hair.*

P: *Yes, with ornaments. . . . Keep it and take a photo of it.*

I feel an aura of emotion surrounding both of us.

After that, she asks me to take a photo of her next to her drawing. She looks at herself in my cell phone, while I look at her look at herself.

In this manner, Lorena shows us a "piggy" side of her experience that starts transforming with the display of anal aspects, put into action but not interpreted at this moment. "Are we going to jump into the mud? Are we both going to jump?" Here Lorena shows the way she uses the analyst in this game.

There is anal content to be explored without feeling that either the analyst or the patient is being destroyed. It is a paradigmatic expression of playing with children in analysis, where we do not always use words, and play shows how we actively immerse ourselves in the anal experiences without getting trapped.

The group believed that there was a path leading from the lonely little pig towards the beautiful "little girl."

Using the phrase "beautiful little girl," the analyst seems to want to reflect and support the child, as well as protect her from her monstrous feelings.

Fears and fantasies

Two aspects the group worked on were fears and fantasies of madness and death.

Lorena's fear of madness is inferred from the very beginning when she says, "There are too many things here also," showing how she feels about excess and that her madness is the result of what she feels are too many things, none of them having their own space.

She needs to refer to her head, as if it were detached from her body, distant, referring to a certain disassociation, a split in the psyche-soma integration: "I'm going to use my small head to decide what toys I want . . . my small head thinks a lot about what I need to do."

In transference, Lorena brings her feelings of non-existence, during a session filled with psychic disorganization. She is spinning like a tornado, inventing words and shouting, "I went crazy because I didn't know who to call. . . . Imagine I'm not here, that I don't exist, and then I say to you 'Boo!'" In a state of intense anguish that disorganizes Lorena and destroys her symbolic possibilities, the experience of not existing leaves her tangled in a state of madness.

Later on in analysis, the patient comes to the session with a storybook:

P: *This is the beginning of the book. . . . We're going to start at the beginning: these are the classrooms, and here we have the school principal who is working. If a child is bad, then they are sent to the principal. . . . The principal writes down whether the child behaves good or bad. . . . I was a bit bad, but they didn't send me to the principal because I was good. What the boy said scares me that I screamed. But if a ghost comes then that also scares me, because I'm thinking that a ghost came to class and it's going to take me to the ghost's classroom; it's a cave with lakes that has ghosts and vampires. I don't want to! . . . Before that painting was without a before, a painter came and painted something scary. I'd better look at a children's painting.*

The working group discusses that there is confusion between the story that Lorena is reading and her fantasies, and some of the group members believe that the word "ghost" marks a tipping point. The girl fears that she will be carried off by killer ghosts and vampires that are not in the book.

The idea triggered a long group discussion about the differences between the child's excessive fantasizing and approaching delirium, as well as whether or not to add medication. This could facilitate a smoother approximation to the "before" that is being "painted" with fear during the analysis.

Body

The working group's observation about the body is especially important in this patient. The body appears robot-like, rigid, and fragile, with a small head that Lorena perceives as detached from her body. Lorena uses her own body as well as the analyst's to express her anguish and conflicts. She brings it to the sessions as something small, large, that defecates and that can go down the toilet along with her feces. It plays in the mud, expressing her anal experiences. It freezes like a statue to defend itself, or it avoids eye contact, etc. Nevertheless, since the beginning of analysis, this body has been able to "loosen up" as soon as she walks into the sessions.

Throughout the process, we see how these experiences change. This happens as the need for her body to achieve "psychic consistency" is expressed to overcome "cutting" structuring experiences relieving the anguishes of liquefaction and fragmentation that invade her at times.

The body, initially rigid, was her means of defence and self-support, and a way to avoid the anguish of a terrifying fall. Gradually, during the sessions, it loosens up and "rocks slowly back and forth like a cradle," using other forms of self-expression such as dance and gymnastics, as freer forms of movement. The analyst can start to see a more feminine patient and less "disguised." A body that showed signs of suffering passively with constant falls becomes active, faced with the possibility of playing, inviting her analyst "to dive into the mud." An important transformation in the patient's psychic-soma integration is observed.

We considered how much she needs to be looked at, and this need had been closely related to her body, since the beginning of her analysis when Lorena avoided eye contact, always bowing her head, until later when she began to look directly into the analyst's eyes. It is during analysis that the girl's desire to "play the game that she never saw" comes up, increasing her desire to see herself mirrored in the other, and with less fear about what she will find. The working group ties this to a mother with flaws in her structuring look over her daughter. The girl displays fears of repetition—in transference—of finding the dis-encounter that makes her mad in the mother's look, in the "face"—look—of the analyst.

Later on, in the course of analysis, during the session described in the vignette, an emotionally intense moment occurs in which the analyst takes a photograph of the drawing, and Lorena asks if they can look at the photograph together. The demand is for an analyst-mother to look at her, look at herself. The analyst reflects the girl with her drawings and starts "putting her together," generating a display of mirroring—that marks a moment of significant transformation.

Family-parent binding interactions

Patterns of interpersonal relationships

The working group used questions from the child's version of the 3-LM to guide the discussion: What is the parents' point of view? What is the relationship with her parents, siblings, and peers?

The group pointed out that changes occur in the entire family over the course of analysis. At the beginning, the parents cannot process the differences between family members. How could they, when the mother feels that Lorena is just like her and that Lorena suffers her brothers and sisters just like she did? Lorena says that nobody knows how to treat her and expresses it angrily—"Nobody knows how to treat me"—opening the way for transference.

The mother says,

> *The same thing happened to me. I was able to make it, doing whatever I could and without therapy. My sister was the beautiful one, and I was the rebel without a cause. My problem was my sister that was just too perfect.*

We discussed the look in the mother's eyes, how she wants to see her daughter, and the anguish she feels in not being able to do so. Intrusion and absence stand out in the relationship. Identifying her history with that of her children, the mother develops intrusion and she cannot respond to her daughter's needs because she cannot see her otherness. We discuss whether the mother needs to "take in" her daughter in order to process her own history.

Based on interviews held exclusively with the mother, aspects of the mother's past that affect the mother–child bond were explored. The mother is able to relocate herself in relation to her own mother and daughter, therefore diminishing projection.

At the end of the process, Lorena's mother acknowledges her daughter's achievements:

> *Lorena wrote me the following for my birthday: "Mom, enjoy your birthday." She was worried about finding her place in the world, and she finally found it. Something clicked. I can see it: she no longer says silly things or talks nonsense. . . . Now she has her feet on the ground, and it's easier to find common ground. . . . Also, I'm trying to stop my mother, because she's in everybody's business; she gets me all worked up.*

During the interviews with both parents, the great difficulties and lack of discrimination in the place of each family member were explored. The effects these had on the child's psyche and her feelings of having "no place" were pointed out.

The father, who previously referred to Lorena with a certain distance and theory, began to approach her differently. Lorena started playing hide-and-seek with him, asking the analyst to join in as "her accomplice."

Shifts in the family allowed increased discrimination and affection between family members, with the possibility of understanding Lorena in a different way, showing how the parents' representation of Lorena was changing.

On one level, we have observations about the child's bonding with her real parents, siblings, or peers that were expressed mainly during interviews with the parents, teachers, and others.

On another level, we have observations that the working group of psychoanalysts explored mainly on the structural interplay "id, ego, superego" (Freud) and the inner world (Klein), along with modifications in the family environment, that occurred possibly as a result of the child's inner changes.

The patient's rigidity and distance from her siblings was of concern. A year into analysis, the parents describe the changes in the relationship with her siblings and peers:

> *Lorena is doing great; she plays with her siblings and enjoys drawing with them. At school, there are also changes with the new friends that she has made. She pretends to be the mother of the new girls in school. . . . She describes all the details. It's a huge change. The same thing happens with her cousins, when she plays with them; now everything is fine. Before she would scream at everybody. Now her cousin hugs her and she doesn't mind.*

Since the drawing of the "beautiful girl" at one and a half years into analysis, the subjective experience gains ground, and the difference between fantasy and reality becomes clearer.

Perhaps the teachers' comments at the beginning of the analysis generated fear of a serious outcome and acted as a shocking warning for the parents.

Level 2: Identification of the main dimensions of change

At this level, the working group analyzes patient transformations according to the diagnostic dimensions using a language close to experience and not saturated with theory.

The model demands that we conceptualize the problem from the patient's point of view. What is the patient struggling against? The question is not asking for theory. Instead, it is asking for the phenomena observed. The patient is their point of reference. The model asks that we avoid psychoanalytic jargon and that we document our perceptions with data collected from the sessions.

The Model's Level 2 leads us to initially consider the child's subjective experience of illness.

In this case, Lorena comes to analysis feeling diminished, extremely small, with a fear of losing herself and disappearing. At times the fear of going mad, overwhelmed by an excess of mental content and not being able to contain herself, takes over and leaves Lorena in a state of serious psychic disorganization. During many sessions, she spins like a tornado, shouts, and speaks incoherently, revealing her great inner confusion: "Imagine that I'm not here, I don't exist, and then I scream 'Boo' at you. . . . Fruitghetti is not food, fruitghetti is food."[3]

The group analyzed the modifications of these aspects that occurred during the treatment. Three years into analysis, there is a variation in the subjective experience. The analyst sees the child as a "beautiful" girl, and more importantly the girl is able to take the image and make it her own, leaving behind her feelings of "small little pig" that she had at the beginning of the analysis.

During her third year of analysis, Lorena is approaching the Oedipal stage of development. We find Lorena concerned about fitting in with her friends, and with fears of exclusion.

P: *I have to tell you something really serious that happened to me . . . it's something unusual. . . . My friend is a bit strange; she says yes to everything, she is very "tapete"*[4] *. . . I gave her all of my snack today; I give her good things and she doesn't. Did you see all the good things I do for her?*

A: *Yes, you do many things to have friends and you are finding things that you don't like, things that make you very mad.*

P: *The red fury, I'm going to draw it with an ugly face.*

Lorena uses verbal language to describe how serious her problems are. She has to deal with jealousy and the rivalry in her group of girlfriends. She is feeling anger, fear of rejection. Her feelings are strong but now with a different intensity, and her psychic apparatus keeps her contained and away from a state of disorganization.

In view of the above vignette, we asked ourselves what would happen to the hostility that the work in analysis could have stirred. Part of the working group believed that some of the "strange" aspects were still there, latent, and projected in her friend. Likewise, the group considered the tension and transition between the dual relationships and the access to Oedipal conflicts (triangulation).

Main defences

The working group considered this an important issue and used the following model questions for discussion: What are the main intrapsychic conflicts (and the related affects)? Are the defences adequate and flexible or predominantly dysfunctional or distorting or restricting the inner and outer experiences? How did these aspects change?

As for the conflicts, the strength of pre-Oedipal aspects and primary failures in the conformation of the psychic apparatus were inferred from the material.

When Lorena was 3 years old, she walked on her toes and flapped her arms, aspects that suggested important flaws in the conformation of her primary identification.

The group believed that the girl used first autistic and manic defences that later evolved into more neurotic-like modalities.

The defence expressed at the beginning of analysis in a "rigid" and "robot-like body" gave way to artistic and creative resources such as dance and gymnastics, among others.

Likewise, the group observed that she was coming into contact with her affects when she expressed the "red fury" with her friends. She also drew them with "ugly faces," in clear contrast with the non-mental defences such as the initial freezing enacted in different types of play.

According to the 3-LM proposal, each dimension implies adopting a new approach to the clinical material, with the aim to observe the transformations from a new perspective triggered by each new question.

Mental functioning and psychic structure

We asked ourselves about the girl's mental functioning and psychic structure using the following questions as guidelines: How capable is Lorena of adequately perceiving her own inner states and those of others? And of recognizing and representing her affects?

Even though at the beginning we saw that the patient was mixed up and lost in her "complications" of being small, big, girl, boy, and her anger and fears, we believe that analysis has allowed the patient to put most of her past in order. She is now able to recognize her affects, to discriminate between sadness and fury, and to integrate and relate them to her process of finding others.

We observe a girl who is struggling to integrate conflicts of Oedipus rivalry, competition, exclusion, and giving to please others; a girl who still feels "tapete," strange, who seeks drawing as a means of expressing this aspect of herself.

P: *M is a bit strange. She never says no. . . . She is very "tapete."*
A: *What does "tapete" mean?*
P: *In* My Little Pony, *Pony is very "tapete," very shy, very good. I can't explain it. I'm going to draw it for you.*

Sensory regulation

To explore this aspect, the group selected a question for their discussions: What is her ability to control the degree, intensity, and nature of her responses to sensory stimuli?

We were interested in the patient's sensitivity to noise and "commotion," as she calls it:

P: *Where are those sounds coming from? I don't want any sounds; the phone, the computer, there's never going to be any sounds. I wasn't the one.*
A: *What are the sounds that worry you like? Are they coming from one of the rooms in the house?*
P: *I know, from the room upstairs, the playroom. I don't know how to control them; I don't know how to control the house [she is playing with a toy house].*

The noise she experiences is too intense for her; she cannot tolerate it and is incapable of controlling it.

We analyzed vignettes of some sessions where we were concerned about aspects of perception and how the child's thinking was affected by them. For example, this was clear when Lorena started describing specific scenes from her book and then shifted towards a narrative with an excess of ghostly content, adding things that were not connected to one another.

Regulation of affects

To explore this issue, the working group uses several questions from the model for discussion: How does the child feel? And does she perceive in others the wide range of affects expected in children of her age? How does the child regulate her impulses and affects in order to foster adaptation, satisfaction, and self-esteem, with flexibility in the use of defences or coping strategies?

The working group observed the continuous work that was done during the analysis on affects regulation.

It took a long journey for the patient to get involved with her different affects and to get her psyche more organized.

At the beginning of analysis, affects disorganized the Lorena's psyche. There were sessions in which she spent time spinning her body like a tornado or using bizarre words or rambling.

After three years in analysis, we saw that she was still using projective mechanisms. However, she could describe her affects differently. She could name fury and jealousy, and she talked about how serious her problems were. There was a change in the way she talked about herself and regulated her affects, keeping in mind the relationship with peers developed during the treatment:

P: *I have to tell you something serious that happened at school. I ended up helping a friend, and she got really angry. It's very strange. She turned red, tomato, apple. V is very strange; today I shared my snack with her, and she didn't.*

A: *You're really angry.*

P: *Yes, like a fire in flames. Fire, plus tomato, and more . . . [laughs].*

A: *We're laughing right now, but you get really angry when V does that to you.*

We observed a stronger tie between words—affects showing how Lorena was able to regulate her affects and impulses, reducing the rigidity of her defences.

The patient resorted to sensory aspects to express anger, such as "red fury," angry, "red, tomato, apple."

Her desire to be the chosen one, as she struggled with duality and triangulation, can be expressed with anger. Although she had improved the drive for control, we asked ourselves how permanent her achievements would be over time.

Attachment with internal and external objects

The group selected for discussion other questions from the model: How profound and stable is the child's relationship with internal and external objects? And how prepared is the patient to make and break off relationships and cope with separations? How does she handle relationships that imply the existence of a third person?

As for transference, the group observed that the analyst respected the time Lorena needed, which was crucial if we considered that construction in the child's play showed her potential to build more stable and safer inner spaces and objects.

The material collected at the beginning of analysis pointed to a good prognosis with respect to bonding, along with fears and doubts about being able to procure a space of containment in the minds of others:

P: *We need a driver; I don't like the idea of only one passenger. Ah! There's no room for this girl; she will have to go somewhere else.*

A: *There is a place for her here. We are getting to know each other. You're probably asking yourself if there is a place for you also, here with me.*

P: *Yes, we're getting to know each other. I have a problem: it falls. . . . I'm going to put things away, but it's such a small box. . . . How are so many toys going to fit in such a small box?*

We believed that, through transference, Lorena was generating abilities that could potentially help her contain herself and have good internal objects that could allow her to bond without feeling like she did in the past, when she was "falling through a black hole."

We referred to a past session in which Lorena leaned on two rigid feminine statues to stop herself from falling. The analyst joined her and pointed out how hard the sculptures were. Lorena said she wanted to draw a girl and later photograph her, as a way of being contained in the mind of the analyst ("save it"), and to be recreated later, in transference, as a photo with cheerful and feminine content.

This transformation from two rigid feminine statues into a colourful girl who could be "saved" in the analyst's psyche shows a containment function destined to be incorporated by the patient.

Nevertheless, the group had its doubts about the stability of the patient's achievements over time in her relationships with internal and external objects, as well as to whether she would be able to cope with the inclusion of a third person.

Level 3: Testing of explanatory hypotheses of transformations

At this level, the working group discussed the theoretical hypotheses explaining the transformations, as well as the possibilities of how and why they occurred. They discussed explicit and implicit theories explaining the observed transformations, starting with those manifested in the analyst's interpretations.

What was the main focus that guided the analyst? What were the analyst's main theories and hypotheses, explicit and implicit, supporting her work? Did they change during the treatment?

Structural flaws gave way to great pain and fantasies of collapsing, that led the working group to infer that, before she was 3 years old, Lorena could have had experiences of "a never-ending fall" (Winnicott, 1971) and fantasies of a "fragmented body."

The analyst worked mainly on the more primary aspects of discrimination between id–not id, and it was only approaching the third year of analysis that we observed Oedipal aspects related to exclusion, jealousy, and rivalry becoming more relevant.

Another point of view discussed was the persistence of an unresolved issue that could be re-enacted during puberty and was linked to the patient's "strange" characteristics: the flapping, and the walking on her toes early on.

The group explored two hypotheses. Some believed that Lorena did everything to feel appreciated, but the anger and feelings of not being loved persisted; meanwhile, others thought that anger did not disorganize her and was not reflected in her body. The analyst's look, which expressed empathy and support, had been essential to the development of Lorena's feelings of being loved.

A "stiff" little girl once arrived at the analyst's office with an inner feeling that she was going mad, unable to cope with her parents' conflicts projected entirely on her, tangled in a serious state of confusion. Then we started seeing transformations in her ability to discriminate herself from her primary objects, giving way to her own resources that were previously "frozen."

From the spectrum of conceptual frameworks underlying the analyst's interventions, we observed that the beginning of the analysis, there was a tendency towards Kleinian theory (1962) (e.g., "You have things that are very good, and you are realizing that there is a friend who is very jealous"). This was followed by a Winnicottian approach with holding and handling playing an important role. There were also signs of Bion (1975), since the analyst attempted to regulate affects permanently, developing an intense reverie function from the beginning.

The Freudian interventions of presence-absence could be conceptualized as Winnicottian also, if we believed that the analyst's aim was to reinforce the presence of a stable object beyond separations: "Like the two of us, we didn't see each other during the holidays and we meet again; with Mom and Dad sometimes you don't see them and afterwards you see them again."

Between the analyst and the patient, there a series of functions was displayed, where the analyst accompanied the patient, mirroring and marking her affects, so that the child could continue becoming more familiar with her own material.

The analyst regulated the affects, supporting them and observing to what extent there was return and synchronization between the two. Of all these functions, support stood out, generating a structure that allowed her to grow up. We pointed out the necessary and important faults related to Winnicott's theory (1962).

During our group discussion it was enlightening to observe how the analyst worked different theoretical approaches and how the theories implicit in her mind operated during the sessions, in transference with the patient.

We saw how she contributed to the development of psychoanalytical and libidinal availability, not only in the child but also in the parents.

During the discussion several alternative hypotheses were discussed.

The weight of transgenerational aspects and their relationship with the transference

The mother seemed to have integrated in her mind that she was a very demanding mother, an aspect that was projected massively onto her daughter.

The group observed that Lorena was struggling with these aspects projected onto her, aiming to find her place as a daughter in the family. This implied parallel work with the parents to relocate the child and allow the parental functions to be re-established, not only in its libidinal aspect but also in cutting and support.

Regarding the cutting function, an observation was made when Lorena said, "Today I brought a penguin; the penguin's name is Pingüi," leaving out the "-no" ending, highlighting the limit in its failed function.[5]

Hypothesis explaining "avoidant attachment"

We explored again the meaning of "oppositional"—to what extent it was related to a disorder present in the patient early in analysis, which consisted of avoidance of eye contact and an avoidant attachment, making it difficult for the child to bond with others.

The place of trauma in Lorena

Previously, we referred to a series of events that the child experienced before she was 3. Since the events were not explained to Lorena, they became part of her traumas. Added to the mother's lack of reverie, they could be considered failures of her maternal function (Bion, 1975) that could have caused a feeling of non-existence in the child.

What is the nature of the changes observed? How profound are they? And what is the stability sought?

We believed that patient's transformations occurred fundamentally at the structural level and allowed improvement in her psychic functions.

As previously mentioned, there was a unique coexistence of evolved aspects with good possibilities of symbolization, along with other aspects of failure in Lorena's psychic structure. Primary failures were a source of intense psychic suffering, experiences of threat, disorganization, and madness that led her to use her primary defences of turning her body into a "robot."

We considered that the Oedipal conflicts were not sufficiently displayed. More work of the analyst was necessary in order to organize her mental functioning and elaborate her traumatic experiences.

An open question remained unanswered of what would happen during the patient's puberty, since she displayed intense psychotic anxieties. We had reasons to believe that we needed to be alert to the coming of puberty and drive reactivation.

Conclusion

The purpose of this chapter was to provide an example of how the 3-LM model works in longitudinal approaches applied to child analyses. It explores the achievements and limitations this process has and opens the floor to discussions.

Summary

This chapter describes how the Three-Level Model (3-LM) was applied to observe the analysis of a girl from 5 to 9 years old. During the observation with the 3-LM, the focus was on intrapsychic, intersubjective, and structural changes. It also included the analyst's work with the child's parents. The purpose of applying the model was to understand whether or not the analytic intervention fostered these changes.

The 3-LM allows analysts to review hypotheses explaining the main reasons that brought the patient to analysis in the first place, jumping back and forth between earlier and later sessions and exploring the clinical material initially at a phenomenological level. At the model's second level, the different dimensions of transformations are considered. At the third level, several are posed: What was the analyst's main focus during the analysis? Which are the official theories inferred in the analysis of interpretations? Finally, we ask ourselves whether other alternative hypotheses, besides those introduced by the analyst, would be possible.

Notes

1 The working group for clinical observation of transformations of a child patient was formed at the Uruguayan Psychoanalytic Association (Asociación Psicoanalítica del Uruguay or APU) in October and November 2015.

Moderator: Marina Altmann de Litvan.

Reporter: Griselda Revella.

Presenter of Clinical Material: Patricia Singer.

Participants: Patricia Arévalo, Tatiana Santander, Luisa Pérez, Gabriela Pouse, Sandra Press, Nahir Bonifacino, Silvia Braun, Fernanda Cubria, Silvia Sapriza, Maria Bauer, Jacqueline Hirschfeld, Adriana Gandolfi, Mariel Brizolara, Claudia Gaione, Ana De Barbieri, Ximena Malmierca, Nancy Delpréstito, and Ilana Luksenburg.

2 For additional information about the 3-LM Model, see References.

3 The patient makes up the word "fruitghetti," combining the words "fruit" and "spaghetti."

4 Later the patient will describe what she means by "tapete."

5 In Spanish the word for "penguin" is *pingüino.*

References

Altmann de Litvan, M., Miller, D., & Bernardi, R. (2014). Three-Level Model for observing child patient transformations. In M. Altmann de Litvan (Ed.), *Time for change: Tracking transformations in psychoanalysis—The Three-Level Model* (pp. 303–319). London: Karnac.

Bion, W. (1975). *Aprendiendo de la experiencia* [*Learning from experience*]. Buenos Aires: Paidos.

Bollas, C. (1987). *La sombra del objeto. Psicoanálisis de lo sabido no pensado* [*The shadow of the object: Psychoanalysis of the unthought known*]. Buenos Aires: Amorrortu.

Freud, S. (1905). Three essays on the theory of sexuality. *S.E. 7* (pp. 123–246).

Freud, S. (1908). On the sexual theories of children. *S.E. 9* (pp. 205–226).

Kernberg, P., Chazan, S., & Normandin, L. (1996). *Cornell Play Therapy Scales.* New York: The New York Hospital Cornell University Medical Center.

Klein, M. (1962). *La técnica psicoanalítica del juego* [*Psychoanalytic play technique*]. Nuevas direcciones en psicoanálisis. Buenos Aires: Paidós.

Nieto, M. (1965). Algunos problemas del analista como investigador [Some problems faced by analysts as researchers]. *Revista de la Asociación Psicoanalítica del Uruguay, 1*(7), 5–27.

Volinsky de Hoffnung, P., Medici C. Sapriza, S., Altmann, M., Braun, S., Cuttinella, O., Ihlenfeld, S., López, C., & Vallespir, N. (1986). El juego en psicoanálisis de niños [Children play in psychoanalysis]. In *El juego en psicoanálisis de niños, 1,* 129–194. Laboratorio de Psicoanálisis de Niños. Asociación Psicoanalítica del Uruguay.

Winnicott, D. W. (1962). La integración del yo en el desarrollo del niño [Ego integration and child development]. In *Los procesos de maduración y el ambiente facilitador* [*The maturational process and the facilitating environment*] (pp. 56–63). London: Hogarth Press.

Winnicott, D. W. (1971). *Realidad y juego* [*Playing and reality*]. Buenos Aires: Granica.

Chapter 13

How does a 5-year-old cope with mourning?

Contributions of the 3-LM for observing child transformations[1]

Marina Altmann de Litvan, Bruno Salesio, and Raquel Andreucci Gomes

Introduction

This chapter aims to show Danilo's case, which was discussed by a clinical observation group using the 3-LM for children (de Litvan, Miller, & Bernardi, 2014). The main topic is the mourning for his mother, who died when Danilo was 2 years old.

Danilo was 5 years old when he started treatment. His father explained in the first session that his wife had passed away more than three years earlier. On Mother's Day at school, children were asked to bring pictures of their mothers. The child picked a picture of him being carried by his mother when he was a baby. When he got home from school, he told his father he missed her. It was then that the father and the grandmother's child decided to take Danilo to therapy to offer him support for his losses.

The family suffered other losses at the time: the maternal great-grandfather and grandfather died, and their old nanny moved out of town. Danilo's father lost his father when he was 13 years old.

When Danilo's mother got sick, they moved to the house of the paternal grandmother and, at the same time, the child got a new nanny. When the mother died, Danilo's father got depressed. He has a daughter with another woman, who is some months younger than Danilo.

The father recalled that his wife had a quiet full-term pregnancy, with a normal delivery, and she breastfed Danilo until he was 6 months old, when she was diagnosed with cancer. He was a calm baby who slept and ate well. He had no toilet training or motor development problems. There were no complaints at school, and he took swimming and judo lessons. His paternal grandmother was very close to him.

The material supplied by the therapist covered four meaningful sessions over a two-year period.

Literature review of bereavement in children

Several studies have found that children respond to loss in the same way as adults in the nature and frequency of their grief reactions, showing an identical chronological pattern of bereavement (Parkes, 1970; Pynoos et al., 1987).

Nevertheless, important differences in childhood symptoms distinguish bereaved children from bereaved adults. There are also studies that prove that loss in the preverbal stages of development has many characteristics unique to infancy (Lieberman, 2003).

Children express different responses that deny reality and thus differ from the mourning experienced by adults, different from Freud's claims. These reactions include unconscious and sometimes conscious denial of the reality of the parent's death; rigid screening out of all affective responses connected with the parent's death; marked increase in identification with and idealization of the dead parent; decrease in self-esteem; feelings of guilt; and persistent unconscious fantasies of an ongoing relationship or reunion with the dead parent. These responses are viewed as being directed toward avoiding the acceptance of the parent's death and the necessity to make the radical reorganization in object attachments that such an acceptance would require (Menes, 1971).

Authors who believe children do undergo mourning when they lose a parent, like Kliman (1969) and Furman (1974), accept this process happens only exceptionally, when facilitated by different kinds of treatment. Moreover, these authors hold the view that children should express sad affect and they do not experience the internal emotional decathexis.

Bowlby (1969, 1973, 1980) used to claim that a child who was separated from the mother went through mourning, but he later followed the position that children react through defensive phenomena to deny the painful event (Menes, 1971). Bowlby developed key concepts such as the connection between mourning and separation anxieties, the desire to retrieve the lost object (by crying and behaving aggressively), and the roles of disorganization and reorganization.

Research on children's reactions to the death of a parent conducted by Wolfenstein (1966), in which data were taken from 42 children aged from early latency to adolescence who had experienced the death of a parent, found that the children continued with their everyday lives, denying the loss, overtly or unconsciously. Also, there was little weeping. By refusing to be emotionally involved in the event, children were found to expect the return of the lost parent, more or less unconsciously.

Also, children have been reported to exhibit depressive symptoms following the loss of a parent. However, despite significant mood disturbances and diminished interest and pleasure, these children were distinguishable from a group of non-bereaved, depressed controls by the absence of feelings of guilt and worthlessness (Clayton, Desmarais, & Winokur, 1968).

Another symptom of bereaved children is a high incidence of separation anxiety, co-mingled with depressive symptoms. Following bereavement, children have been observed to exhibit significantly more anxiety at imagined separations than control; they also manifested more overt, anxious attachment in response to normal separations (Kranzler et al., 1990).

In several studies assessing children's pathology following the early loss of a parent and other trauma, the degree of distress and the level of coping skills in the surviving parent were the most significant mediators of the child's later psychological and behavioural symptoms (Elizur & Kaffman, 1983; Kranzler et al., 1990; Chemtob et al., 2010; Wilson & Durbin, 2010). Maternal and parental depression and other acute or chronic forms of distress have also been observed to affect the child's grieving and recovery and have been associated with negative child outcomes (Weller et al., 1988; Kranzler et al., 1990; Chemtob et al., 2010).

Following the loss of a parent, children show an increase in empathic attunement to the mental well-being of the surviving parent, as well as a heightened need to monitor the parent's recovery. In response to extreme grief reactions in the surviving parent, children tend to inhibit their own grief reactions so as not to increase their parent's distress and anxiety (Pynoos, 1992). Therefore, studies found that when children lose a parent, their mental well-being will reflect that of the surviving parent and they will try to decrease the surviving parent's grief by monitoring it and inhibiting their own. Therefore, the child's externalization or inhibition of affect in relation to the exaggerated or inhibited distress responses of a grieving parent may impede the child's own grieving. Because young children rely on their parents for cognitive, emotional, and behavioural regulation, traumatic stress and distress are best understood within the parent–child system (Yehuda et al., 2008).

Level I

In this level we expect the listening of the clinical material that describes transformations in the child (regarding the child's behaviour, emotions, performance, relationships, personality organization) and in the child's relationship with the analyst. The group selected different moments of the analysis that evidence how Danilo is experiencing loss and mourning and how these aspects change over the two years of analysis in a language close to experience and theoretically non-saturated.

Who is the child and how is he? Five years old, first session

When the first session ended, Danilo asked, "When am I coming back?," and in the following sessions, Danilo tried to control the office's doors when he went in and out, making sure the omnipotent fantasy that the analyst would always be there, even when he came back, was real.

Often the analyst explained the lapses between sessions by finger-counting, telling him that he would come back another day. According to the analyst, Danilo's grief and his attempts to confirm her presence were related to his mother's death and the switching of nannies.

He asked her if he could show her his drawing to his father and his nannies, to which the analyst said yes, thus he went to the waiting room. She told him that she would be waiting for him two days later. It was as though part of the mourning of the separation grief was enacted at the encounters and goodbyes with the analyst.

Throughout the sessions, Danilo still felt worried: he wanted to know who was going to pick him up, what was going to happen later, if he was coming back or not, who was in the waiting room.

It is through the emotional experiences undergone with the analyst and the counter-transference she talked about that we can observe how Danilo developed his potential for symbolic play, like catching a rhinoceros, soldiers who died and came back to life, and airplanes that may have or may have not crashed.

It can be observed how these plays started in the first session. Danilo tried to put a soldier inside an animal transport truck. As he did not manage, he inserted a little rhinoceros instead.

A: *Did you want to leave anything in there, caught?*
P: *So that it can't run away!*
A: *He can't run away nor be lost. He is inside the cage.*

In the same session, only after the interpretation of the game, Danilo started playing with toy soldiers. He sat down and grabbed the soldiers, dividing them into two groups. He asked the analyst to take her group and made her soldiers fight against his. Some of her soldiers died in combat, and he threw them into the paper bin. He was really serious and would not speak. When all her soldiers died, he emptied the bin and started over. Danilo got angry each time the analyst tried to talk during the game, saying, "Stop it! This is a game! Toys can't talk!"

Then, he concluded,

P: *That's it. It's OK. You can talk a little bit.*
A: *[As the soldiers fell into the bin]. We lost; we are falling into the bin.*
P: *But they come back. It's the bin. They die and come back. The bin stinks. It smells of fart!*
A: *They come back because of the smell?*
P: *[Laughs]. Yes. . . .*
A: *Now we can talk about living, fighting, dying. What happens is . . .*

It was at that moment that Danilo was able to feel it was only a game, and then he was not as sad as before, and he could afford to have fun and laugh.

At the end of the session, Danilo lost interest in what he was doing, looked at the box, and asked, "Can we play with the airplane?"

Danilo started playing, making some airplanes attack each other and crash. He asked whether all old airplanes crashed. The analyst replied that they could crash if we no one took care of them, or they could also stop flying when they were too old, but they did not always crash.

P: *But new airplanes can crash too, right?*
A: *They can crash, but that's not usual. If a failure is detected, it can be fixed beforehand. The same happens with animals, cars, people . . .*
P: *Do you know I don't have a mother?*
A: *I do. How do you feel about that?*
P: *I feel ashamed.*

The analyst felt really moved, and he asked her to keep playing with the airplanes as if they were flying.

When the session ended, Danilo closed the door, but the analyst opened it to walk him to the waiting room.

What stands out in that excerpt is that Danilo emphasized how ashamed he felt in comparison to others, because his mother was not alive. The theme of loss, though, was present but not as strongly as expected. Still, the issues Danilo's father himself had faced in the mourning—depression—were evident, so he could not discuss these processes with his son. It was he who was moved by a situation he could not address and discuss with his son, thus "no one talked about it." He entrusted his problems to others, like the analyst, so that they would solve them. As for Danilo, he seemed to be a child who had to bring happiness into his home to keep his father enlivened. When the treatment started, Danilo did not need to talk about his mother. Now we can remember how much "what was not said" was present in the family, both in the difficulty in talking about the mother's death (see the father's depression) and in the hiding of Danilo's other sister.

Balls are round, like bombs: 6 years old, one year and five months of analysis

Danilo talked about his dinosaur fart, a bomb. He said, "Let's play football." Balls are round, like bombs. Danilo was told that his mother "had a disease that was a ball under her arm."

While playing button football, there appeared some sexual content: the ball got under the analyst's legs and Danilo said that he knew that men and women were anatomically different. When they played, he did not want the analyst to lose by many goals, but he did want to win. Maybe he was talking about how masculine he felt, and he was showing his skills and his strength. Nevertheless, he did not want to be so threatening or dangerous and knock out the analyst (through transference, his mother). The hypothesis states that this play somehow reflected his mother's loss.

Playing several consecutive roles: Father, mother, and son

Then, Danilo asked the analyst if he could lie down next to her, for they would go to sleep. The child wanted to sleep hugging a pillow that was in the office and was called Tatá. He had the same one at home. In the morning, a rooster would wake them up with its "cock-a-doodle-doo." While playing, Danilo would ask her to make some coffee and say, "Oh! I'm falling off the bed." The analyst repeated the play a few times. The analyst saw this as the representation of a family, where Danilo played several consecutive roles: the father, the mother, and the son.

Then he had the idea of a cave, where the analyst was the dinosaur mum and he was the little son. The analyst understood this as if she were diving into Danilo's pre-history.

Danilo represented the fantasy suggested by the analyst: Danilo, the little dinosaur, grew up and learned how to hunt; Danilo felt moved by his mother/analyst and was proud as her mum acknowledged his growth. Danilo warned his mother/analyst that the dinosaurs would die, killed by a meteor shower, "and not only because they were old."

A: *We are telling a very ancient story . . . of a dinosaur mum and her little son who were in the cave.*

P: *Come, Mummy [he walks on all fours as if he were a dinosaur].*

A: *I'm getting there [walking like a dinosaur].*

P: *Come inside the cave with me. We must protect ourselves from danger. [Inside the cave: they turned the small sofas upside down].*

P: *Hey . . ., it's dangerous outside.*

A: *The mother is protecting her little dinosaur son from the dangers outside. Maybe you were talking about a mother you had "then," back in the old days, when you were a baby. You were taken care of by her when you lived inside her belly. . . . And, now, we can talk and play games about that.*

P: *[Focused on the game] Shall we see if the danger is gone?*

Playing with balls: 7 years old, two years and five months of analysis

A new stage of the analytic relationship appeared, in which they played with balls: basketball, bowling, football. They talked about his relationship with his father and the fact that they used to play football on the beach. Danilo loved football. This was an activity with a ball that represented life as opposed to the ball that killed his mother. This change in the psychic meaning in Danilo's mind happened through and within a transference. A change in the relationship with the analyst can be observed.

Danilo did not want to miss the session or the game.

Danilo wanted to protect a statue of a saint with her child (a quite modern statue made out of stone of a mother carrying her son on her lap). Later, they talked for a while about a small plasticine ball Danilo had found in a corner of the office, left by the previous patient (the analyst had not seen it). Danilo examined the ball closely and looked at the analyst "inquisitively, almost as if waiting for an answer." They started playing football right away. (Could this have been Danilo's unconscious perception of his out-of-wedlock sister?)

Danilo immediately sat down in front of the analyst and talked about a conversation he had had with his dad about his mother and a mobile made out of little footballs. "My dad says they laughed together as they saw me kicking the balls": the ball that killed Danilo's mother was then transformed into the ball that retrieved early memories in his relationship with the analyst.

There was a transformation through the different plays, which showed the fantasies the child had, not only regarding his mother's illness but also about the life before this illness. And this was a transferential retrieval.

The analyst described the following scene: "I saw his face light up. It was as if I was sharing a dream picture with him, a live photograph. He had never spoken about his mother so straightforwardly." When the analyst tried to talk about the mother, he interrupted her, as always, and said, "Now stop talking. We're going to play."

When the analyst told Danilo that maybe he wanted to show his mother how well he played football, he answered, "At least I can show you." Was this some kind of reparation by transference?

In the following game, Danilo and the analyst hurt themselves touching their feet. Instead of swearing, Danilo tried to throw a ball (the small plasticine ball) out of the window, but he did not do it. The ball seemed to represent something menacing and persecutory as well as something unifying and loving about the family, as the story told by Danilo. The non-persecutory aspects prevailed, and Danilo left the ball inside the office instead of throwing it out of the window.

In another session, before playing football, they played button football: "Let's play button football."

Revealing father's secret: 7 years old, two years and seven months of analysis

The family was told about Danilo's father's secret only a few months after the mother died. Father revealed that he had had another daughter with another woman. The analyst was informed about this two and a half years after treatment started.

Some points led the analyst to reflection: How did the lie or the omission of truth about the father's affair or Danilo's other sister affect Danilo's life? Was this related to the father's depression? The analyst was shocked and tried to understand the unconscious roles (blind spots) of each of them—father, son, analyst—since this was an enacted and shared experience.

The analyst was affected. The group reflected on the question, Which will be my place in the transference of the analyst? Identifying with a betrayed person, or a helpless child, or not idealizing the father anymore?

This information was reflected in the analysis with Danilo's growing capacity to symbolize and transform his silences into words and play.

In the last session, some significant moments appeared that enlightened a ghost. These keys were alive, representing a live transference to solve an enigma. The keys were moving like a ghost, and Danilo told the analyst that he was not afraid of the ghost and then he flatulated—perhaps a bomb to remove the bad smell of the revelation?

Danilo and the analyst started playing darts. The analyst could not find the right game and she could not talk about Danilo's new sister. She thought about the difficulty as the expression of an analytic impasse or perhaps a chronic enactment. They found it hard to hit the target, which was the centre of Danilo's sadness. She had to solve the enigma of the ghost in order to foster the analysis and Danilo's development.

Level 2

This level helps the analyst and training participants in the group discussion to identify the main dimensions along which transformations can or cannot occur.

Through the forms, the analysts assessed the change[2] in the different dimensions of the second level, considering that Danilo's disturbances range from mild or moderate to minimum (3 to 4) in the following aspects.

Subjective experience of illness

Danilo's father brought him to therapy because he argued the child did not talk or avoided talking about his mother's loss.

The group was surprised to find that Danilo was not sick or depressed, in spite of not having a mother or having lost his mother when he was so young. According to the group's evaluation, Danilo did not present the phenomenological appearance of conflict.

Danilo could symbolize his mother's death through play, in an increasingly elaborate and detailed way. The group also observed that the subjective experience of illness was actually more present in Danilo's father than in Danilo. The father thought it better not to have teachers become involved in the analysis process, and, at the same time, the school did not offer professional help.

Interpersonal relational patterns

Danilo had always been a good student and had friends. He had a great relationship, full of love and affection, with his nannies.

With the analyst, Danilo managed to establish patterns of closeness and intimacy and forged bonds that displayed positive affection; visual, verbal, and bodily contact with the analyst. He felt comfortable and relaxed in her presence; he was friendly. There was a reciprocal bond of cooperation and also sometimes of competence, which were expressed by plays and by words.

The analyst put the game scenes into words; her interventions, which dramatized the play, were taken by the child, who related them to his own problems. His need to be protected emerged. There were synchrony and reciprocity. The analyst dramatized the child's fantasies—for example when they played with the dinosaur. In the first sessions, Danilo asked the analyst not to talk during the symbolic play, especially when the "soldiers die and come back to life" play. Little by little, Danilo allowed the analyst to talk, albeit only a little.

He felt also the need to repair damage whenever he thought someone could hurt her. For example, he would help her if he was winning a game by many points or would try not to hit her when playing football. Perhaps this revealed a way of not feeling the threat of the analyst's loss—through transference, his mother.

It can be hypothesized that Danilo was developing the understanding that this was only a game, distinguishing fantasy from reality, and that they could have fun. The activities that once threatened his self, like talking or playing about pain, separations, and death, stopped being this harmful.

The group observed how the child was competing with his father. When he once said he wanted to be taller than his father, he was feeling he would be taller than him because of what the analyst produced in him. More data are required to understand how the father, who was worried about Danilo's well-being, actually treats his son.

Danilo expressed how he feels and asked for help, and the analyst underwent moments of maternal as well as paternal transference. The group observed there were things Danilo's father could not emotionally offer to his son.

No data of how his relationship with his sister was and the "new one."

Main intrapsychic conflicts

Danilo's conflicts were related to the separation anxieties and shame he felt in comparison to his classmates due to the loss of his mother.

The group was surprised to find that Danilo did not present many conflicts. In fact, his father's conflicts were more evident than his.

Mental or personality functioning: Structure

His functioning level and his integrated sense of identity were appropriate for his development stage. Additionally, he had a good perception of self and others and could perceive his internal states and those of others. Danilo's object representations were enabling. Although he wanted to do things by himself, he did not get angry if things were not done as he wished. The patient could feel empathy and tolerance and understand the points of view of the analyst while playing.

Level 3

At this level we shall propose the theoretical perspectives that might explain change or no change in the patient. Which are the analyst's main theories and hypotheses (explicit or implicit) that can be seen in his or her work? Have they changed through treatment? Have these foci of the analytic work changed through the analytic process?

The group discussed how the story of the dinosaur mum showed how Danilo could integrate his own traumatic experiences in a way that was appropriate for his level of development. This was displayed, for example, through the associations with the "cock-a-doodle-doo" rooster and the cave: the analyst explained her theory that they were reviving "a very ancient story . . . of a dinosaur mum and her little son who were in the cave," to which Danilo replied, "Come, Mummy." This made them both vibrate.

Danilo had a healthy self-esteem and had the opportunity to have an analyst who was there for him to play, which helped him express his affect. The connection with an object can become more realistic and whole through a good, trustful relationship.

Nevertheless, the group discussed how important it was to work on these issues with Danilo, his father, and other people of his inner circle, intra- and inter-psychically, so that he could develop emotionally and increase his symbolic capacity, identifying his own self, and connecting with others in a healthy way. The group observed that, even though his conflicts were mainly intrapsychic, Danilo had the structural potential to better develop his defences against grief. At no point were his defences (denial, avoidance) dysfunctional.

Danilo did not display extreme affection or aggressive behaviour; he sometimes said he missed his mother and he had a good affect regulation, which was mainly positive. His functioning level and his integrated sense of identity were appropriate for his development stage.

According to the analyst, Danilo needed to create, through analytic dialogue, a narrative and a meaning for his own feelings ("longing").

One focus of the analyst was that Danilo had suffered many losses, and thus many mourning processes in the wake of his mother's loss. The analyst and Danilo had to work on this together, yet it did not happen as expected, challenging the theory that the mourning processes experienced are repeated in the transference.

Another focus of the analyst was Danilo's separation anxieties. The analyst believed that Danilo would not allow her to close the door because he wanted to control the separation between them, so that "they would not lose each other."

Another focus was Danilo's growth. The father, the nanny, Danilo, and the analyst participated in a session in which the analyst worked on Danilo's growth.

In the counter-transference the analyst felt that Danilo seemed to be searching for a special look, like the look a mother gives to her child when she proudly tells others about their growth.

Which other explanatory hypotheses of change could be suggested from different theoretical perspectives?

A blind spot that the analyst did not manage to work with was Danilo's half-sister, the family secrets, and ghosts regarding this issue.

Throughout the analysis, the main relationship was between Danilo and his analyst. The group discussed the need to work more with the father or the family.

Discussion and final comments

The observations of the group and the analyst showed that Danilo was not traumatized by having lost his mother at a young age.

The group discussion emphasized the "shame" in Danilo's discourse, because he felt different from his friends, and, indeed, this was what caused his grief rather than the pain of mourning for his mother. Moreover, the group provided the analyst with great help showing this aspect.

Shame, from a developmental perspective, is related to a pre-Oedipal situation (Rothstein, 1994). The fantasy of shameful disapproval may be associated with ideas of being laughed at, ridiculed, humiliated, or rejected. Thus, the conscious experience of shame is more often associated with the idea of the external shaming object (Rothstein, 1994).

We did not find in Danilo the reactions mentioned in the literature (Menes, 1971): unconscious and sometimes conscious denial of the reality of the parent's death; rigid screening out of all affective responses connected with the parent's death; marked increase in identification with and idealization of the dead parent; decrease in self-esteem; feelings of guilt; and persistent unconscious fantasies of an ongoing relationship or reunion with the dead parent.

Danilo's responses did not seem directed toward avoiding acceptance of his mother's death, and he managed to reorganize his object attachments adequately. In Danilo's case, his nannies and his grandmother played a vital role in helping the patient.

We can observe the connection between object and separation anxiety in this case, because Danilo put the mourning and separation processes on the same level, as we could see in the child's play with dinosaurs and at the end of the session, when saying goodbye to the analyst.

This was a kind of mourning that differed with our explicit theories.

Is it necessary to internalize the object in order to mourn? Is this why little children who lost a parent do not experience the grief of mourning as adults do?

The mourning process in children seemed different from mourning in adults. Danilo suffered the fear of losing the integrity of the self to shame, since he felt different from his friends—as a result of his mother's death. Danilo wanted to cheer his family up in order to take care of his father's survival (in the face of depression) and he was worried about his grandmother (airplanes play). After all, they were his most significant protective figures.

Notes

1 Clinical Observation Group: Sao Paulo Psychoanalytic Society, September 2018.
Moderators: Marina Altmann de Litvan and Bruno Salesio
Presenter: Raquel Andreucci Pereira Gomes
Discussants: A. M. de Almeida Camargo, D. A. Cilurzo Neto, E. Guimarães Oliveira, I. Garcia de Barros, L. Gnatos Lombardi, L. Pinto Chaves, L. M. Chacon de Freitas, L. Todescan Lessa Mattos, M. C. Andreucci Pereira Gomes, M. C. Brisighello Boarati, M. da C. Câmara Barone, M. U. Lambrecht, M. C. Antonácio Povedano, M. Dias Vianna Braga de Sá, N. F. Monteiro Duarte, P. E. Bertini S. Rossetti, R. Andreucci Pereira Gomes, R. Jales Leitão de Carvalho, R. E. Lordello Coimbra, and W. A. Hamad Leoncio

2 Resorting to mode, the value that appears among analysts most often.

References

Bowlby, J. (1969). *Attachment and loss* (Vol. 1). London: Hogarth.
Bowlby, J. (1973). *Attachment and loss* (Vol. 2). New York: Basic Books.
Bowlby, J. (1980). *Attachment and loss* (Vol. 3). New York: Basic Books.

Chemtob, C. M., Nomura, Y., Rajendran, K., Yehuda, R., Schwartz, D., & Abramovitz, R. (2010). Impact of maternal posttraumatic stress disorder and depression following exposure to the September 11 attacks on preschool children's behavior. *Child Development, 81*(4), 1129–1141.

Clayton, P., Desmarais, L., & Winokur, G. (1968). A study of normal bereavement. *American Journal of Psychiatry, 125*(2), 168–178.

de Litvan, M. A., Miller, D., & Bernardi, R. (2014). Three-Level Model for observing child patient transformations. In M. Altmann de Litvan (Ed.), *Time for change: Tracking transformations in psychoanalysis—The Three-Level Model.* London: Karnac.

Elizur, E., & Kaffman, M. (1983). Factors influencing the severity of childhood bereavement reactions. *American Journal of Orthopsychiatry, 53*(4), 668–676.

Furman, E. (1974). *A child's parent dies: Studies in childhood bereavement*. New Haven: Yale University Press.

Kliman, G. (1969). Facilitation of mourning during childhood. Draft presented at American Orthopsychiatric Association, New York, April.

Kranzler, E. M., Shaffer, D., Wasserman, G., & Davies, M. (1990). Early childhood bereavement. *Journal of the American Academy of Child & Adolescent Psychiatry, 29*(4), 513–520.

Lieberman, A. F. (Ed.). (2003). *Losing a parent to death in the early years: Guidelines for the treatment of traumatic bereavement in infancy and early childhood.* Washington, D.C.: Zero to Three.

Menes, J. B. (1971). Children's reactions to the death of a parent: A review of the psychoanalytic literature. *Journal of the American Psychoanalytic Association, 19*, 697–719.

Parkes, C. M. (1970). "Seeking" and "finding" a lost object: Evidence from recent studies of the reaction to bereavement. *Social Science & Medicine, 4*(2), 187–201.

Pynoos, R. S. (1992). Grief and trauma in children and adolescents. *Bereavement Care, 11*(1), 2–10.

Pynoos, R. S., Nader, K., Frederick, C., Gonda, L., & Stuber, M. (1987). Grief reactions in school-age children following a sniper attack at school. *Israel Journal of Psychiatry and Related Sciences, 24*(1–2), 263–277.

Rothstein, A. M. (1994). Shame and the superego: Clinical and theoretical considerations. *Psychoanalytic Study of the Child, 49*(1), 263–277.

Weller, E. B., Weller, R. A., Fristad, M. A., Cain, S. E., & Bowes, J. M. (1988). Should children attend their parent's funeral? *Journal of the American Academy of Child & Adolescent Psychiatry, 27*(5), 559–562.

Wilson, S., & Durbin, C. E. (2010). Effects of paternal depression on fathers' parenting behaviors: A meta-analytic review. *Clinical Psychology Review, 30*(2), 167–180.

Wolfenstein, M. (1966). How is mourning possible? *Psychoanalytic Study of the Child, 21*, 93–123.

Yehuda, R., Bell, A., Bierer, L. M., & Schmeidler, J. (2008). Maternal, not paternal, PTSD is related to increased risk for PTSD in offspring of Holocaust survivors. *Journal of Psychiatric Research, 42*(13), 1104–1111.

Part VII

Improving clinical evidence

Chapter 14

Assessing strengths and limitations of clinical evidence in a psychoanalytic clinical material

Ricardo Bernardi and Luisa Pérez Suquilvide, with discussion by Charles Hanly

Introduction

This chapter aims to reflect on the criteria used to evaluate the degree of certainty or weight of the evidence offered by clinical material to support certain theoretical hypotheses or techniques related to a case. When analysts are faced with a clinical case, whether their own or of another person, they must answer a multitude of questions, both theoretical and technical. Therefore, they must decide which aspects of the material they can rely on to answer them. The material may provide support for more than one hypothesis, and we must then decide which is the most grounded, that is, evaluate the nature and degree of evidence offered by the material. By "evidence" we do not mean an absolute proof or an unquestionable truth. We refer to the clinical reasons that lead us to consider that an inference about a patient is better than some other inference (see Boesky, 2002). This evaluation involves examining not only the strengths of the evidence or findings that emerge from clinical observations but also the omissions or biases that limit its value.

Psychoanalysis, as a method of research, therapy, and theory, relies heavily on clinical observation. As Freud pointed out, speculative theoretical hypotheses "are not the foundation of science, upon which everything rests: that foundation is observation [*Beobachtung*] alone. They are not the bottom but the top of the whole structure, and they can be replaced and discarded without damaging it" (Freud, 1914, p. 77). This does not mean disregarding the theoretical conceptions, because they help us to bring order and clarity to the raw material of observations (Freud, 1933). However, theoretical conceptions very easily become paradigmatic models that, while helping to perceive and think about the clinical material based on certain premises, make it difficult or impossible to see it in the light of other approaches (Bernardi, 1989). For this reason, although current pluralism allowed the emergence of diverse theoretical and technical approaches, it did not manage to promote true scientific controversies (Bernardi, 2002).

Psychoanalysis is essentially a complex clinical discipline and encompasses both scientific and hermeneutic approaches (Bernardi, 2015). In the clinical field, it must address the questions raised by the formulation of a clinical case, namely, what the patient's problems are, what they are due to, what their treatment is, and the benefits obtained (Bernardi, 2016; Rodríguez Quiroga de Pereira et al., 2018). Therefore, they essentially refer to the therapeutic process and its results.

There is an agreement on the need to map evidence. However, emphasis on what the central aspects of evidence are vary, as shown in the controversy over "What does the presentation of case material tell us about what happened in an analysis and how does it do this?" (Blass, 2013; Boesky, 2013; Da Rocha Barros, 2013; Chabert, 2013). Boesky focuses on the interpretations and in explaining what the rationale is. Evidence understood as the information that the analyst can adduce to justify that his or her hypothesis gives a better account of the clinical situation than an alternative hypothesis that arises from the contextualization of the patient's associations in the development of central hypotheses. This brings certain aspects to the fore, such as the application by the pathologist of a particular dye determines the structures that can be made visible (Blass, 2013, p. 1131). Validating an interpretation based only on the patient's reactions immediately after its formulation, without considering the context, would be, for this author, to rely on a fallacious assumption. Given that some hypotheses explain the available data better than others do, one of the most serious problems we face is to resolve and refine the arguments for agreeing or disagreeing on how to make such comparisons. On the other hand, Da Rocha Barros emphasizes the emotional context, the transmission of the living experience of the analytical encounter, and the need for a poetics that can give an account through metaphorical expression. Nevertheless, he proposes that the repetition of specific patterns of mental functioning would be a useful initial form for mapping evidence. Chabert considers that what is important in a clinical material lies in expanding associative thinking, revitalizing a dialogue that would put us in touch with the dialogue that has been maintained in the analysis, a process that is inherently linked to the theoretical models from which we think. The 3-LM shows that some aspects of these three positions can be used as complementary perspectives in a sequential analysis of the clinical material.

Evidence-based practice

The search for evidence criteria is different in psychoanalytical clinical material and extra-clinical research. A systematic empirical investigation of the process and outcomes of psychoanalytic or psychotherapeutic treatments faces problems similar to those of evidence-based medicine

(EBM). This current orientation of health practices seeks the integration of evidence from the best available research with clinical expertise and patient values and preferences (Sackett et al., 1997). The APA Presidential Task Force on Evidence-Based Practice (2006) reaffirms these criteria in the field of psychotherapy and emphasizes that evidence can come from many different areas of both quantitative and qualitative methods. Practice-based evidence (PBE) complements EBM. PBE aims to gather scientific evidence from the clinician's routine practice settings (Barkham & Mellor-Clark, 2003).

A cornerstone of EBM is a hierarchical system of classifying evidence according to the level or weight of the available evidence. Therefore, a treatment's recommendation can range from high to moderate, low, or very low (or similar categories in other classifications) evidence. When the strength of a recommendation is weak, shared decision-making is especially important.

While the assessment of the levels of evidence was conducted with the utmost methodological rigour, many studies were found to be contradictory or non-replicable. This drew attention to the need to practise extreme care in exposing biases and omissions, intentional or unintentional, that could go unnoticed. In our field, Shedler (2015), Leichsenring et al. (2015), and other authors showed biases that could lead to favouring certain psychotherapies over others. This also led to highlighting the importance of the "Discussion" section in scientific work and the need to carefully outline not only the contribution of the undertaken research but also all the factors that may limit its scope (Ioannidis, 2007; Avidan, Ioannidis, & Mashour, 2019).

The degree of psychoanalytic clinical evidence

The path taken by the EBM suggests some topics of reflection for clinical psychoanalytic research. First, it is useful to make our criteria of evidence explicit when examining clinical material. Freud believed that not all clinical cases allowed the same advance of knowledge:

> Something new can only be gained from analyses that present special difficulties, and to the overcoming of these, a great deal of time has to be devoted. Only in such cases do we succeed in descending into the deepest and most primitive strata of mental development and in gaining from there solutions for the problems of the later formations.
>
> (1918, p. 10)

We would like to emphasize this idea: it is necessary to evaluate to what extent the analysis has managed to bring out the central problems of the patient.

Freud also believed that there was an inseparable bond between research and cure (*juntkim* is the word Freud uses to describe the relationship between research and healing). However, the relationship between increased knowledge and therapeutic benefit is complex. The effectiveness of a treatment can be effective as the result of factors other than those invoked by the psychoanalyst (e.g., "common factors," present in different psychotherapeutic approaches). There are "third variables," such as confounders or moderators, that influence both the assumed cause and the effects. In clinical research, we have to carefully examine the way we relate the changes in the analytic process to the changes in the internal world and in the life of the patients.

It is difficult to compare competing hypotheses in single cases. We cannot treat the same patient in two different ways. However, we can advance making our clinical reasoning and the assumed mechanisms of change traceable. In this way, we also expose the strengths and flaws of our hypotheses and "test" them through thought experiments and counterfactual thinking. Thought experiments are a conceptual tool that, although commonly used, has not been methodically employed enough. Thought experiments designate, in science and philosophy, the imaginary scenarios used to conceptually investigate inaccessible phenomena. This type of experiment does not provide factual results but allows us to understand the scope and consistency of our models better. They have always been used by philosophy and sciences such as physics, history, or economics, and the interest in them has increased recently in the philosophy of science (Brown & Fehige, 2019). However, in a rudimentary form they are present, for example, when we try to predict the effect of an interpretation. In that sense, they show the operational models that guide our actions. We will return to this point later, as we consider that their explicitness helps give replicability and traceability to our clinical reasoning.

Empirical research and EBM, as Tuckett says, forces clinicians to try to describe more rigorously and accurately what they see, and to draw out precisely both the viewpoint of observation and the inferential processes that follow (Tuckett, 1995, 1998). It helps us to see more. "Evidence-based psychoanalysis, seen in this way, is an opportunity as well as an imperative" (Tuckett, 2001, p. 214).

We will focus on the criteria for evaluating clinical evidence. These problems are different, whether we consider a cross-sectional—i.e., one session or a few sessions—or a longitudinal study of a treatment and the changes in a long-term perspective. First, we will discuss evidence in both situations, and then we will refer to the problem of biases and omissions that limit the evidence provided by the material. Finally, we will propose, as an outline, a summary table that seeks to prioritize the main criteria set out in the chapter.

The clinical evidence in the session

When thinking about what evidence is available to evaluate the degree of certainty provided by clinical material, the interpretations and their effects present themselves as the observable elements that can bring us closer to the subject. In this sense, two aspects are closely related: the inferential process that leads the analyst to formulate an interpretation and the way in which the patient responds to such formulation, that is, how an interpretation is validated or not. Paul, quoted by Ramzy and Shevrin (1976), points out the need to make a distinction between the psychoanalyst's evaluation of a situation and the interpretation. The analyst's silent and uncommunicated evaluation of the situation constitutes a hypothesis, while the interpretation refers to the communication to the patient of all or part of this hypothesis. Sand (1983) raises the need to discriminate between the formation of hypotheses (how an idea is obtained) and what corresponds to their confirmation (how this idea is proven to be correct), in order to avoid confusion of categories.

Isaacs (1939) raised a controversial issue when she pointed out the need to discuss the tests and verifications to which analysts submit the views they hold in their interventions. At that time, she stressed the practical importance, for analysts and non-analysts alike, of establishing criteria to test the validity of interpretations when thinking about the progress or non-progress of the patients. However, the discussion has focused mostly on what, how, and when to interpret rather than on the validation of the interpretation (Schmidl, 1956). Ramzy and Shevrin (1976) raise with surprise the issue of the scarcity of publications on this subject (fewer than 20) in a period of 50 years. The strength, firmness, or veracity of the interpretations constitutes a central point in the psychoanalytic clinical work. Still, the issue of their confirmation (or not) has not been reflected in an in-depth discussion from the theoretical point of view (Sand, 1983).

Searching for truth in clinical psychoanalysis, Hanly (2009) states that the three criteria of the truth of philosophy—coherence, correspondence, and pragmatism—are not in disagreement with each other, but rather work together in psychoanalysis. In the session, the coherence criterion will bring the patient's previous clinical situations closer to the analyst's memory based on the similarity, consistency, and affection that unites them, and will guide our first ideas in the choice of interpretation. The correspondence criterion (the hypothesis that we formulate in relation to what is happening at that moment in the patient's mind and between analyst and patient) will guide the choice of interpretation. These criteria, together with the pragmatic criterion (if the interpretation is clinically useful), will help to decide on the adequacy of the interpretation based on the changes in associations, affects, and transference of the patient.

According to Isaacs (1939), an interpretation may be correct or incorrect. It can be incorrect in two ways: by being false (it is not related to what is in the patient's mind) or by being incomplete (some aspects are not taken into account by the analyst or one aspect is weighed too much to the detriment of another). If the interpretations have no relation to what is in the mind of the patient, they leave the patient cold or indifferent and are dismissed without any movement of affection. However, incomplete interpretations or those that emphasize one aspect of the material more than on another, "falsely emphasized," can provoke intense responses from the patient. Glover (1931) warns of the suggestive effect of inexact interpretation in the context of strong authority.

As Isaacs stated, the main points to confirm correct interpretations are:

1 The patient consciously elaborates images and meanings that were implicit in their associations or behaviours.
2 They contribute with other associations specifically linked to the interpretation, by amplifying the unconscious attitude or the interpreted fantasy.
3 The associations change, or the patient changes his or her attitude, actively rejecting the analyst's hypothesis by highlighting the defence.
4 In the following sessions, the patient can bring dreams that continue, elaborate on, and clarify the fantasy or unconscious aspect that was interpreted.
5 The patient recovers memories of real experiences from the past.
6 New material emerges that evokes a change at the level of the unconscious fantasy.
7 There is a reduction or transformation of specific anxieties (e.g., paranoid).

In our opinion, these criteria constitute a landmark. The new contributions, instead of questioning these criteria, aimed to broaden the perspective.

To determine the validity of an interpretation, Schmidl (1956) proposes to observe whether there is an analogy ("relationship identity" or at least "relationship similarity") between the proposition to be interpreted and the given interpretation. Each one has a specific gestalt, and both gestalts fit together so closely that there can be no doubt about their joint membership. First, it is necessary to ask ourselves if the gestalt of the proposition to be interpreted (e.g., a dream or a symptom) and the gestalt of the material used for the interpretation are sufficiently determined by concrete elements and their interconnection to justify their meaning. Second, we must ask ourselves if the gestalts fit one into the other—e.g., approach the implicit theory in the analyst's mind as closer to the real patient.

In order for the patient to test an interpretation for its content of truth or falsehood, it should be formulated precisely, clearly, and unambiguously and not include more than one hypothesis (Etchegoyen, 1986, 2001). Long and complex interpretations, in addition to offering more than the patient may think, are difficult to test. Providing them in parts favours waiting for the answer at each step and adjusting the course accordingly. Etchegoyen warns about the risk of arbitrariness and whims of our theories and even our conflicts if the patient's response to the interpretation is not taken into account, not only in its informative and heuristic value but also in its evaluation. Verbal, para-verbal, and non-verbal associations and the insistence of certain signifiers of the patient allow the analyst to test hypotheses within the session. The repetition in the transference allows the analyst to do so throughout the process. The validity of the process is reached at the point of convergence where the findings of the session are prolonged in the slow and persistent changes that appear in it, an aspect that the 3-LM has been able to show.

From an intersubjective and a field perspective, M. and W. Baranger (2008) point out, as process and non-process indicators, the convergence of the variability of the patient and analyst languages, the enrichment of the patient's story, and the affective exchange and the alternation with blocking moments.

From a dyadic and interactive conception, Jiménez (2009) suggests that in the analyst's mind there is continuous decision-making influenced by the patient's reactions and actions and the "implicit" use of explicit theories as mini working models. The task of the analyst is not explanatory but predictive, i.e., to evaluate how the patient reacts if the analyst intervenes in one way or another. During the session, the analyst's mind moves between theoretical and practical reasons. Theoretical reasons allow the analyst to understand and explain the interaction on the basis of knowledge acquired—the implicit use of explicit theories. The practical reasons seek to answer, out of a series of alternatives, which would be the best in clinical utility. The singularity of the encounter in the here-and-now of the session marks the decision to intervene. It constitutes an "ideographic, creative, and ineffable" (p. 236) moment in which the analyst assumes a risk that might not be fully explained by theory. The validation or refutation of the analyst's interventions takes place in the course of this interaction where analyst and patient continuously interpret and negotiate, agreeing or constraining their differences in what they observe and what they consider "clinical facts" and their signification.

Then, the construction of an interpretation constitutes a complex silent and non-communicated evaluation, in which different aspects intervene. On the one hand, the unconscious and preconscious perception of the patient's mental states through free associations, transference, and counter-transference, change in affects, and para-verbal and non-verbal expressions intervene. On the other hand, the theoretical knowledge, the explicit theories, are used implicitly as mini operational models at the time of the session. It does not constitute an isolated process in the analyst's mind, but it occurs in an interactive, intersubjective context and within a dynamic field (Baranger & Baranger, 1961). In this way, the analyst elaborates a hypothesis in correspondence with what is happening in the patient's mind and formulates it so that the patient can evaluate it in its degree of truth or falsehood.

Summarizing, the criteria formulated above by Isaacs remain accurate as evidence to validate the interpretation. It has to be complemented with an interactional and field perspective focused on the evidence necessary to make decisions about what to interpret from a pragmatic and predictive clinical perspective.

Clinical evidence of changes over extended periods of analysis: The 3-LM

The efficacy of psychodynamic therapy in many mental disorders has been confirmed using the methodology of EBM (randomized control trials, meta-analysis) (Leichsenring et al., 2015). Systematic single case research (Kächele et al., 2008) uses a multi-level observational strategy using tape-recorded material. It combines traditional clinical observation with the application of assessment instruments applied by independent researchers, aiming at a systematic description of the aspects and dimensions of the psychoanalytic process. In this way, it combines traditional clinical understanding and the requirements of greater objectification.

The Three-Level Model (3-LM) to observe the patient's transformations (Altmann de Litvan, 2014; Bernardi, 2014a, 2014b) uses only the clinical perspective. We will not present this model here, but we will point out some aspects related to the issue of evidence. The 3-LM constitutes a guide or heuristic to refine and systematize observation of the patient's transformations from the perspective of multiple analysts with different theoretical approaches. Therefore, it seeks, in three successive steps or levels, to find in the clinical material the evidence that allows for identifying, conceptualizing, and formulating explanatory hypotheses about the patient's changes.

The empirical basis on which the 3-LM is based is given by the resonance of a transcribed or tape-recorded clinical material in a group of analysts who listen to it, making use of the "third psychoanalytic ear." This means making full use of the subjective and intersubjective empathic understanding. It is, therefore, an "observation of observation," where the participants take a "second look" at the patient, the analyst, and their own reactions in the group and in an observer–participant attitude. In this sense, it attempts to objectively describe phenomena that are essentially subjective and intersubjective. It moves "bottom up," from the experience as the analyst perceives it from an analytical phenomenological perspective, towards conceptualizations and explanatory hypotheses of a higher level of abstraction. The shared group resonance of the clinical material is the first source of evidence.

At the second level, evidence rises from the critical descriptive analysis of the clinical material, taking into account its group resonances in the previous level. The group is required to adopt a descriptive-analytical attitude in order to conceptualize the dimensions in which the patient's transformations occurred. The questions posed by the 3-LM are based on the diagnostic dimensions of patients' changes, which have been operationalized by manuals such as the *OPD-2* and *PDM-2*. These dimensions encounter several problems. On the one hand, the operationalization is controversial inside psychoanalysis, which makes the use of shared diagnostic criteria difficult. On the other hand, data required by the assessment of the 3-LM dimensions are not always available in the clinical material. It is important to be also aware of other potential limitations. Initial psychoanalytic interviews are often of an exclusively associative type and do not include exploratory aspects, which does not allow for adequate investigation of aspects that the patient splits or omits. The limited number of sessions examined favours selection bias. The analyst does not always select sessions according to the criteria of qualitative research, showing both evidence in favour of the existence of changes and no changes. The greatest restriction appears when the material does not comply with Isaacs's criteria of clinical evidence and contextual information is insufficient.

The clinical material is convincing when the anchor points underlined by the discussion group converge with the foci of the interventions of the analyst, with the patients' structural changes, and with their assimilation and insight about their problematic experiences (see Chapter 4, the discussion of John's case). The clinical material is less convincing if the analyst's assumptions are not confirmed by relational episodes inside and outside the analysis, which show the changes in the patients' vision of their own self and of the others at both the real and fantasy levels. The importance of functioning at the level of the self and with others, highlighted in current psychodynamic manuals, has also been hierarchized by the World Health Organization to define personality disorders in its new classification of illnesses (ICD-11) (World Health Organization, 2018) and by the *DSM-5* in its alternative model, section III (American Psychiatric Association, 2013).

The third level seeks to formulate explanatory hypotheses about the patient's changes or no changes. The aim is to find the best possible explanation of the changes observed in the analytic process with those that occurred in the functioning of the patient's personality. Since these hypotheses are speculative, it is important to compare them through thought experiments. In this way, the rationale of each is exposed, making it possible to examine the internal consistency of the analyst's working models and implicit theories and their correspondence with the clinical facts. The 3-LM long-term perspective has a positive effect on the search for evidence. On the one hand, participants make contact with the clinical material by following the way in which the events occurred, that is, from before to after. During the group discussion, it is also possible to examine this first impression a posteriori. The perspective from the "after" on the "before" allows participants to check the predictions and to examine factors that may have influenced the evolution of the analysis.

It is possible to extend this view over time. Often the 3-LM groups help analysts to change their interpretative strategy and to observe the consequences. Other times it is possible to discuss a material again after some time. In both cases, the new information facilitates reviewing the validity of the initial conclusions.

Systematic single-case research and the 3-LM have been used in a complementary way, which favours the increase of clinical and extra-clinical evidence available (Rodríguez Quiroga de Pereira, 2018). This type of research can contribute significantly to the development of psychoanalytic practice-based evidence.

Limitations, omissions, and biases

It is as important to discover and prioritize the evidence provided by clinical material, as it is used to identify where this evidence is not sufficient or not reliable. As we said in relation to EBM, something similar occurs in the field of health sciences. The study of errors in medical decision-making has increased recently, after the beginning of the patient safety movement (Henriksen & Brady, 2013). Of particular interest is the systematic error, when biases or omissions of significant information are recurrent.

In the field of psychoanalysis, perhaps the strongest criticism came from Grünbaum (1984), who argued that the patient's response to the analysis could be explained as an effect of suggestion and response to the analyst's expectations. This provoked multiple responses, some of which are very recent (Azcona, 2019). Phenomena of suggestion and indoctrination can occur in analysis, but this does not mean that they always occur, nor that it is easy to produce them in all cases. This suggests reversing the burden of proof and studying when and in what analysis suggestion occur. Evidence is greater when the material shows answers from the patient that confirm in an unexpected and surprising way the hypotheses of the analyst. However, multiple other factors can distort clinical evidence and oblige practitioners to adopt a cautious attitude regarding them.

Recently, research on EBM focused on situations when available studies provide only low or limited level of evidence (Detterbeck et al., 2018). In such cases, they suggest weighing the evidence according to an explicit framework and countering the temptation to think it is more robust than it actually is. They propose to use a framework that includes (1) the degree of confounding in non-randomized comparisons; (2) the uncertainty involved in extrapolation from indirect evidence; (3) the plausibility of a rationale; and (4) the systematization of clinical casuistic. These criteria are useful for clinical studies. Confounders, i.e., factors that influence both the intervention and the outcome, can mislead the attribution of causality. For example, better outcomes can be attributed to a high frequency of sessions, without examining if high-frequency patients are at the same time more motivated, have less stressful events, etc., which can also affect the outcome. Extrapolation using indirect evidence is frequently used, e.g., when a famous case is adopted as a general model for other cases without examining their similarities and differences. Sometimes a clinical conclusion rests on a rationale based on theoretical principles without consideration of reasonable alternative explanations. Clinical experience and clinical intuition are a valuable source of hypotheses, but they also are vulnerable to numerous biases.

A bias is an a priori tendency that leads to favouring a certain type of conclusion over other possible ones. They can occur intentionally or unintentionally. More than 50 types of cognitive biases and more than a dozen affective biases have been identified in the field of medical diagnosis (Croskerry, 2009).

Psychoanalysis has extensively studied counter-transference and the effects that the patient may exert consciously or unconsciously on the analyst, as well as the reactions or enactments of the analyst. The extent to which counter-transference can be an obstacle and/or an instrument for the progress of analysis has been also discussed at length. However, the study of other types of biases or omissions has not received similar attention, so, without intending to carry out a systematic study here, we would like to draw attention to their importance.

Biases are present in all fields of human knowledge, and the study of their role in decision-making in situations of uncertainty acquired greater notoriety from the work of D. Kahneman (2011), psychologist and economist, who received the Nobel Prize for his research on these topics.

The "confirmation bias" (also called "my side bias") that leads to looking at clinical phenomena from only one theoretical perspective is frequent in psychoanalysis. The influence of theoretical assumptions has been considered an insurmountable obstacle to achieve a clinical common ground between analysts with different theoretical affiliations (Green, 2005). Although the confirmation bias is usually considered a cognitive bias, from a psychoanalytic point of view, the intense emotions related to professional and personal identity that are usually associated with belonging to psychoanalytic schools cannot be ignored. This leads to the exclusion of hypotheses based on different theoretical premises. The groupthink phenomena reinforce an attitude in which freedom of thought is limited by the need to maintain agreement with the rest of the group. Confirmatory biases favour circular reasoning and "illusory correlations" or "apophenia," biases that lead to the establishment of an association between unrelated phenomena. For example, narratives that relate certain problems of the patient to specific childhood events or maternal attitudes are often considered an indisputable causal, although a closer examination shows that there are other equally defensible hypotheses.

The path followed by the 3-LM as it moves from experience to theoretical hypotheses and includes participants with diverse theoretical affiliations decreases this type of confirmatory bias. Instead, it promotes the search for specific models adjusted to the patient. It cannot prevent the emergence of other types of biases, such as groupthink, selection biases that lead to the omission of clinically meaningful material, and anchoring biases, which deem the information that arrives first more important, and to the "halo effect" that leads to the initial impressions spreading to other areas.

For that reason, it is key that clinical discussions are attentive to such biases. Kahneman (2011) used the acronym WYSIATI (What You See Is All That Is) to describe the belief that the information available is sufficient when it is not, because we see only a part of the problem. Some types of bias, such as "congruence bias," "selection bias," "memory bias," and "authority bias," are more frequent when setting aside a broader contextual perspective and attention is focused only on certain aspects of the material. Confirmation biases and omissions of information reinforce each other.

The importance and pervasiveness of biases and omissions have led several researchers in the field of psychotherapy to question whether the therapist can reliably assess a patient's progress. Lilienfeld et al. (2014) note that the combination of biases may lead to (1) perceiving changes that do not exist; (2) if they do exist, attributing them to the treatment when in fact they are due to other causes; or (3) relating them to specific factors in a therapeutic approach, when in fact they are due to common or nonspecific factors. For this reason, many authors render evaluation through tests and questionnaires more important than the opinion of the therapist (Hannan et al., 2005; Lilienfeld, 2007; Hatfield et al., 2010).

Without denying the usefulness of triangulating the therapist's opinion with other forms of assessment, our interest here is to improve clinical evidence, reducing biases and achieving wider and more reliable clinical information. In the field of health sciences, Wilson and Brekke (1994) consider cognitive bias "mental contamination" and de-biasing "mental correction." A crucial issue is the awareness of the direction and magnitude of biases and the motivation to correct biases. This is also the direction taken by this chapter. Kahneman suggests that there are two types of systems of thinking. "Fast thinking" is an automatic, frequent, emotional, stereotypic, and not conscious heuristic for problem-solving, used most of the time. "Slow thinking," on the contrary, implies logical, calculating, and conscious reasoning, which leads to more reliable although more effortful decisions. Clinical discussion groups force implementation of this second system of thinking. The 3-LM expands Baranger, Baranger, and Mom's (1983) "second look" concept by combining analysis of the analytical field during the sessions with a prolonged observation in time and with the contribution of participants with diverse theoretical approaches. This broadening of the perspective does not eliminate, as we said, the possibility of bias, but favours critical thinking.

The critical review of the strengths and limitations of the evidence offered by clinical material should be part of clinical papers. Their publishing in psychoanalytic journals does not usually include discussions of this kind. Usually authors present their perspective as the only one possible. When taking into account divergent authors, it is frequent that the work highlights the complementary aspects, without discussing the contradictory aspects or discussing the arguments for or against each of them. This situation does not promote the scientific development of the discipline.

The "Discussion" section of a scientific paper should fulfill two main functions. First, it should offer authors the opportunity to present the value of their results and proposals. At the same time, authors should acknowledge the limitations of their study. That means to mention where the results are inconclusive or present weaknesses or limitations in their scope. For editors and reviewers, the inclusion of a realistic and adequately self-critical description of these limitations is not a weakness but a strength of a clinical paper.

This is not an exclusive problem of psychoanalysis. Ioannidis (2007), in a paper provocatively entitled "Limitations are not properly acknowledged in the scientific literature," shows the consequences of this lack of critical appraisal. The acknowledgment of limitations, in his opinion, has to go beyond identification of systematic errors and validity problems. It requires an interpretation of its meaning and influence on the published findings. Knowledge and discussion of limitations are essential for credibility and genuine scientific progress. Insufficient acknowledgment of limitations contributes to the current crisis of conceptual reproducibility of scientific findings. However, sometimes authors are not aware of the limitations of their papers. For this reason, Avidan, Ioannidis, and Mashour (2019) suggest the inclusion of independent external reviewers in the "Discussion" section of scientific papers. In psychoanalytic publications, it would be ideal for authors to expose the inner path they took to reach their conclusions, showing both the arguments that convinced them of their conclusions and those that raised doubts or suggested alternatives. The 3-LM discussions are brainstorming processes where alternative hypotheses are confronted. The challenge is to include this kind of deliberation in the clinical papers.

Towards a framework for evaluating clinical evidence

What follows is a first attempt to offer a framework for evaluation of the level of evidence (high, moderate, or low) provided by clinical material. We are putting together the criteria that clinical psychoanalysis has always taken into consideration and we examined in the previous paragraphs. The result is a multidimensional assessment that helps critical reflection about clinical judgments and theory building.

Quality of the analytical process: Transformations in the session

The weight of evidence provided by an analysis increases when significant transformations occurred in the patient and in the therapeutic relationship.

This implies, first, evaluating the short-term effect of the analyst's interpretations. The criteria proposed by Isaacs (1939) remain unquestioned. They underline unconscious answers from the patient, which limit the most direct effects of the suggestion or the expectations of the analyst. In this sense, the importance of the manifestation of unexpected effects that are surprising for the analyst and for the patient themselves should be emphasized. When the clinical material meets the criteria indicated by Isaacs, with the required contextual information, we can affirm that the level of evidence it offers as support for hypotheses is high. On the contrary, the level of evidence is low or absent when we do not find answers of this type from the patient but rather conscious answers to the analyst's interpretations, in which the analyst's theoretical orientation is perceptible. When the analyst remains mostly silent, it is necessary to examine to what extent this leads to the patient's free association or to increase a defensive discourse.

The weight of the evidence increases if, following Baranger and Baranger's (2008) descriptions, we consider a dynamic field co-created by the patient and the analyst, which allows visualizing with more clarity of the progress of the analytical process and the shared resistances (bastions, enactments) or the sequences of ruptures and repairs of the link. The level of evidence increases when the analyst is able to identify these phenomena and predict the effect of the interpretations that will be effective. In this way, it is possible to verify that there is a real exchange and attunement between patient and analyst.

On the contrary, the level of evidence is low when the analyst's thread of argument is possible to discover only through interpretations, while on the patient's side we only find repetitive or conscious topics, which sometimes do not even clearly show what leads them, at a conscious and unconscious level, to continue the analysis.

Between clear cases of high and low evidence, there are intermediate degrees that can be classified as moderate evidence.

The transformations that take place during long-term periods of analysis

We find a second criterion of high-level evidence in changes at the patient's level of psychopathology and personality throughout the treatment. The second level of the 3-LM seeks to evaluate those changes. The weight of the evidence increases when there is a follow-up of the case or added evaluation tools from single-case research.

Evidence increases when patients' changes can be related to the analytic process through specific hypotheses about possible mechanisms of change. When there is no explanation of how the analytical process had an effect on the existence or non-existence of changes, evidence should be considered moderate or low. Evidence is also low when changes are described in terms of purely behavioural or symptomatic modifications without showing connections with changes in the patient's inner world and personality functioning. It is important to include contextual information about other factors that could have influenced patients' changes.

Discussion of alternative hypotheses

As already explained, clinical material can usually be interpreted from more than one theoretical perspective. Evidence is greater when different interpretative hypotheses are confronted and the strengths and limitations of each are critically compared. Each hypothesis should account for neglected aspects that are highlighted by competing hypotheses. This is the function of mental thought experiments. Although they do not provide direct factual evidence, they force the working models that seek to account for the situation to be formulated more precisely. This allows listeners to put their similar experiences into play, evaluating which hypothesis is more convincing, thus reinforcing the level of evidence. The discussion of alternative hypotheses helps to reduce omissions in the presentation of the case.

Table 14.1 Assessment of the weight of evidence provided by the clinical material for answering 3-LM third-level questions

	High evidence	*Moderate or low evidence*	*Very low evidence*
1 Clinical information about treatment foci	• Initial Interviews combine associative and exploratory aspects. • There is contextual information about the experience of illness, stressful events, trait/state, conflict/structure, and severity markers.	• The patient's subjective suffering is clearly described at Level 1 of the 3-LM, but there are omissions and insufficient information about Level 2 dimensions.	• Clinical descriptions are insufficient at both Levels 1 and 2. • Clear bias (availability, confirmatory, selection, etc.).
2 Relationship between analyst's interventions and patient's change process	• There is clear evidence of an interactive dialectical process and its progress during the sessions, and it is linked to long-term changes. • Hypotheses are a coherent and plausible explanation of the process.	• Weak relationship between interpretations and change process.	• Changes cannot be linked to interpretations (without evidence in favour of a non-linear system model).
3 Inferential processes. Consideration of alternative hypotheses	• Hypotheses are clearly linked to the clinical material and reasonable alternative hypotheses are discussed. • Clinical reasoning and arguments or thought experiments are carefully described.	• Hypotheses are theory-driven and insufficiently grounded in the clinical material • Alternative hypotheses are discarded on the basis of theoretical preferences • An insufficient conceptual analysis. Alternative hypotheses are deemed complementary.	• Strong confirmation bias. One-sided or authority arguments.

Evidence levels decrease when the severity of the dysfunctions and split-off aspects of the self and the object are not investigated, or the duration, extension, and severity of the problems are not mentioned. Sometimes the clinical material does not allow for the distinction of a transitory state from a permanent personality trait, or problems related to unconscious conflicts from failures in integrating the structural aspects of psychic functioning. The assumption that exclusive attention to free association leads to better capture of unconscious phenomena leads to highlighting only aspects of the material in agreement with the previous theoretical premises, i.e., to a "my side bias."

Thoughtful discussion of alternative hypotheses led to a better understanding of the context. We agree with Boesky (2013) when he says, "We need to know how and why certain material was deemed meaningful" (p. 1138), and

> How we think about "evidence" is inseparable from how we think about contextualization. At issue is a call for wider recognition of the problems we perpetuate in continually denying the profound epistemological penalties we have incurred by our neglect of this gap in our methodology, how we gather and evaluate our contextualizing criteria. . . . We cannot continue to delay the necessity of facing this problem
>
> (p. 1142)

Table 14.1 summarizes some of the characteristics that allow us to evaluate the weight of evidence of clinical material. This attempt to establish a gradation should be considered preliminary and necessarily incomplete.

References

Altmann, M. (2014). *Time for change: Tracking transformations in psychoanalysis—The Three-Level Model*. London: Karnac.

American Psychiatric Association. (2013). *Diagnostic and statistical manual of mental disorders* (5th edn). Arlington: American Psychiatric Association.

APA Presidential Task Force on Evidence-Based Practice. (2006). Evidence-based practice in psychology. *American Psychologist, 61*(4), 271–285.

Avidan, M. S., Ioannidis J. P. A., & Mashour, G. A. (2019). Independent discussion sections for improving inferential reproducibility in published research. *British Journal of Anaesthesia, 122*(4), 413–420.

Azcona, M. (2019). Hacia una redefinición del problema de la sugestión en psicoanálisis: minimizando el efecto Pigmalión [Towards a redefinition of the problem of suggestion in psychoanalysis: Minimizing the Pygmalion effect]. *Perspectivas en Psicología, 16*(2), 98–107.

Baranger, M., & Baranger, W. (1961). La situación analítica como campo dinámico [The analytical situation as a dynamic field]. *Revista Uruguaya de Psicoanálisis, 4*.
Baranger, M., & Baranger, W. (2008). The analytic situation as a dynamic field. *International Journal of Psychoanalysis, 89*(4), 795–826.
Baranger, M., Baranger, W., & Mom, J. (1983). Process and non-process in analytic work. *International Journal of Psychoanalysis, 64*, 1–15.
Barkham, M., & Mellor-Clark, J. (2003). Bridging evidence-based practice and practice-based evidence: Developing a rigorous and relevant knowledge for the psychological therapies. *Clinical Psychology & Psychotherapy, 10*, 319–327.
Bernardi, R. (1989). The role of paradigmatic determinants in psychoanalytic understanding. *International Journal of Psychoanalysis, 70*(2), 341–357.
Bernardi, R. (2002). The need for true controversies in psychoanalysis: The debates on Melanie Klein and Jacques Lacan in the Rio de la Plata. *International Journal of Psychoanalysis, 83*, 851–873.
Bernardi, R. (2014a). The assessment of changes: Diagnostic aspects. In M. Altmann (Ed.), *Time for change: Tracking transformations in psychoanalysis—The Three-Level Model* (pp. 263–278). London: Karnac.
Bernardi, R. (2014b). The Three-Level Model (3-LM) for observing patient transformations. In M. Altmann (Ed.), *Time for change: Tracking transformations in psychoanalysis—The Three-Level Model* (pp. 3–44). London: Karnac.
Bernardi, R. (2015). What kind of discipline is psychoanalysis? *International Journal of Psychoanalysis, 96*, 731–754.
Bernardi, R. (2016). La formulación clínica del caso: su valor para la práctica clínica [The clinical formulation of the case: Its value for clinical practice]. In R. Bernardi, B. Varela, D. Miller, R. Zytner, L. de Souza, & R. Oyenard (Eds), *La formulación psicodinámica de caso. Su valor para la práctica clínica* [*The psychodynamic formulation of a case: Its value for clinical practice*] (pp. 25–24). Montevideo: Grupo Magro Editores, Universidad Católica del Uruguay.
Blass, R. B. (2013). Psychoanalytic controversy. Introduction: What does the presentation of case material tell us about what actually happened in an analysis and how does it do this? *International Journal of Psychoanalysis, 94*, 1129–1134.
Boesky, D. (2002). Why don't our institutes teach the methodology of clinical psychoanalytic evidence? *Psychoanalytic Quarterly, 71*(3), 445–475.
Boesky, D. (2013). What does the presentation of case material tell us about what actually happened in an analysis and how does it do this? *International Journal of Psychoanalysis, 94*(6), 1135–1143.
Brown, J. R., & Fehige, Y. (2019). Thought experiments. In Edward N. Zalta (Ed.), *The Stanford Encyclopedia of Philosophy Archive* (Winter 2019 Edition). https://plato.stanford.edu/archives/win2019/entries/thought-experiment/.
Chabert, C. (2013). Psychoanalytic controversy. Response: What does the presentation of case material tell us about what actually happened in an analysis and how does it do this? *International Journal of Psychoanalysis, 94*, 1153–1162.
Croskerry, P. (2009). A universal model of diagnostic reasoning. *Academic Medicine, 84*(8), 1022–1028.
Da Rocha Barros, E. (2013). Psychoanalytical controversy: What does the presentation of case material tell us about what actually happened in an analysis and how does it do this? *International Journal of Psychoanalysis, 94*, 1145–1152.

Detterbeck, F. C., Gould, M. K., Lewis, S. Z., & Patel, S. (2018). Extending the reach of evidence-based medicine. *Chest, 153*(2), 498–506.

Etchegoyen, R. H. (1986). *Los fundamentos de la técnica psicoanalítica* [*The basics of psychoanalytic technique*]. Buenos Aires: Amorrortu.

Etchegoyen, R. H. (2001). Algo más sobre el testeo del proceso clínico [Something else about testing of the clinical process]. *Subjetividad y Procesos Cognitivos, 1*, 34–59.

Freud, S. (1914). On narcissism. *S.E. 14*, 67–102.

Freud, S. (1918). From the history of an infantile neurosis. *S.E. 17*, 1–12.

Freud, S. (1933). New introductory lectures on psychoanalysis. *S.E.* 22, 1–182.

Glover, E. (1931). The therapeutic effect of inexact interpretation: A contribution to the theory of suggestion. *International Journal of Psychoanalysis, 12*, 397–411.

Green, A. (2005). The illusion of *common ground* and mythical pluralism. *International Journal of Psychoanalysis, 86*(3), 627–632.

Grünbaum, A. (1984). *The foundations of psychoanalysis: A philosophical critique.* Berkeley: University of California Press.

Hanly, C. (2009). On truth and clinical psychoanalysis. *International Journal of Psychoanalysis, 90*(2), 375–383.

Hannan, C., Lambert, M. J., Harmon, C., Lars Nielsen, S., Smart, D. W., & Shimokawa, K. (2005). A lab test and algorithms for identifying clients at risk for treatment failure. *Journal of Clinical Psychology in Session, 61*, 155–163.

Hatfield, D., McCullough, L., Frantz, S. H. B., & Krieger, K. (2010). Do we know when our clients get worse? An investigation of therapists' ability to detect negative client change. *Clinical Psychology and Psychotherapy, 17*, 25–32.

Henriksen, K., & Brady, J. (2013). The pursuit of better diagnostic performance: A human factors perspective. *BMJ Quality & Safety*, 22, ii1–ii5.

Ioannidis, J. P. A. (2007). Limitations are not properly acknowledged in the scientific literature. *Journal of Clinical Epidemiology, 60*, 324–329.

Isaacs, S. (1939). Criteria for interpretation. *International Journal of Psychoanalysis, 20*, 148–160.

Jiménez, J. P. (2009). Grasping psychoanalysts' practice in its own merits. *International Journal of Psychoanalysis, 90*(2), 231–248.

Kächele, H., Schachter, J., & Thomä, H. (2008). *From psychoanalytic narrative to empirical single case research: Implications for psychoanalytic practice.* New York: Routledge.

Kahneman, D. (2011). *Thinking, fast and slow.* New York: Farrar, Straus and Giroux.

Leichsenring, F., Luyten, P., Hilsenroth, M. J., Abbass, A., Barber, J. B., Keefe, J. R., Leweke, F., Rabung, S., & Steinert, C. (2015). Psychodynamic therapy meets evidence-based medicine: A systematic review using updated criteria. *Lancet Psychiatry, 2*, 648–660.

Lilienfeld, S. O. (2007). Psychological treatments that cause harm. *Perspectives on Psychological Science,* 2(1), 53–70.

Lilienfeld, S. O., Ritschel, L. A., Lynn, S. J., Cautin, R. L., & Latzman, R. D. (2014). Why ineffective psychotherapies appear to work: A taxonomy of causes of spurious therapeutic effectiveness. *Perspectives on Psychological Science, 9*, 355–387.

Ramzy, I., & Shevrin, H. (1976). The nature of the inference process in psychoanalytic interpretation: A critical review of the literature. *International Journal of Psychoanalysis, 57*, 151–159.

Rodríguez Quiroga de Pereira, A. (2018). La formulación psicodinámica de caso. Su valor para la práctica clínica [Psychodynamic case formulation: Its value for clinical practice]. *International Journal of Psychoanalysis, 99*(1), 266–271.
Rodríguez Quiroga de Pereira, A., Borensztein, L., Corbella, V., & Marengo, J. C. (2018). The Lara case: A group analysis of initial psychoanalytic interviews using systematic clinical observation and empirical tools. *International Journal of Psychoanalysis, 99*(6), 1327–1352.
Sackett, D. L., Straus, S. E., Richardson, W. S., & Rosenberg, W. (1997). *Evidence-based medicine: How to practice & teach EBM*. New York: Churchill Livingstone.
Sand, R. (1983). Confirmation in the Dora case. *International Review of Psychoanalysis, 10*, 333–357.
Schmidl, F. (1956). The problem of scientific validation in psycho-analytic interpretation. *International Journal of Psychoanalysis, 36*, 105–113.
Shedler, J. (2015). Where is the evidence for "evidence-based" therapy? *Journal of Psychological Therapies in Primary Care, 4*, 47–59.
Tuckett, D. (1995). The conceptualization and communication of clinical facts in psychoanalysis. *International Journal of Psychoanalysis, 76*, 653–662.
Tuckett, D. (1998). Evaluating psychoanalytic papers: Towards the development of common editorial standards. *International Journal of Psychoanalysis, 79*, 431–448.
Tuckett, D. (2001). Evidence-based psychoanalysis. *International Forum of Psychoanalysis, 10*(3–4), 211–215.
Wilson, T. D., & Brekke, N. (1994). Mental contamination and mental correction: Unwanted influences on judgments and evaluations. *Psychological Bulletin, 116*, 117–142.
World Health Organization. (2018). *International classification of diseases for mortality and morbidity statistics* (11th rev.). https://icd.who.int/browse11/l-m/en.

Commentary: Perspectives from the Philosophy of Science—Charles Hanly

In their study, Bernardi and Pérez Suquilvide are seeking to strengthen two aspects of psychoanalytic knowledge: the objectivity of its clinical base and the implications of reliable clinical facts for psychoanalytic theory. This is an important step because psychic processes are often over-determined, e.g., Oedipal fantasies are phallic and narcissistic. As a result, theoretical differences have arisen over causal explanations that are compatible, or, with modifications, can be shown to be so. There are also theories or components of different theories that are incompatible, e.g., "the Oedipus complex is instinctual" as opposed to "the Oedipus complex is caused by narcissistically inadequate parenting." In assessing evidence for evaluating interpretations and the theories they imply, the sorting out of such issues is essential. Bernardi and Pérez Suquilvide have usefully explored the need to estimate the relevance and degree of evidence for and against alternative psychoanalytic theories. This undertaking is an essential aspect of the 3-LM's contribution to finding ways to integrate compatible theories and to find evidence to logically test contrary or contradictory alternative theories (Hanly, 2019). The authors take up Freud's empiricist premise that what happens and does not happen in an analysis is epistemologically fundamental to psychoanalytic knowledge. In this spirit, the "discussions" in this book entertain alternative assumptions and perspectives, not as a priori principles but as hypotheses to be tested against clinical verbatim material (Hanly, 1983). Bernardi and Pérez Suquilvide tackle the problems of how to find and evaluate the evidence for this important undertaking for the future of psychoanalysis.

Their basic position is addressed in the structure of the Three-Level Model. When it comes to validating (and falsifying) psychoanalytic hypotheses, there are three basic clinical phenomena to consider: the patient's presenting problems embedded in the patient's symptoms and inhibitions, and expressed (made evident) in the patient's feelings about the analysis and the analyst (referred to as "anchor points" in the model); their treatment in an analytic process of empathic interpretation; and the gains or lack of gains in these aspects of the treatment measured by the extent and durability of the amelioration of the symptoms and inhibitions after the treatment has ended. This is the core of the 3-LM method.

Psychoanalysis is a clinical discipline. Although it has powerful implications for the humanities and social sciences, the truth of its findings is vouchsafed only by clinical experience or what Grünbaum has called the tally argument. Grünbaum's critique of the tally argument can be shown to be fallacious, although I agree with his inductivism in the construction of knowledge. Grünbaum's critique should not deter us from being guided by the core idea of the tally argument (Hanly, 1988, 1992). In the extent to which psychoanalysis can genuinely and durably ameliorate symptoms, inhibitions, and related psychic incapacities is evidence that the interpretations that have brought about this amelioration do "tally" with what had caused them in the patient. Bernardi and Pérez Suquilvide tackle the fundamental problems of how to assemble and assess this clinical evidence.

The authors propose that a core problem of psychoanalytic clinical evidence is that analysts can be subject to bias. Although ideas are required for intelligently organized observation (Hanly, 1995), ideas need not, but may, fail to yield unbiased observation. An observational science must address and solve these problems of reliability as much as possible. For example, the personal analysis is supposed to facilitate a sufficient degree of clinical objectivity. But it may fail, for example, if the training analyst fails to analyze the candidate's idealizing transference, leaving the candidate predisposed to over-value the analyst's theoretical ideas and to devalue ideas that are contrary to them (Hanly, 1982). The unanalyzed idealizing transference turns theory into ideology and inhibits the open-minded skepticism needed to entertain ideas from alternate perspectives and to allow the details of what happens to the patient in the analysis to decide what theory is most probable. Ideological ideas are not subject to criticism on the basis of clinical facts, i.e., evidence. Nor do they favour the ability to carry out the thought experiments described by Bernardi and Pérez Suquilvide that allow analysts to check out the bearing of clinical facts on alternative theories by contextualizing the facts (i.e., in interpretation sequences that have brought about real symptom reduction). The importance of being able to employ alternative perspectives in the history of human knowledge is evident in Copernicus's revolutionary speculation about what we would see if the observer rotated and the sun stood still. Or much later Freud's question "What if sexuality had its onset with birth?" What Cooper (2008) identifies as "theoretical and technical dogmatism" may also be rooted in the analyst's idealizing transference to his or her own analyst and the aggression repressed by the idealization becoming attached to alternative theories causing the analyst to miss evidence in associations and transferences. The analyzed psyche of the analyst employing the methods of free association, transference observation, and interpretation is the only instrument we have to learn about the nature of the psychic unconscious of our patients. Along with their extensive scholarship, the authors explore how reliable evidence for deciding questions of theory can be evaluated even while facing this daunting fact.

In their search for the nature of authentic psychoanalytic evidence and the difficulties that stand in the way of gaining it, Bernardi and Pérez Suquilvide may attribute too much to Boesky's (2008) idea of contextualization. Boesky does strongly share the goal of finding reliable clinical evidence for and against psychoanalytic theories. Moreover, there is a fairness and a respect for others as well as an important cognitive value in making sure that we have understood an interpretation, or its absence, by clarifying and understanding its theoretical context. Contextualization is an essential part of the exploration of an analyst's explicit, public, formally espoused theories and the implicit theories that actually inform his analytic work (Sandler, 1992; Canestri, 2012). Bernardi and Pérez Suquilvide make good use in the chapter of Boesky's idea of contextualization. The 3-LM requires us to use clinical detail to understand the meaning of the associations and transferences of the patient and of the analyst's interpretations communicated to the patient. For these purposes its value cannot be exaggerated. However, contextualization is not in itself adequate for meeting Cooper's (2008) wish for a method that can identify two or more logically inconsistent alternative theories and find out which interpretive strategy tallies best with the causes of the patient's neurosis because it heals symptomatic and inhibited functioning and restores normal functioning.

Boesky's idea of contextualization requires that we find the theory that makes an interpretive strategy fully meaningful, when any other contextualization would deprive the interpretations of their meaning or even distort their meaning. To this one must surely concur. But nothing in this procedure provides evidence for whether or not an interpretation tallies with what was causing the symptoms and inhibitions in a patient that have undergone change in an analysis. Contextualization establishes only that the interpretation is coherently related to essential components of a theory, be it Freudian, Kleinian, relational, self-psychological, etc., the effectiveness of which in any particular clinical situation is left up in the air. The results of contextualization, treated as evidence itself, leaves psychoanalytic knowledge divided in isolated mutually untestable, solipsistic bodies of knowledge. The coherence involved is a necessary but not a sufficient criterion for reliable evidence. Contextualization does not provide the evidence we need to work toward a more integrated psychoanalytic theory composed of the most probable knowledge we now have, open to fresh evidence to further improve it and methods for doing so. For this work we need contextualization but also factual, objective evidence of significant beneficial changes in patients in analysis and the interpretative strategies that caused them. Only with these clinical facts in hand can we then test theories.

Bernardi and Pérez Suquilvide significantly address the problems of assessing the merit and weight of evidence for the efficacy of interpretations. Freud's tally argument and his use of it to falsify the universality of his initial seduction theory, and which also provided evidence for Freud's hypotheses of pre-pubertal sexuality and the power of unconscious fantasy, establishes the link between the therapeutic efficacy of interpretation and the probability of their correspondence with the psychological processes at work in the patient. This link is the pragmatic evidence for the probable correspondence of psychoanalytic interpretations with the patient's difficulties, and therefore evidence for theories they imply, to which Bernardi and Pérez Suquilvide refer in their chapter.

Given the importance of this pragmatic evidence, it might be useful to comment further on the philosophical and scientific definitions of pragmatism (Hanly, 2009). James (1907) held that a belief is true if it coheres with and enriches a person's other beliefs and experience of life. Hence, a belief in God that gives meaning and purpose to an individual's life is treated by James as evidence of its truth, although all that it proves is that a belief that there is a beneficent God is beneficial to the person whose belief it is. This definition relies in part on the idea that coherence is a sufficient criterion of truth. Freud's idea of pragmatic evidence is very different in being an idea of scientific pragmatism. Let us briefly consider the evidence that caused Freud to modify but not altogether reject the seduction theory. Release from the symptoms of hysteria caused by interpretations based upon a theory of their origin (sexual seduction theory) using a treatment method specific to the theory (cathartic method) would provide sufficient evidence that the theory is true. When the symptomatic relief does not occur or is not durable, although it does work for some cases of the neurosis, we have pragmatic evidence that the theory is true of some but not of all cases of hysteria. The theory is not, as Freud had believed, universal. Some other factors would have to be at work. Freud correctly inferred that patients must have experienced fantasies of being seduced and, therefore, these children must have had a sexual life and had known some form of sexual excitation and pleasure during their childhood. Bringing about, partially bringing about, and failing to bring about a specific change (in 3-LM in an anchor point) is a pragmatic test of the interpretations used and the theory that accredits them. The coherence of belief with other beliefs and experience is not enough.

Bernardi and Pérez Suquilvide have given us a useful (pragmatic in the scientific sense) perspective on assessing, among other sorts of evidence, pragmatic evidence in psychoanalysis. The 3-LM is on the path that leads to the use of scientific pragmatism to test interpretations and theories (here contextualization plays an important part) by realizing, despite difficulties, the potential for objectivity and intersubjectivity (competently trained observers see what is there to be seen for the most part and, hence, are able to agree about the facts) in the clinical observation of change, degrees of change, and no change in specified areas of a patient's functioning. The model is on its way to finding the causal links of sets of interpretations to ameliorative change and, hence, to the evaluation of theories.

The authors' thoughtfully skeptical and demanding study of psychoanalytic evidence is a welcome antidote to the subjectivistic and individualistic "arts and crafts" approach to psychoanalytic knowledge currently in vogue with some analysts. Theirs is a robustly demanding approach to the epistemological, methodological, and logical problems of evidence in a necessarily observational science.

References

Boesky, D. (2008). *Psychoanalytic disagreements in context*. Lanham: Jason Aronson.

Canestri, J. (2012). *Putting theory to work: How are theories actually used in practice?* London: Karnac Books.

Cooper, A. M. (2008). Psychoanalysis today: A plurality of orthodoxies. *Journal of the American Academy of Psychoanalysis, 36*, 235–253.

Hanly, C. (1982). Narcissism, defence and the positive transference. *International Journal of Psychoanalysis, 63*, 427–444.

Hanly, C. (1983). A problem of theory testing. *International Review of Psychoanalysis, 10*, 393–405.

Hanly, C. (1988). The foundations of psychoanalysis: A philosophical critique. *Journal of the American Psychoanalytic Association, 36*, 521–528.

Hanly, C. (1992). Inductive reasoning in clinical psychoanalysis. *International Journal of Psychoanalysis, 73*, 293–301.

Hanly, C. (1995). On facts and ideas in psychoanalysis. *International Journal of Psychoanalysis, 76*, 901–908.

Hanly, C. (2009). On truth and clinical psychoanalysis. *International Journal of Psychoanalysis, 90*(2), 363–373.

Hanly, C. (2019). The problem of pluralism in psychoanalysis. In P. Cesar Sandler and G. Pacheco Costa (Eds), *On Freud's "The Question of Lay Analysis"* (pp. 135–167) Abingdon: Routledge.

James, W. (1907). *Pragmatism: A new name for some old ways of thinking*. Cambridge, MA: Harvard University Press, 1975.

Sandler, J. (1992). Reflections on developments in the theory of psychoanalytic technique. *International Journal of Psychoanalysis, 73*, 189–198.

Part VIII

Three-Level Model

Chapter 15

Guidelines for organizing 3-LM Groups

Margaret Ann Fitzpatrick Hanly,
Ricardo Bernardi, and
Marina Altmann de Litvan

The 3-LM is a flexible model that has evolved over time. The model is used as a guide in clinical groups, in various settings, to explore a psychoanalytic clinical material and can be adapted to meet the needs of our different institutions (see Chapter 10). The model's aim is to ask more and more useful, cogent, and accurate questions that help to understand the changes in patients in analysis. For this reason, we present here ideas and methods updated in the current version (still evolving), which present the model's objectives, various ways of organizing discussion groups and questions formulated to guide the 3-LM discussion groups.

About the 3-LM

This description of the Three-Level Model, written as a proposal by Ricardo Bernardi in May 2011, is updated into a current 3-LM Manual by Margaret Ann Fitzpatrick Hanly, Ricardo Bernardi, and Marina Altmann de Litvan.

Method of analysis of clinical observation: Three-Level Model for Observing Patient Transformations

The aim of the Project Committee on Clinical Observation is to promote a more accurate and systematic clinical observation, useful for theory testing and theory building. The committee's first book on the Three-Level Model, *Time for Change: Tracking Transformation in Psychoanalysis—The Three-Level Model* (2014) presents a full account of the model and the thinking behind it.

The model aims to enrich and refine clinical observation, analyzing its functioning and different levels of clinical practice, focused on the transformation that occurs in the patient during analysis. The transformation in the psychoanalytic patient is prioritized, although the model takes into account the fact that change occurs in the context of the mutual relationship between patient and analyst.

The transformations that occur during analysis have multiple facets and raise a wide range of questions: What changes? How does change occur? When? Why? These problems have been discussed extensively in the literature. The aim here is not to answer the questions themselves but to study ways in which a better clinical observation can contribute to advance the study of their answers.

The guidelines for the Three-Level Model that are presented here outline a method for heuristic evaluation of change and no change in psychoanalysis, ways to refine, systematize, and conceptualize clinical observations. The model can be used in personal reflections or in group deliberations, when the analyst feels that it is necessary to take a "second look" (Baranger et al., 1983) at the session material. The model can also be used as an open guide for analysts in discussion groups who want to enhance clinical observation through systematic analysis of a clinical material. The committee is especially interested in fostering these discussion groups in local IPA societies.

The three levels or steps considered in the model are the following:

Level I: Phenomenological description of the transformations

The first aim of the model is to refine the description of the transformations that took place in an analysis over several years, through a group discussion using the phenomenological descriptions of the analysis—that is, using ordinary language and quoting passages from the verbatim sessions taken at intervals over the course of the analysis. The presenting analyst includes in the clinical material a brief history and five or six detailed verbatim sessions, selecting sessions in a spontaneous way that allows the analyst to transmit the psychoanalytical meaning and resonance of her or his experience. (Other materials, such as tape-recorded sessions, can be used.) The 3-LM clinical material should include notes on the patient's experiences, and tones also conveyed (preconsciously) in the analyst's reading, as well as the analyst's key counter-transference reflections, and other clinical phenomena that can support inferences about the underlying unconscious processes.

The analytic sessions selected during two or more points in the analysis permit a focus on the appraisal of the transformations at a macro level. The individual sessions describe transformations that occur in the interaction between patient and analyst at a micro level, with details of the patient's response to an interpretation.

Aims of the group discussion at Level I

Listening as a group to the analytic session material read by the analyst and sorting out the main presenting problems and changes in the patient can help participants increase their sensitivity to unfamiliar clinical situations and make them more aware of blind spots and subtleties in the clinical material.

Level 2: Identification of the main diagnostic dimensions of change

The aim in the second-level discussions is to identify the main "dimensions," conceptually, along which the transformations in the patient occur. A systematic and valid description of change requires that at least two points of reference be compared, and requires that the group refer to sufficiently ample data concerning the initial problems of the patient, in his or her mental and interpersonal functioning, as well as intrapsychic conflicts.

The following dimensions are considered indispensable for adequate understanding of psychic transformations:

1 Patient's subjective experience of illness and concept, and expectations of change.
2 Patterns of interpersonal relationships in the external world and in the transference–counter-transference relationship
3 Main intrapsychic conflicts.
4 Mental functioning and psychic structure: (a) capacity for self and other perception; (b) regulation (of impulses, affects, and self-esteem); (c) internal and external communication (including aspects related with bodily self); (d) attachment with internal and external objects.
5 Type of personality disorder (if any).
6 Therapeutic foci: analyst's view of the aspects that play a central role in the psychodynamics of the clinical picture, causing or maintaining the disturbances and that require treatment.
7 Follow-up information about the evolution between and after the chosen points of reference.

Aims of the group discussion at Level 2

First, to contextualize the transformations of the patient, finding a more comprehensive description of what is wrong in the patient. Second, to analyze changes in the patient according to diagnostic dimensions (using questions from Level 2 selected by the moderator) described in a language that is experience-near and theoretically unsaturated. Given the multiplicity of theories, it is a good idea to start the discussion using a phenomenological language based on words that comprise the smallest common denominator of the diverse existing theoretical versions of these concepts. (At Level 3 there will be the opportunity to reformulate and develop these theoretical aspects from multiple perspectives.)

Level 3: Hypotheses on links between interventions and observed changes

Transformations during analysis are brought about by interpretive strategies that are related to different explanatory theoretical models and approaches. Level 3 explores which problems the analyst focused on in the clinical material, and any changes in the focus over time. Questions lead to observations about the effect on the patient of specific interventions. At Level 3, participants deliberate on possible change mechanisms or curative factors brought about by interventions in this analysis. The Level 3 discussion also engages in an enquiry into aspects of the clinical material that were not addressed by the analyst. Hypotheses can then be made concerning alternative interpretations related to passages in the verbatim sessions, which could have addressed problems observed in the patient or process.

The aim of the discussion at this level is not to make decisions about whether an alternative interpretation would have worked better, but to examine the clinical support for each hypothesis. "Testing" a hypothesis should be understood as attempting to enhance the observational base of theoretical hypotheses, thereby developing the capacity to link theoretical concepts with clinical data, and to make predictions or conjectures that can stimulate new clinical observations.

Aims of the group discussion at Level 3

To observe what the interpretations address in the clinical material, patterns of interpretations, and the effects on the patient of interpretations. To test and enhance the observational base of theoretical hypothesis about how the interpretations facilitate change.

The three levels of group discussion could properly be regarded as contributing an expert validation of clinical inferences concerning change and observations on how change happens.

Practical guidelines for 3-LM clinical observation groups—Marina Altmann de Litvan, chair 2011–2017, and Margaret Ann Fitzpatrick Hanly, chair 2017–2021

The Committee on Clinical Observation welcomes all analysts who are interested in the creation of one or more IPA Clinical Observation Groups in their own psychoanalytic societies, and encourages them to follow the steps described in this guide.

The practical guidelines presented here aim to give groups of analysts a method to apply the Three-Level Model for Observing Patient

Transformations to psychoanalytic clinical material. Should your group find any difficulty, please do not hesitate to contact us through our IPA e-mail address: ipa.clinical.observation@gmail.com.

There are many adaptations of the 3-LM format for groups that can be made. 3-LM groups have been moderated for candidates in one and a half- or two-hour seminars over several weeks of a course or for professional development groups once a month for six or seven months.

Please contact us and ask us for our latest version of the Three-Level Model for Observing Patient Transformations (3-LM).

About the clinical material

General considerations

The 3-LM has been designed to evaluate change in the patient. The presenter is asked to include material that shows the changes as well as material that could question these changes (respecting qualitative research criteria). The presenter is asked to include in the report the motives that lead her or him to present this specific material, to reflect on whether expectations were met. When a follow-up is possible, after the 3-LM group discussion the analyst will report on whether there has been an effect (positive or negative) on the analyst's work with the patient.

The analyst's doubts about change in the analysis

All psychoanalytic clinical materials raise questions about how and how much the patient has changed, since all analyses have limitations. The analyst may have in mind certain doubts about the gains the patient has made when choosing the material, but is asked not to make these explicit until the relevant moments in the group process.

Specifics on sessions to be selected

The clinical material will be chosen in a way that allows a good description of the opening situation for patient and analyst and transformations through the course of the analysis. The analyst is asked not to give her or his theoretical ideas but a brief history of the session material.

3-LM clinical material:

1 A brief history, with an account of the patient (such as stated reasons for coming to analysis, kinds of suffering known or indirectly communicated, childhood events told at the onset, crises, family trauma, etc.) and the characteristics of the setting (frequency, use of the couch, etc.).

2 Verbatim session material from the first and second sessions (or an early important session), and one or two sessions from two, possibly three, later phases of the analysis (that show significant aspects of the process) (Verbatim session material is a detailed transcription ("he said/she said") made by the analyst during and after an analytic session, with the associations of the patient and interpretations of the analyst, differentiating them with notations P and A.).
3 A general analytic context for the sessions when needed, in order to introduce a session or give some key information about the periods between the selected sessions.
4 After the presenter selects the clinical material, he/she discusses it with the moderator.
5 The clinical material for the group discussion is usually 20–25 pages, with pages and lines numbered.

Confidentiality

The confidentiality rule means that the presenter will have carefully modify all information that could identify the patient. The presenter of the clinical material takes the responsibility to respect the confidentiality rule, deleting or changing any biographical information that could enable the patient's identification in any way (names of people, educational institutions, enterprises, etc., but also any participation in well-known events or other identifiable situations). The presenter will judge if she or he needs to have consent from the patient. Participants will not use or disseminate the material without the presenter's explicit consent.

Notes on moderating a 3-LM group

Committee members and moderators have worked consistently to improve the art of moderating the clinical observation groups. The task of the moderator is to facilitate the group discussion while bringing pertinent open-ended questions from each level of the model to guide discussion. Here are some notes on different methods.

The moderator hands out the 3-LM questions and the Forms to the group.

1 A brief introduction to the 3-LM and outline of the schedule.
2 Level 1

   a The presenter reads the entire material and opens group discussion with Level-1 questions, or
   b The presenter reads the material in three segments (history and opening sessions; mid-analysis sessions; late analysis sessions) with brief discussion in between (bringing in the Leve-1 questions as relevant).

3 First report
The reporter reviews the anchor points and change points discussed by the group. The group makes corrections and additions to the summary on anchor points and change points.

4 Level 2
The moderator opens Level 2, selecting first the questions that help to conceptualize those areas of difficulty and change most discussed from the different dimensions of Level 2. Thus, Level 2 moves organically from Level-1 discussion with its points of consensus and its debates.

5 Second report
The reporter makes a second report after the second main break that summarizes the group consensus and debate on main difficulties and change and no change observed in the material. The group discusses briefly, making corrections and additions.

6 Level 3
The moderator reads the first three questions in Level 3.

a The moderator opens a free discussion on foci of the interpretations, theories behind them, and hypotheses on alternative interpretations, or
b The moderator begins by reading just the interpretations in some sessions to recall the group's ideas on opening, middle, and end phase interpretations and effects on the patient, or:
c The moderator reads question four at Level 3 and opens discussion of mechanisms of change, hypotheses on theories of therapeutic action behind the interpretations, and hypotheses on possible alternative interpretations grounded in the clinical material.

7 Final report
The moderator helps reporter with suggested revisions for the final report, which is sent to the group.

Summary of the reporter's roles

1 The reporter writes a brief report summing up the discussion on anchor points and change points at Level 1 and reads the report to the group.
2 The reporter takes notes as the group gives feedback on any points of group discussion that need to be corrected or added.
3 The reporter makes a second brief report on the second phases of group discussion and on the group process, conceptualizing the problems and changes and absence of changes, which is discussed, revised, and added to by the group.

4 The reporter writes up a final report (based on the first two reports, and on the further observations of the 3-LM group at Level 2 and Level 3). Two or three weeks later, the report is sent to the moderator for suggested revision, then to the presenting analyst and then sent to the group.

Questions for group discussion: Adults

Current Version, 2020

Box 15.1 Questions about Level 1: Phenomenological description of transformations

1 Which parts of the clinical material had special resonance for the group participants and can be considered as anchor points that make it possible to track changes in the patient? What is the relationship of these anchor points to the foci of the analyst's interpretations?
2 Are there changes in the analytic process in (a) how the patient uses the analyst and his or her interventions?; (b) how the patient uses his or her own mind and body during the session? Are there noticeable changes in the course of one session? And through time, between different sessions?
3 In which of the following areas is it possible to observe changes? (a) Capacity to love and sexuality; (b) Family and social relationships; (c) Occupation and leisure; (d) Interests and creativity; (e) Symptoms and subjective well-being. Which is the patient's perspective regarding his changes?
4 What aspects of the material suggest the existence of positive changes, negative changes, or the nonexistence of changes? Which prevail?

Box 15.2 Questions about Level 2: Dimensions of change

1 Subjective experience of illness and contextual factors

a What are the patient's subjective experiences, beliefs and expectations about his/her problems and treatment? How much does the patient recognize his or her problems? How much does the patient foresee possibilities of change? To what extent do patient and analyst agree on the expected transformations?

b Are there contextual factors that affect the therapeutic process? (For example, crises, traumatic experiences, somatic illnesses, drugs, etc.? How capable is the patient of facing these situations?)

c How have these aspects changed? How much has the patient's understanding of his or her problems and therapeutic possibilities changed?

2 Patterns of interpersonal relationship and how they have changed

a What are the interpersonal relationships of the patient like, especially in the bonds that imply closeness and intimacy?

b How does the patient experience others, and how does the patient experience himself or herself in relation to others? How do others experience the patient, and how do they experience themselves in relation to the patient (in transference–counter-transference and in other meaningful bonds)?

c To what extent can I relate the patient's current relational patterns to the experiences lived in his or her childhood and with the bonds that the patient establishes with the analyst?

d How have these aspects changed?

3 Main intrapsychic conflicts and how they have changed

a What are the main conflicts (e.g., individuation vs. dependency; submission vs. control; need for care vs. self-sufficiency; self-worth, guilt, Oedipal conflict, identity conflict)? Which are the dominant unconscious fantasies that can be inferred from conflicts and relational patterns?

b Are the prevailing defences adequate and flexible or dysfunctional, distorting, or limiting internal and external experiences?

c How have these aspects changed?

4 Structural aspects of mental functioning

a What is the level of mental functioning in the following areas? Are there signs of change?

1) Perception of self and others; identity
How capable is the patient of adequately perceiving his or her own internal states and those of others? Is the patient able to empathize, tolerating and understanding different points of view? Does the patient have an integrated

feeling of his or her own identity, open to the possibility of unconscious aspects? What are the characteristics of the identifications (especially pathological ones)? Does the patient manage to connect with his or her past and give direction to his or her life, with a sense of agency and short- and long-term wishes and goals?

2) Affective regulation
Is the patient able to adequately regulate impulses, affects, and self-esteem? Do the patient's ideals and values help him or her to handle his or her emotions? Does the patient manage to regulate his or her need for self-esteem when facing internal and external demands? How much does the patient achieve an adequate balance between his or her own interests and those of the others?
3) Internal and external communication; symbolization
How rich is the dialogue with the patient and others, based on affective experiences, bodily self, fantasies, dreams, sexuality, symbolic representations, and capacity to play and creativity?
4) Attachment with internal and external objects
How deep and stable and differentiated are the relationships with internal and external objects? How much can the patient start and end relationships and tolerate separations? How does the patient handle relationships that imply the existence of a third person? How have these aspects changed?

5 Type of disorder

a Is it possible to identify a type of personality disorder or other kind of mental or bodily disorder?
b How severe are the disturbances in personality functioning? How much is the analytic work conditioned by the structural vulnerabilities in mental functioning?
c How have these aspects changed?

Box 15.3 Questions about Level 3: Hypotheses on links between interventions and observed links

1 What were the foci of the analyst's interventions? How did the foci change over the course of the analysis?

2 What can be observed about the impact on the patient of the different foci of interventions, in different phases in the analysis?
3 Do you consider that some interventions were especially effective? Which ones?
4 Which aspects of the analysis facilitate inner processes that lead to change in the patient (mechanisms of change/curative factors)? (The group should be that the analyst's intentions in giving certain interventions—what the analyst is aiming it—may be different from what we outside observers see as factors in the change observed.)
5 What parts of the clinical material did the analyst not address? And what other kinds of intervention could the 3-LM group hypothesize might have been useful?

Questions for group discussion: Children—Adapted by Marina Altmann de Litvan, Delfina Miller, and Ricardo Bernardi, 2014

Level I: Phenomenological description of transformations

1 Which aspects of the material (supplied by the child, parents, teachers, or other informants) suggest the existence of positive or negative transformations, or the absence of transformations?
2 Which of these changes may be attributed to the growth of the child regarding the development patterns that were highlighted in the material presented (for example, dream, feeding, sphincter control, psychomotor development, relationships)?
3 Which may be attributed to changes in the environment (family events such as separations, divorce, death, newborns, accidents, moving, etc.).
4 As noted, we give a special place to the child's play. First, we observe whether it is adequate to the child's age, and which phase of libidinal development it refers to.
Regarding these aspects, we shall note transformations or the absence of them, taking as a model the evaluation of play proposed by Kernberg, Chazan, and Normandin (1996):

a Type of play (sensory-motor, exploration, construction, phantasy)
b Narrative (originality, elaboration, organization, sequence)
c Subjects (presentation, elaboration, processing)

   d Affects (which and how many, with which intensity and adequacy, level, and way of regulation)
   e Expressed relationships (with the analyst, among characters within the game)

5 Which transformations can be observed in the course of one session? And through different moments in time?
6 In which of these areas are meaningful changes perceived showing transformations in the functioning and well-being of the child?

   a Symptoms and subjective well-being
   b Relationship within child's family, and with peers, teachers, etc.
   c School performance and interests

7 Changes in treatment regarding

   a How does the child accept the treatment (for example, attitude regarding the setting)?
   b How does the child use the therapist?
   c How does the child use the therapist's interventions?
   d How does the child use his or her own mind and body during the session?
   e How does the child use the mind and body of the child's caregivers?

8 How have therapist and patient participated in the transformational process? Which is the perspective of each of them about transformations? What is the perspective from the child's caregivers and teachers in this regard? What relations can be established between the transformations and the characteristics of the analytic process?
9 Which parts of the clinical material have a special resonance in participants regarding the transformational process?

Level 2: Dimensions of change

The following questions seek to identify the dimensions in which transformations could occur. They are based mainly on *OPD-2* (OPD2 Task Force, 2008) and *PDM* (2006) proposals.

Subjective experience of illness

1 Which are the patient's main problems and symptoms, according to the analyst? What subjective experience does the child have of them? Which are the child's beliefs regarding what occurs and his or her expectations of treatment?
How much is the patient aware of his or her problems? What is the parents' perspective about the child's problems? What is the teachers' perspective about them? How much does the child see the ways

that could lead him or her to a change? And parents? How much do analyst, patient, and parents (other informants could correspond, too) agree about the expected transformations?

2 How did these aspects change? How much has changed the understanding of problems in the child and the expectancy of transformation possibilities? How has this been modified in parents (or caregivers, teachers, etc.)?
3 Are there contextual factors that affect the therapeutic process (e.g., crises, traumatic experiences, somatic illnesses, etc.)? How capable is the patient of facing these situations?

Patterns of interpersonal relationships

RELATIONAL PATTERNS OUTSIDE ANALYSIS

1 How are the patient's interpersonal relationships, especially in bonds that imply closeness and intimacy? Do they have depth, range, and consistency?
2 How does the child experience others? How does the child experience himself or herself in relation to others (e.g., does the child feel comfortable and relaxed in the presence of the adult)? Is the child friendly, avoidant, or does the child seek for excessive attention? How is his or her visual, verbal, and bodily contact? How do others (mother, father, siblings, peers) experience the child and themselves in relation to the child? How is the child's relationship with them? How are these aspects observed in the sessions?

RELATIONAL PATTERNS WITH THE ANALYST

1 What characteristics does the transferential–counter-transferential relationship have? For example, how is the relationship with the therapist? Is it comfortable and relaxed? Does the child show hesitancy to connect at the beginning? Is the child's play isolated and solitary in the analysis? Are the child's bonds in the play reciprocal, of co-operation? Of competence? Is there inhibition? Do the child relate in a close and intimate way? Can this relating be expressed through words?
2 How have these relational patterns changed?

MAIN INTRAPSYCHIC CONFLICTS

1 Which are the main conflicts and affects related to them (for example, individuation, self-esteem, guilt, oedipal conflict, identity conflict)? Which are the prevailing unconscious phantasies that can be inferred from conflicts? How much consciousness does the child have of them?

And the parents? Can they calm down and provide adequate measures for containment and facing of the conflict? To regulate anxiety, to acknowledge, to tolerate, and to soothe, helping to encode conflicts with the internal and external reality as enduring resolution?

2 Are defences against conflicts adequate and flexible or mainly dysfunctional (distorting or restricting internal and external experiences)?

3 Which affects accompany this dynamics? For example, does the child manifest aggression? Caution? Fear? Pleasure? Joy? Reactions of frustration? Anger? Rage? Surprise? Uneasiness? Sadness? Feeling lost? Is the child able to control himself or herself? Is the child worried about the effects of these on others?

4 How have these aspects changed?

MENTAL OR PERSONALITY FUNCTIONING: STRUCTURE

1 What is the level of the child's mental functioning in the following areas?

   a Self-perception and perception of others. Identity.
   How capable is the child, according to the expected level of development, to adequately perceive his or her own internal states and those of the others? Can the child feel empathy, tolerating and understanding different points of view? Does the child have an integrated sense of his or her own identity that corresponds to the expected level of development? Can the child integrate in his or her identity or past, especially the traumatic experiences in the way that would be expected considering the child's level of development? Which are the characteristics of the prevailing identifications?
   How is the child's self-perception and self-representation (integrated/contradictory, adequate/inadequate, dystonic/syntonic)? How are the child's affective states in this regard? Does he or she feel disdain, appreciation, shame, pride, for himself or herself?
   How are the child's object representations (e.g., enabling, persecutory, idealized, devaluated, fragile)?
   How are the child's manifestations regarding the dependency and autonomy expected for his or her level of development? For example, does the child show goodwill and want to do things independently? Does the child insist on things being done as he or she wants? Does the child get angry if it is not like that? Does the child get angry if he or she does not achieve what he or she wants?)
   Does the child act freely according to his or her desires and obligations? Does the child act reactively (e.g., does the child present oppositional manifestations)?

Does he or she show flexibility or stubbornness and obstinacy? Does the child show pleasure in success only when approval is shown to him or her?
How have these aspects changed?

b Sensory regulation
Considering the expected level for the child's development, how is his or her ability to control the degree, intensity, and nature of his or responses to sensory stimuli (e.g., excessive response with fear, anxiety, negativism, stubbornness, self-absorption)? How does the child react to different stimuli (sounds, lights, touch) (e.g., lack of response, excessive response, etc.)? Does the father or mother have the capacity to provide a feeling of vitality and enthusiasm? Can the father/mother regulate physiological states (sleep, hunger, activation, sedation, pain, temperature)? How much do parents manage to understand what is happening to the child and have an answer that helps him or her?
What is the child's general level of activity? How much does it vary?
Can the child focus of attention on one activity or interaction? What average time does he or she devote to one specific toy or activity? Is the child frequently distracted?
Regarding the psyche-soma integration, we can wonder: How does the child feel his or her body? Does the child like it? Are there signs in bodily posture that call one's attention? And in his or her way of walking?
Does the child have organic illnesses? Does he or she frequently become ill?
Which are the child's manifestations and experiences about them? What are parents' experience about the child's illness? Has this incidence of somatic factors revealed any situation? If so, has he or she been able to discover in analysis the factors that precede his or her psyche-soma disorganization, such as apathy, depression, withdrawal?
How strong is the influence of factors depending on the context (e.g., changes linked to development, somatic illnesses, medication, acute or chronic stressors, traumatic situations, etc.) and how capable is the patient of facing these difficulties? How do parents influence these aspects?

c Affective regulation
Which attachment style and reflexive capacity does the child show? And the parents? What regulation model was suggested and approved? For example, we consider the following aspects regarding his father or mother: does the parent have the capacity as an adult for tenderness, for erogeneity inhibited in its end? Does the parent have the capacity to take into consideration the

reasons behind actions from others? To consider the feelings, mental states, and desires of his or her child? To anticipate danger and neglect? To regulate the child's anxiety and anguish? Does the father or mother have the capacity to build a bond of safe attachment, including tolerance of both early dependence and growing autonomy?

Taking the above into account, we define the following.

How does the child feel in himself or herself and perceive in others the wide range of affects expected at his or her age? How much does the child manage to process impulses and emotional experiences in a way that favours his or her adaptation and satisfaction?

Do the child's norms and ideals help acknowledging and tolerating his or her emotional experiences in the face of adversities, keeping a stability in accordance with his or her level of emotional development?

Can the child regulate his or her self-esteem when facing internal and external demands? Can the child balance his or her interests and those of the others protecting him or her and his or her bonds?

Can the child regulate relationships with others (capacity for intimacy, reciprocity, taking care of himself or herself and the other in relationships)?

How much is the child able to integrate positive and negative feelings towards himself or herself and others?

How would you place the child with regard to the level of development expected for his or her age? And regarding the model received from the family?

How have these aspects changed?

d Internal and external communication and symbolization

In this regard, we ask, How rich is the dialogue of the child with himself or herself and others, based on affective experiences, phantasies, dreams, sexuality, bodily self, and symbolic representations? How would you place it regarding the level of development expected for the child's age?

Does the child count on the necessary tools and has he or she adequately developed them? For instance, is his or her vocalization and speech production adequate for his or her age? Does the child understand others' speech well? Is the primary thought process and/or verbalisations in the play expected for his or her age? How does the child use the information to resolve problems?)

Can the father or mother help in this process?

How have these aspects changed?

e Bonds with internal and external objects

How deep and stable are the child's relationships with internal and external objects? How much can he or she create relationships of intimacy and reciprocity based on stable representations and on representations differentiated between himself or herself and others? How does the child handle the relationships that imply the existence of a third?
How capable is the child of initiating and finishing relationships and facing separations?
How would you place the child regarding the expected level of development for his or her age?
How have these aspects changed?

Level 3: Testing of explanatory hypotheses of change

Therapeutic foci

1 Which aspects have received special attention from the analyst in his or her interventions, that one can suppose the analyst considers play a central psychodynamic role in the clinical case, originating or maintaining conflicts? How much do analyst, child, caregivers, and teachers coincide on the need to work around them?
2 Have these foci of the analytic work changed through time? Why?

Level and type of disorder

1 Do the child's symptoms integrate in one syndrome? Is it possible to identify a type of development disorder, personality disorder, or any other kind of disorder?
2 Is the level of personality organization orientated towards a functioning that is healthy, neurotic, border, or psychotic?
Could the therapeutic work be centred in neurotic conflicts, or was it necessary to previously, or at the same time, attend to structural failures in the functioning and psychic integration that affected the stability of conflicts and therapeutic work? How have these aspects changed?

Explanatory hypotheses of change

1 Which are the main theories and hypotheses from the analyst (explicit or implicit) that can be seen in his or her work? Have they changed through treatment?
2 Which other explanatory hypotheses of change could be suggested from different theoretical perspectives? Which are the most and least convincing aspects of each of these different hypotheses and how could they be refined in order to better adjust to the clinical material?

Forms 1, 2, and 3

Instructions for moderators

These forms serve several purposes. They seek to gather information about changes in the psychoanalytic treatments discussed by the groups. They also collect information on the operation of the 3-LM in the group discussion. Finally, they are intended to help personal reflection and group on central questions posed by the model.

Form 1

Form 1 is to be completed individually by participants after they have read all the clinical material and at any time before group discussion begins. Their initial personal opinion is of interest, as it will allow the investigation of personal opinions and the effect of the group discussion on them.

Form 2

To be completed by the moderator, after the three levels have been worked on, in discussion with group members. First, the moderator will investigate how many participants agree on overall assessment of the changes in the patient, using the same questions posed in Form 1. Second, the moderator will explore the number of agreed on changes in the severity of the disturbances at the beginning and end of treatment. The two kinds of question complement each other.

The moderator will try to have the group reach as much consensus as possible (with reference to data discussed) and record it according to the instructions on Form 2. The group consensus on the changes is fundamental, as it will serve as a criterion for the classification of cases.

Form 3

The moderator will ask participants to complete Form 3 individually before leaving. The aim of this form is to record the individual assessment of the changes in the patient after group discussion. Both the overall (or global) assessment (using the same questions as in Form 1) and assessments in each of the dimensions of change identified in Level 2, are of interest. The form also asks how useful the participants consider the discussion of each of the 3-LM levels to be.

Select bibliography

Altmann, M. (2013). Tracking transformations in a psychoanalytic process: Unconscious and explicit. *International Journal of Psychoanalysis, 94*(6), 1191–1193.

Altmann de Litvan, M. (Ed.). (2014). *Time for change: Tracking transformations in psychoanalysis—The Three-Level Model*. London: Karnac.

Altmann de Litvan, M. (Ed.). (2015). *Tiempo de cambio: Indagando las transformaciones en psicoanálisis: El Modelo de los Tres Niveles*. London: Karnac.

Altmann de Litvan, M. A. (2015). Panel report, IPA Congress Boston 2015: Metaphors and the use of analyst as tools to improve our clinical practise. Panel and small discussion group organized by The IPA Project Committee on Clinical Observation. *International Journal of Psychoanalysis, 96*(6), 1651–1654.

Baranger, M., Baranger, W., & Mom, J. (1983). Process and non-process in analytic work. *International Journal of Psychoanalysis, 64*, 1–15.

Bernardi, R. (2013). Observing transformations in patients: The assessment of mental functioning. *International Journal of Psychoanalysis, 94*(6), 1170–1172.

Bernardi, R. (2015a). Investigación clínica e investigación empírica sistemática: ¿Qué nos enseñan las controversias actuales? *International Journal of Psychoanalysis (en español), 1*(3), 836–866.

Bernardi, R. (2015b). What kind of discipline is psychoanalysis? *International Journal of Psychoanalysis, 96*(3), 731–754.

Bernardi, R. (2017). A common ground in clinical discussion groups: Intersubjective resonance and implicit operational theories. *International Journal of Psychoanalysis, 98*(5), 1291–1309.

Bernardi, R. (2018). Discussion of "Ending Analysis: The Case of Karl." *International Journal of Psychoanalysis, 99*(6), 1444–1452.

Bernardi, R. (2019). About the criteria for evaluating patient transformations in "Ending Analysis: The Case of Karl," The International Journal of Psychoanalysis 99: 1424–1457. *International Journal of Psychoanalysis, 100*(5), 1041–1042.

Bernardi, R., & de León de Bernardi, B. (2019). Commentary on Bruce Fink's "On the value of the Lacanian approach to analytic practice." *International Journal of Psychoanalysis, 100*(2), 333–340.

Duarte, A. L., Glover, W., Gullestad, S., Salesio, B., de Litvan, M. A., & Bernardi, R. (2015). Informe de Panel, Congreso de la IPA Boston 2015: Las metáforas y el uso de analista como herramientas para mejorar nuestra práctica clínica Panel y pequeño grupo de debate organizados por: Comité de Proyectos de observación clínica IPA. *International Journal of Psychoanalysis (en español), 1*(6), 1957–1962.

FEPAL. (2019). Rutas de investigación. Comité de Observación Clínica—El Modelo de los 3 niveles [Research routes. Clinical Observation Committee—The Model of the 3 Levels]. www.fepal.org/es/rutas-de-investigacion-3/ (interview with Marina Altmann and Ricardo Bernardi).

Fitzpatrick Hanly, M. A. (2019). Panel on: "Transformations in female bodily experiences and bodily metaphors." *International Journal of Psychoanalysis, 100*(5), 1031–1033.

Glover, W. (2017). Panel report, IPA Congress Buenos Aires 2017: Transformations in the fear of intimacy. *International Journal of Psychoanalysis, 98*(6), 1770–1773.

IPA Project Committee on Clinical Observation. (2011). Three-Level Model for Observing Patient Transformations (3-LM). www.youtube.com/watch?v=2R4a1vFAG78.

IPA Project Committee on Clinical Observation and Testing. (2009). Home page. https://sites.google.com/site/clinicalobservation/.

Kernberg, P., Chazan, S., and Normandin, L. (1998) The Children's Play Therapy Instrument (CPTI): Description, development, and reliability studies. *Journal of Psychotherapy Practice and Research*, 7(3), 196–207.

OPD Task Force (2008). *Operationalized Psychodynamic Diagnosis (OPD-2)*. Cambridge, MA: Hogrefe & Huber.

PDM-2 Task Force (2017). *Psychodynamic Diagnostic Manual (PDM)*. New York: Guilford Press.

Rodríguez Quiroga, A. (2018). La formulación psicodinámica de caso. Su valor para la práctica clínica [Psychodynamic case formulation: Its value for clinical practice]. *International Journal of Psychoanalysis, 99*(1), 266–271.

Rodríguez Quiroga de Pereira, A., Borensztein, L., Corbella, V., & Marengo, J. C. (2018). The Lara case: A group analysis of initial psychoanalytic interviews using systematic clinical observation and empirical tools. *International Journal of Psychoanalysis, 99*(6), 1327–1352.

Appendix 15.1

Form 1 Individual conclusions before group discussion

Case identification (moderator):__________________________
Name of participant:____________________________________
Place:__________________________ Date:__________________________

Please let us know your personal opinion after reading the material and before group discussion:

Comparison of initial interviews with later moments of analysis	*No change or worse*	*Slight positive changes*	*Moderate changes*	*Major changes*
Global change of the patient				
Changes in the patient's "use" of the analyst and his or her interpretations				
Changes in the patient's use of his or her own mental and bodily resources for the analysis				

Comments:____

Appendix 15.2

Form 2 Group consensus after discussion

Identification of the case:____________________
Name of participant:____________________
Place:____________________Date:____________________

Group conclusion on the global changes of the patient

At the end of the group discussion, the moderator will ask if the group can reach consensual conclusions about the changes. Only the options where more than half of the group agree will be marked with a cross.

Comparison of initial interviews with later moments of analysis	*No change or worse*	*Slight positive change*	*Moderate changes*	*Major changes*
Global change of the patient				
Changes in the patient's "use" of the analyst and his or her interpretations				
Changes in the patient's use of his or her own mental and bodily resources for the analysis				

Comments:____________________

Global Personality Organization (PDM-2)

The moderator will ask if there is majority agreement in the group about the level of organization of the personality at the beginning and in the last sessions, taking into account mental functioning in aspects such as identity, object relationships, defences, reality testing, etc.

Beginning of the analysis

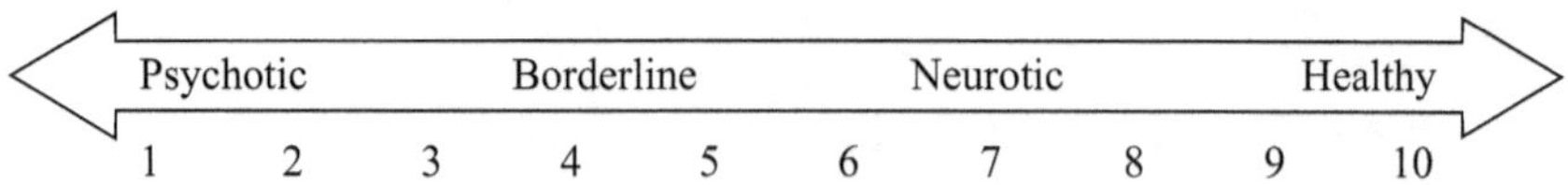

Level at the beginning (more than half of the participants must agree):_____
(Two consecutive levels can be marked if the point of agreement is between the two)
Number of participants who agree on that opinion:____________________

Number of participants present:________________________________
No majority agreement (mark here with an X):____________________
Clarifications:____

Final sessions

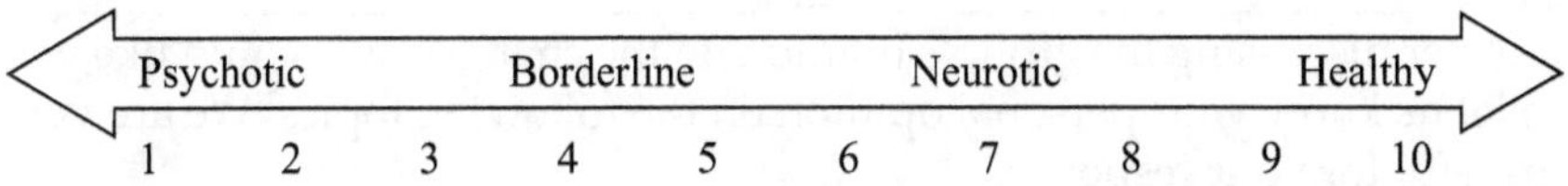

Level in the last sessions (more than half of the group must agree):______
(Two consecutive levels can be marked if the point of agreement is between the two)
Number of participants who agree on that opinion:__________________
Number of participants present:________________________________
No majority agreement (mark here with an X):____________________
Clarifications:____

Definitions

Healthy personality: Characterized by mostly 9–10 scores in mental functions. Life problems rarely get out of hand, and enough flexibility to accommodate to challenging realities. (Use 9 for people at the high-functioning neurotic level.)

Neurotic level: Characterized by mostly 6–8 scores; basically a good sense of identity, good reality testing, mostly good intimacies; fair resiliency, fair affect tolerance and regulation; rigidity and limited range of defences and coping mechanisms; favours defences such as repression, reaction formation, intellectualization, displacement, and undoing. (Use 6 for people who go between borderline and neurotic levels.)

Borderline level: Characterized by mostly 3–5 scores; recurrent relational problems; difficulty with affect tolerance and regulation; poor impulse control, poor sense of identity, poor resiliency; favours defences such as splitting, projective identification, idealization/devaluation, denial, omnipotent control, and acting out. (Use 3 for people who go between psychotic and borderline levels.)

Psychotic level: Characterized by mostly 1–2 scores; delusional thinking; poor reality testing and mood regulation; extreme difficulty functioning in work and relationships; favours defences such as delusional projection, psychotic denial, and psychotic distortion.

(There are no sharp cutoffs between categories. Use your clinical judgment.)

Appendix 15.3

Form 3 Individual conclusions after group discussion

(Form to be completed before leaving)
Name of participant:____
Place:_________________________Date:____________________________

After discussing the group's opinion on the changes, we would like you to let us know your personal opinion on the following topics. We are very grateful for your response.

Level 1: Phenomenological. Global description of changes

Comparison of initial interviews with later moments of analysis	*No changes or worse*	*Slight positive changes*	*Moderate changes*	*Major changes*
Global change of the patient				
Changes in the patient's "use" of the analyst and his or her interpretations				
Changes in the patient's use of his or her own mental and bodily resources for the analysis				

Level 2: Main dimensions of change (OPD-2)

Score 1–10 (1 = maximum disturbances; 10 = minimum or imperceptible disturbances)
0 = No data/doesn't apply

Dimensions	*Initial moment*	*Later moments*
Experience of illness: understanding of difficulties and hints of possible changes		
Relational patterns outside the analysis		
Relational patterns with the analyst		
Defences and conflicts		
Self-perception, sense of identity and integrity of the self		
Perception of the others. Empathy		
Regulation of impulses, affects, and self-esteem		
Regulation of the relationship with others (self-care and care of the other, reciprocity)		
Internal communication and symbolization (bodily and mental self)		

Dimensions	*Initial moment*	*Later moments*
Communication with others (depth and richness of affects and representations)		
Bonds with internal objects		
Bonds with others. Capacity to establish and end bonds, to face separation, and the existence of a third		

Evaluation of group discussion

Usefulness of the model in observing and understanding changes	*Not much, or not at all*	*Somewhat*	*Quite*	*Very*
How useful did you find the group activity in refining your observation of the material?				
How useful did you find the 3-LM group to conceptualize the dimensions of change?				
How satisfactory was the discussion on linking interventions with observed changes?				

Other comments you would like to add:______________________

Index

Page numbers in **bold** denote information in tables.

For Product Safety Concerns and Information please contact our EU representative GPSR@taylorandfrancis.com
Taylor & Francis Verlag GmbH, Kaufingerstraße 24, 80331 München, Germany

www.ingramcontent.com/pod-product-compliance
Lightning Source LLC
LaVergne TN
LVHW021118300926
849160LV00010B/766